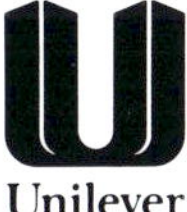

CONTACT URTICARIA SYNDROME

CRC Series in
DERMATOLOGY: CLINICAL AND BASIC SCIENCE
Edited by Dr. Howard I. Maibach

The CRC Dermatology Series combines scholarship, basic science, and clinical relevance. These comprehensive references focus on dermal absorption, dermabiology, dermatopharmacology, dermatotoxicology, and occupational and clinical dermatology.

The intellectual theme emphasizes in-depth, easy to comprehend surveys that blend advances in basic science and clinical research with practical aspects of clinical medicine.

Published Titles:

Bioengineering of the Skin: Cutaneous Blood Flow and Erythema
Enzo Berardesca, Peter Elsner, and Howard I. Maibach

Bioengineering of the Skin: Water and the Stratum Corneum
Peter Elsner, Enzo Berardesca, and Howard I. Maibach

Bioengineering of the Skin: Methods and Instrumentation
Enzo Berardesca, Peter Elsner, Klaus P. Wilhelm, and Howard I. Maibach

Dermatologic Research Techniques
Howard I. Maibach

Hand Eczema
Torkil Menne and Howard I. Maibach

Handbook of Mouse Mutations with Skin and Hair Abnormalities:
Animal Models and Biomedical Tools
John P. Sundberg

Health Risk Assessment: Dermal and Inhalation Exposure and Absorption of Toxicants
Rhoda G. M. Wang, James B. Knaak, and Howard I. Maibach

Pigmentation and Pigmentary Disorders
Norman Levine

Protective Gloves for Occupational Use
Gunh Mellström, J.E. Walhberg, and Howard I. Maibach

Skin Cancer: Mechanisms and Human Relevance
Hasan Mukhtar

Human Papillomavirus Infections in Dermatovenereology
Gerd Gross and Geo von Krogh

Bioengineering of the Skin: Skin Surface, Imaging, and Analysis
Klaus P. Wilhelm, Peter Elsner, Enzo Berardesca, and Howard I. Maibach

Contact Urticaria Syndrome
Smita Amin, Arto Lahti, and Howard I. Maibach

Forthcoming Titles:

Handbook of Contact Dermatitis
Christopher J. Dannaker, Daniel J. Hogan, and Howard I. Maibach

CONTACT URTICARIA SYNDROME

Edited by

Smita Amin, M.D.
Department of Medicine
Division of Dermatology
University of Toronto
Toronto, Canada

Arto Lahti, M.D., Ph.D.
Department of Dermatology
University of Oulu
Oulu, Finland

Howard I. Maibach, M.D.
Department of Dermatology
University of California
School of Medicine
San Francisco, California

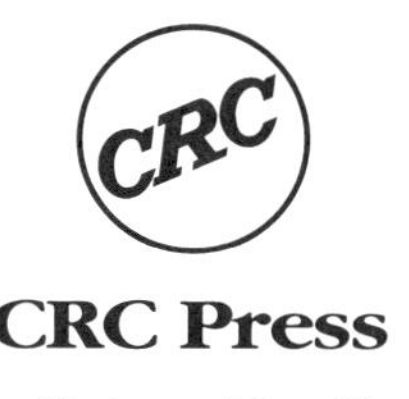

CRC Press

Boca Raton   New York

Senior Editor: Paul Petralia
Project Editor: Debbie Didier
Cover design: Denise Craig
PrePress: Kevin Luong

Library of Congress Cataloging-in-Publication Data

Contact urticaria syndrome / edited by Smita Amin, Arto Lahti, Howard
    I. Maibach.
        p.   cm. -- (CRC series in dermatology)
    Includes bibliographical references and index.
    ISBN 0-8493-7352-2
    1. Contact dermatitis.   2. Urticaria.   I. Amin, Smita.
II. Lahti, Arto.   III. Maibach, Howard I.   IV. Series.
    RL244.C66   1997
    616.5′1--dc21   97-12227
                                                                                      CIP

Contributors

Smita Amin, M.D.
Department of Medicine
Division of Dermatology
University of Toronto
Toronto, Canada

David I. Bernstein, M.D.
Department of Internal Medicine
Division of Immunology
University of Cincinnati College of
  Medicine
Cincinnati, Ohio

Jonathan A. Bernstein, M.D.
Department of Internal Medicine
Division of Immunology
University of Cincinnati College of
  Medicine
Cincinnati, Ohio

I. Leonard Bernstein, M.D.
Department of Internal Medicine
Division of Immunology
University of Cincinnati College of
  Medicine
Cincinnati, Ohio

Jonas Brisman, M.D.
Department of Occupational Medicine
Sahlgrenska Hospital
Gothenburg, Sweden

Christopher J. Dannaker, D.O., M.P.H.
Department of Dermatology
University of California
School of Medicine
San Francisco, California

Flora B. de Waard-van der Spek, M.D.
Department of Dermatology and
  Venereology
University Hospital Rotterdam
Rotterdam, The Netherlands

Rebecca J. Dearman, Ph.D.
Zeneca Central Toxicology Laboratory
Macclesfield Cheshire, United Kingdom

Tuula Estlander, M.D., Ph.D.
Section of Dermatology
Finnish Institute of Occupational Health
Helsinki, Finland

Matti Hannuksela, M.D., Ph.D.
South Karelia Central Hospital
Lappeenranta, Finland

Jurij J. Hostýnek, Ph.D.
Euromerican Technology Resources, Inc.
Lafayette, California
and
Department of Dermatology
University of California
San Francisco, California

Tami Ichikawa, M.D.
Mashiko Dermatology Clinic
Fukuoka Prefecture, Ohkawa City, Japan

Erika Isolauri, M.D.
Department of Pediatrics
Universities of Tampere and Turku
Finland

Riitta Jolanki, D.Tech.
Section of Dermatology
Finnish Institute of Occupational Health
Helsinki, Finland

Lasse Kanerva, M.D., Ph.D.
Section of Dermatology
Finnish Institute of Occupational Health
Helsinki, Finland

Ian Kimber, Ph.D.
Zeneca Central Toxicology Laboratory
Macclesfield Cheshire, United Kingdom

Arto Lahti, M.D., Ph.D.
Department of Dermatology
University of Oulu
Oulu, Finland

Antti I. Lauerma, M.D., Ph.D.
Department of Dermatology
Helsinki University Central Hospital
Helsinki, Finland

Timo Leino, M.D.
Department of Occupational Medicine
Finnish Institute of Occupational Health
Helsinki, Finland

Howard I. Maibach, M.D.
Department of Dermatology
University of California
School of Medicine
San Francisco, California

Jason D. Morrow, M.D.
Departments of Pharmacology and
  Medicine
Vanderbilt University
Nashville, Tennessee

Hideo Nakayama, M.D.
Nakayama Dermatology Clinic
Shinagawa-ku, Tokyo, Japan

Arnold P. Oranje, M.D., Ph.D.
Department of Dermatology and
  Venereology
University Hospital Rotterdam
Rotterdam, The Netherlands

Bianca Maria Piraccini, M.D., Ph.D.
Department of Dermatology
University of Bologna
Bologna, Italy

L. Jackson Roberts II, M.D.
Departments of Pharmacology and
  Medicine
Vanderbilt University
Nashville, Tennessee

Päivikki Susitaival, M.D., Ph.D.
Kuopio Regional Institute of
  Occupational Health
Kuopio, Finland

Kyllikki Tarvainen, M.D., Ph.D.
Department of Dermatology
North Karelia Central Hospital
Joensuu, Finland

Jouni Toikkanen, M.Soc.Sc.
Department of Epidemiology
Finnish Institute of Occupational
  Health
Helsinki, Finland

Antonella Tosti, M.D.
Department of Dermatology
University of Bologna
Bologna, Italy

Kristiina Turjanmaa, M.D.
Department of Dermatology
Tampere University Hospital
and
Medical School of University of Tampere
Tampere, Finland

Outi Tupasela, M.Sc.
Department of Occupational Medicine
Finnish Institute of Occupational
  Health
Helsinki, Finland

Ronald van Ree, Ph.D.
Department of Allergy
Central Laboratory of the Netherlands
  Red Cross Bloodtransfusion Service
Amsterdam, The Netherlands

Joanna Wallengren, M.D., Ph.D.
Department of Dermatology
University Hospital Lund
Lund, Sweden

Table of Contents

Introduction

Smita Amin and Howard I. Maibach

CONTENTS

INTRODUCTION

Contact urticaria syndrome (CUS) (immediate contact reaction) comprises a heterogeneous group of inflammatory reactions that usually appear within minutes after contact with the eliciting substance.

The epidemiology of these reactions is inadequately documented. The first such studies were performed in Hawaii (Elpern, 1985a, 1985b, 1986), Poland (Rudzki and Rebandel, 1985), Sweden (Nilsson, 1985), Denmark (Veien et al., 1987), Finland (Turjanmaa, 1987), and Switzerland (Weissenbach et al., 1988). These studies suggested that immediate contact reactions are common in dermatologic practice. Some substances cause immediate reactions in almost everyone at the first contact (methyl nicotinate), but others need a period of sensitization (latex rubber). Kanerva et al. (1994; 1997, in press) provides convincing data of its high frequency in the occupational setting.

The contact urticaria syndrome, first defined as a biologic entity in 1975 (Maibach and Johnson, 1975), has attracted increasing interest in clinical medicine and biology. Numerous cases have been and continue to be published and provide information on the etiologies and the clinical and pathophysiologic features of the syndrome.

TABLE 1   Staging of Contact Urticaria Syndrome

Cutaneous (skin) reactions only:	
Stage 1:	Localized urticaria (redness and swelling)
	Dermatitis (eczema)
	Nonspecific symptoms (itching, tingling, burning)
Stage 2:	Generalized urticaria
Extracutaneous reactions:	
Stage 3:	Bronchial asthma (wheezing)
	Rhinitis, conjunctivitis (runny nose, watery eyes)
	Orolarngeal symptoms (lip swelling, hoarseness, difficulty swallowing)
	Gastrointestinal symptoms (nausea, vomiting, diarrhea, cramps)
Stage 4:	Anaphylactoid reactions (shock)

SYMPTOMS

Immediate contact reactions appear on normal or eczematous skin within minutes to an hour or so after agents capable of producing this type of reaction have been in contact with the skin. They disappear within 24 hours, usually within a few hours. The symptoms can be classified according to morphology and severity: itching, tingling, or burning accompanied by erythema are the weakest types of immediate contact reaction, and these symptoms are often produced by cosmetics (Emmons and Marks, 1985) and fruits and vegetables. Local wheal-and-flare is the prototype reaction of contact urticaria (Table 1). Generalized urticaria after a local contact is uncommon. Tiny vesicles may rapidly appear on the fingers in protein contact dermatitis. In some cases, immediate contact reactions can be demonstrated only on slightly or previously affected skin, and it can be part of the mechanism responsible for maintenance of chronic eczemas (Hannuksela, 1980; Maibach, 1976; Veien et al., 1987).

There has been confusion in using terms such as contact urticaria, immediate contact reactions, atopic contact dermatitis, and protein contact dermatitis. Immediate contact urticaria includes both urticarial and other reactions, whereas protein contact dermatitis means allergic or nonallergic eczematous dermatitis caused by proteins or proteinaceous materials.

Extracutaneous symptoms may also occur as part of a more severe reaction. These symptoms may include rhinoconjunctivitis and orolaryngeal or gastrointestinal dysfunctions.

Finally, anaphylactoid reactions may occur as the most severe type of manifestation of CUS.

ETIOLOGY AND MECHANISMS

The mechanisms underlying contact reactions are divided into two main types, namely, immunologic (IgE-mediated) and nonimmunologic immediate contact reactions (Lahti and Maibach, 1987). However, there are substances causing immediate contact reactions whose mechanism (immunologic or not) remains unknown.

REFERENCES

Elpern, D. J. 1985a. The syndrome of immediate reactivities (contact urticaria syndrome). An historical study from a dermatology practice. I. Age, sex, race and putative substances. *Hawaii Med. J.,* 44:426–439.

Elpern, D. J. 1985b. The syndrome of immediate reactivities (contact urticaria syndrome). An historical study from a dermatology practice. II. The atopic diathesis and drug reactions. *Hawaii Med. J.,* 44:466–468.

Elpern, D. J. 1986. The syndrome of immediate reactivities (contact urticaria syndrome). An historical study from a dermatology practice. III. General discussion and conclusions. *Hawaii Med. J.,* 45:10–12.

Emmons, W. W. and Marks, J. G. 1985. Immediate and delayed reactions to cosmetic ingredients. *Contact Dermatitis,* 13:258–265.

Hannuksela, M. 1980. Atopic contact dermatitis. *Contact Dermatitis,* 6:30.

Kanerva, L., Jolanki, R., and Toikkanen, J. 1994. Frequencies of occupational allergic diseases and gender differences in Finland. *Int. Arch. Occup. Environ. Health,* 66:111–116.

Kanerva L. et al. 1997. in press.

Lahti, A. and Maibach, H. I. 1987. Immediate contact reactions: contact urticaria syndrome. *Semin. Dermatol.,* 6:313–320.

Maibach, H. I. 1976. Immediate hypersensitivity in hand dermatitis: role of food contact dermatitis. *Arch. Dermatol.,* 112:1289–1291.

Maibach, H. I. and Johnson, H. L. 1975. Contact urticaria syndrome: contact urticaria to diethyltoluamide (immediate type hypersensitivity). *Arch. Dermatol.,* 111:726–730.

Nilsson, E. 1985. Contact sensitivity and urticaria in "wet" work. *Contact Dermatitis,* 13:321–328.

Rudzki, E. and Rebandel, P. 1985. Occupational contact urticaria from penicillin. *Contact Dermatitis,* 13:192.

Turjanmaa, K. 1987. Incidence of immediate allergy to latex gloves in hospital personnel. *Contact Dermatitis,* 17:270–275.

Veien, N. K., Hattel, T., Justesen, O., and Norholm, A. 1987. Dietary restrictions in the treatment of adult patients with eczema. *Contact Dermatitis,* 17:223–228.

Weissenbach, T., Wutrich, B., and Weihe, W. H. 1988. Allergies to laboratory animals. An epidemiological, allergological study in persons exposed to laboratory animals. *Schweiz. Med. Wochenschr.,* 118:930–938.

1

Nonimmunologic Contact Urticaria

Arto Lahti

CONTENTS

1.1 DEFINITIONS, CONCEPTS, AND SYMPTOMS

Nonimmunologic contact urticaria (NICU) and other nonimmunologic immediate contact reactions (NIICRs) of the skin comprise a group of inflammatory reactions that appear within minutes to an hour after contact with the eliciting substance and usually disappear within a few hours. These reactions can also be called immediate-type irritancy. NIICRs occur without previous sensitization in most exposed individuals, and they are the most common type of immediate contact reaction.[1]

Symptoms of NIICRs are heterogeneous, and the intensity of the reaction typically varies depending on the concentration, the vehicle, the skin area exposed, the mode of exposure, and the substance itself.[2] Itching, tingling, or burning accompanied by erythema are the weakest type of reaction. Sometimes only local sensations without any visible change in the skin are reported. The redness is usually follicular at first and then spreads to cover the whole application site. A local weal and flare suggest a contact urticarial reaction. Generalized urticaria after contact with NICU agents is a rare phenomenon but has been reported more often after contact with agents eliciting immunologic IgE-mediated contact urticaria. Repeated applications of NICU agents may cause eczematous reactions. Quickly appearing microvesicles are frequently seen after contact with food products in protein contact dermatitis, which can be caused by nonimmunologic (irritant) or immunologic (allergic) mechanisms.[3-4]

In NICU reactions, the symptoms usually appear and remain in the contact area. In addition to local skin symptoms, other organs are occasionally involved causing conjunctivitis, rhinitis, an asthmatic attack, or anaphylactic shock. This is called the contact urticaria syndrome, and it mostly involves immunologic mechanisms.[5] In some cases, NICU reactions only appear on slightly affected skin and can be part of the mechanism responsible for the maintenance of chronic eczemas.

The usage of the terms "immediate contact reaction," "contact urticaria," "immediate type irritancy," "contact urticaria syndrome," "protein contact dermatitis," and "atopic contact dermatitis" varies in the literature. Immediate contact reaction is the broadest concept, which covers both immunologic (allergic) and nonimmunologic (irritant) reactions, but does not say anything about the appearance of the reaction. Contact urticaria can be allergic or irritant. The redness of skin appearing within tens of minutes after contact with the eliciting substance cannot be regarded as contact urticaria unless at least some persons get urticarial reactions at the application site. Protein contact dermatitis is caused by proteins or proteinaceous materials, and it means allergic or irritant dermatitis, which has characteristic features of acute or chronic eczema.[1] Atopic contact dermatitis is a historical term and means an immediate type (IgE-mediated) allergic contact reaction in an atopic person.[6] It is included in the concept of allergic protein contact dermatitis (Table 1.1).

1.2 MECHANISMS OF NONIMMUNOLOGIC IMMEDIATE CONTACT REACTIONS

The mechanisms of NIICRs, similarly to other irritant reactions, are not well understood. It was previously assumed that substances eliciting NIICRs result in nonspecific histamine release from mast cells. However, it has been shown that H_1-antihistamines, hydroxyzine and terfenadine, do not inhibit reactions to benzoic acid, cinnamic acid, cinnamic aldehyde, methyl nicotinate, or dimethyl sulfoxide, though they inhibit reactions to histamine in prick tests.[2,7] These results suggest that histamine is not the main mediator in NIICRs to these well-known contact urticants.

The NIICRs to benzoic acid, cinnamic acid, cinnamic aldehyde, methyl nicotinate, and diethyl fumarate can be inhibited by peroral acetylsalicylic acid and

TABLE 1.1 Definitions and Terms

Immediate contact reaction	Immunologic (allergic) or nonimmunologic (irritant), urticarial or non-urticarial reactions. Does not define the appearance of the reaction.
Contact urticaria	Allergic and nonallergic urticarial reactions.
Immediate-type irritancy	Nonallergic urticarial or nonurticarial reactions.
Protein contact dermatitis	Allergic or nonallergic eczematous reactions caused by proteins or proteinaceous material.
Contact urticaria syndrome	Local reactions in the skin and systemic symptoms in other organs, usually allergic.

indomethacin[8,9] and by a topical application of diclofenac or naproxen gels.[10] The duration of inhibition by a single dose of acetylsalicylic acid can be as long as 4 days.[11] The mechanism by which nonsteroidal anti-inflammatory drugs inhibit NIICRs in human skin has not been defined, but it is probably ascribable to the inhibition of prostaglandin metabolism.

The role of skin nerves in NIICRs has been studied using capsaicin (trans-8-methyl-*N*-vanillyl-6-nonenamide), which is known to induce a release of bioactive peptides, such as substance P, from the axons of unmyelinated C-fibers of sensory nerves. Pretreatment of the skin with capsaicin inhibits erythema reactions in histamine prick tests,[12] but does not inhibit either erythema or edema elicited by benzoic acid or methyl nicotinate.[13] This suggests that NIICRs to these model substances are not a type of neurogenic inflammation of the skin. Topical anesthesia inhibits erythema reactions to histamine, benzoic acid, and methyl nicotinate, but it is not known whether the inhibitory effect is due to the influence on the sensory nerves only or whether the anesthetic also affects other cell types or regulatory mechanisms of immediate-type skin inflammation.[13]

NIICRs to benzoic acid and methyl nicotinate can be inhibited by exposure to ultraviolet B and A light. The inhibition lasts for at least 2 weeks.[14] The reactions on nonirradiated skin sites also decrease, suggesting the possibility that UV irradiation may have "systemic effects."[15] The mechanism of UV inhibition is not known, but it does not seem to be due to thickening of the stratum corneum, as has been speculated.[16]

Molecular structure is important for the irritant properties of a NIICR agent. Pyridine carboxaldehyde (PCA) has three isomers, 2-, 3-, and 4-PCA, depending on the position of the aldehyde group on the pyridine ring. It has turned out that 3-PCA is a strong and 2-PCA a weak irritant in both human and animal skin (guinea pig ear swelling test). A slight change in the molecular structure of a chemical may substantially alter its capacity to produce NIICRs.[17]

1.3 ANIMAL TESTING METHODS

Animal test methods for determining NIICRs are needed to screen for putative agents and to clarify the mechanisms. At the moment, the guinea pig ear swelling test is the best animal test available for studying NIICRs.[18,19] A positive reaction in the guinea pig ear lobe comprises erythema and edema. Quantification of the edema by measuring the change in ear thickness is an accurate, quick, and reproducible method. Similar to human skin, the swelling response in the guinea pig ear lobe depends on the concentration of the eliciting substance. The maximal response is a roughly 100% increase in ear thickness and it appears 40–50 min. after the application, depending on the vehicle.

A decrease in reactivity to NIICR agents is noticed after reapplication on the following day.[20] This tachyphylaxis phenomenon is not specific to the substance which produces it, and reactivity to other agents also decreases. The length of the refractory period is 4 days for methyl nicotinate, 8 days for diethyl fumarate and cinnamic aldehyde, and 16 days for benzoic acid, cinnamic acid, and dimethyl sulfoxide.

The guinea pig ear lobe resembles human skin in many respects, including the morphology of the reaction, the timing of the maximal response, the concentrations of the eliciting substances needed to produce the reaction, the tachyphylaxis phenomenon, and the lack of an inhibitory effect of antihistamines on the NIICRs.

1.4 HUMAN TESTING METHODS

Special tests for NIICRs are needed, because these reactions are not seen in ordinary tests for irritancy and contact allergy. The most frequently used tests are the open test and the chamber test.

In the open test, 0.1 ml of the test substance is spread on a 3×3 cm area of the skin of the upper back, on the extensor aspect of the upper arm, or on the forearm. There are marked differences between skin sites in the reactivity to NIICR substances. The face, especially the cheek, the antecubital space, the upper back, the upper arm, the volar forearm, the lower back, and the leg constitute a rough order of decreasing reactivity.[1,16,21] A 10 µl dose to a 1×1 cm area is often used if a greater number of substances are to be tested at the same time. Petrolatum and water were the most often used vehicles 15 years ago,[1] but it has been shown that the use of alcohol vehicles and the addition of propylene glycol to the vehicle enhance the sensitivity of the test to detect marginal immediate irritant reactions.[22,23] The test is usually read at 20, 40, and 60 min. in order to see the maximal response. In visual grading, scores for the erythema and edema components of the reaction (+ weak, ++ moderate, +++ strong) have been used,[22] but objective measurement of erythema using chroma meters and laser Doppler flowmeters is strongly suggested.[9,24] The test is usually performed on normal-looking skin, but it is sometimes useful to test suspected irritants on slightly or previously affected skin areas or on skin sites suggested by the patient's history. For example, if an immediate irritant reaction to a cosmetic cream has appeared on the face, we may see nothing if the test is performed on the back, but the reaction can be elicited by reapplication to the previously affected skin of the face. Repeated open tests on the same test site may be needed to detect weak immediate irritant reactions.[25] In a use test, the suspected product or substance is used in the same way as it was when the symptoms appeared.

The chamber test is a routine method of patch testing for contact allergy, but it can also be used to study NIICRs. The test substances are applied in small aluminium chambers (Finn Chamber, Epitest Ltd, Hyrylä, Finland) and fixed to the skin with porous acrylic tape. The occlusion time is 15 min. and the test is read at 20, 40, and 60 min. Occlusion enhances percutaneous penetration and may increase the sensitivity of the test. The advantage of the chamber test is that a smaller skin area is needed than in the open test.[2,26]

The concentration of a NIICR agent needed in a skin test may be difficult to define, as it is in case tests with classical, delayed-type irritants. Therefore, dilution series are recommended. They make it possible to determine the threshold irritant concentration for that particular patient and skin area. Examples of the concentrations often used in dilution series in alcohol vehicles are 250, 125, 62, 31 mM for benzoic acid and 50, 10, 2, and 0.5 mM for methyl nicotinate.[7,27]

It is known that oral[9] and topical[10] nonsteroidal anti-inflammatory drugs efficiently suppress NIICRs and may therefore cause false negative results in testing. The minimum refractory period is 3 days.[11] Tanned skin has decreased reactivity to NIICR agents,[16] and both UVB and UVA irradiation suppresses these reactions for 2 to 3 weeks.[14,15] Skin sites which are washed repeatedly may have a lowered threshold for immediate irritancy to NIICR agents.[27] The importance of the selection of the test site and the testing method has already been mentioned. These sources of false results should be kept in mind when tests for immediate irritancy are performed and the results of such tests are interpreted.

REFERENCES

1. Lahti, A., Immediate contact reactions, in *Textbook of Contact Dermatitis*, Rycroft, R. J. G., Menné, T., and Frosch, P. J., Eds., Springer-Verlag, Berlin, 1995, Chap. 2.3.
2. Lahti, A., Nonimmunologic contact urticaria, *Acta Dermatol. Venereol. (Stockh.)*, 60, 1, 1980.
3. Hjorth, N. and Roed-Petersen, J., Occupational protein contact dermatitis in foodhandlers, *Contact Dermatitis*, 2, 28, 1976.
4. Hannuksela, M., Contact urticaria from foods, in *Nutrition and the Skin*, Roe, D. A., Ed., Alan R. Liss, New York, 1986, Vol. 10, 153.
5. Maibach, H. I. and Johnson, H. L., Contact urticaria syndrome. Contact urticaria to diethyltoluamide (immediate-type hypersensitivity), *Arch. Dermatol.*, 111, 726, 1975.
6. Hannuksela, M., Atopic contact dermatitis, *Contact Dermatitis*, 6, 30, 1980.
7. Lahti, A., Terfenadine (H1-antagonist) does not inhibit nonimmunologic contact urticaria, *Contact Dermatitis*, 16, 220, 1987.
8. Lahti, A., Oikarinen, A., Viinikka, L., Ylikorkala, O., and Hannuksela, M., Prostaglandins in contact urticaria induced by benzoic acid, *Acta Dermatol. Venereol. (Stockh.)*, 63, 425, 1983.
9. Lahti, A., Väänänen, A., Kokkonen, E-L., and Hannuksela, M., Acetylsalicylic acid inhibits nonimmunologic contact urticaria. *Contact Dermatitis*, 16, 133, 1987.
10. Johansson, J. and Lahti, A., Topical non-steroidal anti-inflammatory drugs inhibit nonimmunologic immediate contact reactions, *Contact Dermatitis*, 19, 161, 1988.
11. Kujala, T. and Lahti, A., Duration of inhibition of nonimmunologic immediate contact reactions by acetylsalicylic acid, *Contact Dermatitis*, 21, 60, 1989.
12. Bernstein, J. E., Swift, R. M., Keyoumars, S., and Lorincz, A. L., Inhibition of axon reflex vasodilatation by topically applied capsaicin, *J. Invest. Dermatol.*, 76, 394, 1981.
13. Larmi, E., Lahti, A., and Hannuksela, M., Effects of capsaicin and topical anesthesia on nonimmunologic immediate contact reactions to benzoic acid and methyl nicotinate, in *Current Topics in Contact Dermatitis*, Frosch, P. J., Dooms-Goossens, A., Lachapelle, J-M., Rycroft, R. J. G., and Scheper, R. J., Eds., Springer-Verlag, Berlin, 1989, 441.
14. Larmi, E., Lahti, A., and Hannuksela, M., Ultraviolet light inhibits nonimmunologic immediate contact reactions to benzoic acid, *Arch. Dermatol. Res.*, 280, 420, 1988.

15. Larmi, E., Systemic effect of ultraviolet irradiation on nonimmunologic immediate contact reactions to benzoic acid and methyl nicotinate, *Acta Dermatol. Venereol. (Stockh.),* 69, 269, 1989.

16. Gollhausen, R. and Kligman, A. M., Human assay for identifying substances which induce non-allergic contact urticaria: the NICU-test, *Contact Dermatitis,* 13, 98, 1985.

17. Hannuksela, A., Lahti, A., and Hannuksela, M., Nonimmunologic immediate contact reactions to three isomers of pyridine carboxaldehyde, in *Current Topics in Contact Dermatitis,* Frosch, P. J., Dooms-Goossens, A., Lachapelle, J-M., Rycroft, R. J. G., and Scheper, R. J., Eds., Springer-Verlag, Berlin, 1989, 448.

18. Lahti, A. and Maibach, H. I., An animal model for nonimmunologic contact urticaria, *Toxicol. Appl. Pharmacol.,* 76, 219, 1984.

19. Lahti, A. and Maibach, H. I., Species specificity of nonimmunologic contact urticaria: guinea pig, rat and mouse, *J. Am. Acad. Dermatol.,* 13, 66, 1985.

20. Lahti, A. and Maibach, H. I., Long refractory period after one application of nonimmunologic contact urticaria agents to the guinea pig ear, *J. Am. Acad. Dermatol.,* 13, 585, 1985.

21. Larmi, E., Lahti, A., and Hannuksela, M., Immediate contact reactions to benzoic acid and the sodium salt of pyrrolidone carboxylic acid. Comparison of various skin sites, *Contact Dermatitis,* 20, 38, 1989.

22. Ylipieti, S. and Lahti, A., Effect of the vehicle on nonimmunologic immediate contact reactions, *Contact Dermatitis,* 21, 105, 1989.

23. Lahti, A., Poutiainen, A-M., and Hannuksela, M., Alcohol vehicles in tests for non-immunological immediate contact reactions, *Contact Dermatitis,* 29, 22, 1993.

24. Lahti, A., Kopola, H., Harila, A., Myllylä, R., and Hannuksela, M., Assessment of skin erythema by eye, laser Doppler flowmeter, spectroradiometer, two-channel erythema meter and Minolta chroma meter, *Arch. Dermatol. Res.,* 285, 278, 1993.

25. Hannuksela, A., Niinimäki, A., and Hannuksela, M., Size of the test area does not affect the result of the repeated open application test, *Contact Dermatitis,* 28, 299, 1993.

26. Hannuksela, M., Skin tests for immediate hypersensitivity, in *Textbook of Contact Dermatitis,* Rycroft, R. J. G., Menné, T., and Frosch, P. J., Eds., Springer-Verlag, Berlin, 1995, Chap. 10.4.

27. Lahti, A., Pylvänen, V., and Hannuksela, M., Immediate irritant reactions to benzoic acid are enhanced in washed skin areas, *Contact Dermatitis,* 33, 177, 1995.

2

Immunologic Contact Urticaria Definition

Smita Amin and Howard I. Maibach

CONTENTS

2.1 IMMUNOLOGIC CONTACT URTICARIA

Immunologic contact urticaria (ICU) is the form of contact urticaria that is less frequently encountered in clinical practice. Generally, persons with an "atopic" background (personal or family history of eczema, hayfever, and/or asthma) are more predisposed to ICU. A unique and serious clinical feature of ICU is the ability of the reaction to spread beyond the site of contact and progress to generalized urticaria, involvement of internal organs, and/or anaphylaxis.

The mechanism of ICU is a type 1 hypersensitivity immunologic reaction mediated by specific IgE antibodies in the patient's serum made against the causative agent. This mechanism requires that the person has previously been exposed to the causative agent and has become "sensitized" (i.e., has produced specific IgE antibodies). The route of sensitization can be via the skin (natural latex and some foods), mucous membranes, or via other organs, such as the respiratory and gastrointestinal tracts. The specific IgE antibodies can be detected in the serum by using an assay called the radioallergoabsorbent test (RAST).

In skin challenge, the molecules of a contact reactant penetrate the epidermis and react with specific IgE molecules attached to mast cell membranes. Cutaneous symptoms and signs (pruritis, erythema, and edema) are elicited by vasoactive substances, mainly histamine released from mast cells. The role of histamine is important, but other mediators of inflammation, such as prostaglandins, leukotrienes, and kinins, may also influence the intensity of response. However, little is known regarding the dynamics of their interplay in clinical situations. More is known about the mediators of nonimmunologic contact urticaria (NICU).

Not only do mast cells and circulating basophils have Fc-receptors for IgE molecules, but eosinophils (Capron et al., 1981), peripheral B and T lymphocytes (Yodoi and Iskizaka, 1979), platelets (Joseph et al., 1983), monocytes (Melewicz and Spiegelberg, 1980), and alveolar macrophages (Joseph et al., 1980) can also bind IgE. These findings make the issue of immunologic contact urticaria (ICU) more complicated than was believed earlier.

Patients with atopic dermatitis, but no other atopics or normal controls, have IgE on their epidermal Langerhans cells (Barker et al., 1988; Bruynzeel-Koomen, 1986; Bruynzeel-Koomen et al.,1986). This finding may provide an explanation for the high frequency of positive patch-test reactions to inhalant allergens, such as house dust mites, birch and grass pollen, and animal danders, in these patients (Adinoff et al., 1988; Leung et al., 1987; Mitchell et al., 1986; Reitamo et al., 1986; Tiga-lonowa et al., 1988). An important function of epidermal Langerhans cells is antigen presentation in delayed-type contact allergic reaction, but it can be hypothesized that protein allergens (inhalant, food, etc.) for type I immediate contact reactions bind to specific IgE molecules present on epidermal Langerhans cells, which become apposed to mononuclear cells (Najem and Hull, 1989) and induce a delayed-type hypersensitivity reaction resulting in eczematous skin lesions. This may be the mechanism whereby repeated immediate contact reactions lead to more persistent eczematous skin lesions.

Contact urticaria to rubber latex is a typical example of immediate immunologic contact reaction and is common (Estlander et al., 1987; Pecquet and Leynadier, 1993; Turjanmaa, 1987; Turjanmaa and Reunala, 1988; Wrangsjo et al., 1986). Anaphy-lactic symptoms and generalized urticaria have occurred after contact with surgical (Axelsson et al., 1988; Carrillo et al., 1986; Spaner et al., 1989; Turjanmaa et al., 1988a) and household rubber gloves (Seifert et al., 1987). These reactions have been shown to be immediate, allergic, and IgE-mediated (Frosch et al., 1986; Seifert et al., 1987; Turjanmaa and Reunala, 1989; Turjanmaa et al., 1989). The allergens are among the proteins that constitute 1–2% of natural latex. Allergy to latex can be established by open application, skin prick tests (Turjanmaa et al., 1988c), and by latex radioallergosorbent test (RAST) (Turjanmaa et al., 1988b).

Veterinary surgeons can contract contact urticaria on the hand after contact with cows' amnion fluid, but they do not acquire reactions to cows' dander in clinical provocation tests or in skin prick tests with cows' epithelium extracts. RAST inves-tigations have shown that antibodies to cows' amnion fluid and serum, but not to epithelia, can be found in the sera of veterinary surgeons. The allergen causing contact urticaria in these cases is a compound of amnion fluid and serum but not of the epithelium of cows (Kalveram et al., 1986).

Foods are the most common causes of immediate allergic contact reactions (Table 2.1). The orolaryngeal area is a site where immediate reactions are provoked by food allergens, frequently among atopic individuals. Of 230 patients allergic to birch pollen, 152 (66%) gave a history of itching, tingling, or edema of the lips and tongue and hoarseness or irritation of the throat when eating raw fruits and vegetables such as apple, potato, carrot, and tomato (Hannuksela and Lahti, 1977). Plum, peach, cherry, kiwi, celery, and parsnip can also elicit immediate contact reactions in birch pollen-allergic people. Positive results ("scratch-chamber" test) with suspected raw fruits and vegetables were noted in 36% of 230 patients. Apple, carrot, parsnip, and potato elicited reactions more often than swede (rutabaga), tomato, onion, celery, and parsley. The clinical relevance of the skin test results with apple, potato, and carrot was 80–90%. Only 7 of 158 (4%) atopic patients who were not allergic to birch pollen had positive skin test reactions to any of the fruits and vegetables.

RAST and RAST-inhibition studies have confirmed the cross-allergy between birch pollen and fruits and vegetables. All immunological determinants in apple, carrot, and celery tuber appeared to be present also in birch pollen but not vice versa (Halmepuro and Løvenstein, 1986; Halmepuro et al., 1984).

2.2 DIAGNOSTIC TESTS

The diagnosis of immediate contact reactions is based on a full medical history and on skin tests with suspected substances.

2.2.1 Tests for Both Immunologic and Nonimmunologic Contact Urticaria

The simplest test is the open test. For this test the suspected substance (fish, apple, carrot) is applied and gently rubbed on either normal-looking or slightly affected skin, usually the hand. The test site is observed for 60 minutes (Hannuksela, 1986). A positive result is seen as an edema and erythema reaction or as tiny intraepidermal spongiotic vesicles typical of acute eczema.

The use test requires the patient to handle the suspected agent precisely as handled when symptoms appeared. Wearing surgical gloves on wet hands to provoke contact urticaria to latex is a typical use test.

In the open test, 0.1 ml of the test substance is spread on a 3×3 cm area of the skin of the upper back or on the extensor side of the upper arm. The test should first be performed on nondiseased skin and then, if negative, on previously or currently affected skin (Lahti and Maibach, 1986). Even in immunologic contact urticaria there may be a marked difference between skin sites in their capacity to elicit contact urticaria (Maibach, 1986). This is typical of nonimmunologic contact urticaria. The face has been considered the most sensitive skin area (Gollhausen and Kligman, 1985). Often it is desirable to apply contact urticants to skin sites suggested by the patient's history. The immunologic contact reactions usually appear within 15–20 minutes and nonimmunologic ones within 45–60 minutes after application. A positive reaction comprises a wheal and flare reaction and sometimes a vesicular

TABLE 2.1 Agents Producing Immunologic Contact Urticaria (ICU)

Animal products

Amnion fluid
Blood
Brucella abortus (Trunnel et al., 1985)
Cercariae
Cheyletus malaccensis (Yoshikawa, 1985)
Chironomidae, Chironomus thummi thummi (Mittelbach, 1983)
Cockroaches
Dander (Agrup and Sjostedt, 1985; Weissenbach et al., 1988)
Dermestes maculatus Degeer (Lewis-Jones, 1985)
Gelatine (Wahl and Kleinhans, 1989)
Gut
Hair
Listrophorus gibbus (Burns, 1987)
Liver
Locust (Monk, 1988; Tee et al., 1988)
Mealworm, *Tenibrio molitor* (Bernstein et al., 1983)
Placenta
Saliva (Valsecchi and Cainelli, 1989)
Serum
Silk
Spider mite, *Tetranychus urticae* (Reunala et al., 1983)
Wool

Food

Dairy
Cheese
Egg
Milk (Boso and Brestel, 1987; Salo et al., 1986)

Fruits
Apple (Halmepuro and Løwenstein, 1985; Pigatto et al., 1983)
Apricot
Banana
Kiwi
Mango
Orange
Peach
Plum

Grains
Buckwheat (Valdivieso et al., 1989)
Maize
Malt
Rice (Lezaun et al., 1994)

TABLE 2.1 (continued)   Agents Producing Immunologic Contact Urticaria (ICU)

Wheat
Wheat bran

Honey
Nuts/Seeds
Peanut
Sesame seed
Sunflower seed

Meats
Beef
Chicken
Lamb
Liver
Turkey

Seafood
Fish (Kavli and Moseng, 1987; Melino et al., 1987)
Prawns
Shrimp (Nagano et al., 1984)

Vegetables
Beans
Cabbage
Carrot (Muñoz et al., 1985)
Celery (Kremser and Lindemayr, 1983; Wuthrich and Dietschi, 1985)
Chives
Cucumber
Endive
Lettuce
Onion
Parsley
Parsnip
Potato (Larkö et al., 1983)
Rutabaga (swede)
Tomato
Soybean

Fragrances and flavorings

Balsam of Peru
Menthol
Vanillin

Medicaments

Acetylsalicylic acid
Antibiotics
    Amoxicillin, Ampicillin

TABLE 2.1 (continued)   Agents Producing Immunologic Contact Urticaria (ICU)

Bacitracin
Cephalosporins
  Cefotiam dihydrochloride (Mizutani et al., 1994)
  Cephalotin
Chloramphenicol (Schewach-Millet and Shpiro, 1985)
Cloxacillin
Gentamicin
Iodochlorhydroxyquin
Mezlocillin (Keller and Schwanitz, 1993)
Neomycin
Nifuroxime (Aaronson, 1969)
Penicillin (Rudzki and Rebandel, 1985)
Rifampin
Rifamycin (Grob et al., 1987)
Streptomycin
Virginiamycin (Baes, 1974)
Benzocaine (Kleinhans and Zwissler, 1980)
Benzoyl peroxide
Clobetasol 17-propionate (Gottmann-Lückerath, 1982)
Dinitrochlorobenzene (Valsecchi et al., 1986; van Hecke and Santosa, 1985)
Etophenamate (Pinol and Carapeto, 1984)
Fumaric acid derivatives (de Haan et al., 1994)
Mechlorethamine
Pentamidine (Belsito, 1993)
Phenothiazines
  Chlorpromazine (Lovell et al., 1986)
  Levomepromazine (Johansson, 1988)
  Promethazine
  Pyrazolones
  Aminophenazone (Lombardi et al., 1983)
  Methamizole
  Propylphenazone
Tocopherol (Kassen and Mitchell, 1974)

Metals

Cobalt, Gold, Mercury, Tin, Zinc (Hostynek, 1997)
Copper (Shelley et al., 1983)
Nickel (Valsecchi and Cainelli, 1987)
Platinum, Rhodium, Palladium, Iridium, Rutherium (Nakayama, 1997)

Plant products (Lahti, 1986b)

Abietic acid (El-Sayed et al., 1995)
Algae
Birch
Camomile
Castor bean

TABLE 2.1 (continued)   Agents Producing Immunologic Contact Urticaria (ICU)

Chrysanthemum (Tanaka et al., 1987)
Cinchona (Dooms-Goossens et al., 1986a)
Colophony (Rivers and Rycroft, 1987)
Corn starch (Assalve et al., 1988; Fisher, 1987)
Cotoneaster
Emetin
Fennel (La Rosa et al., 1986)
Garlic
Grevillea juniperina (Apted, 1988a)
Hakea suaveolens (Apted, 1988b)
Hawthorn, *Crataegus monogyna* (Steinman et al., 1984)
Henna
Latex rubber (Axelsson et al., 1987; Frosh et al., 1986; Morales et al., 1989; Spaner et al.,
  1989; van der Meeren and van Erp, 1986; Wrangsjö et al., 1988)
Lichens
Lily (Lahti, 1986a)
Lime (Picardo, 1988)
Limonium tataricum (Quirce et al., 1993)
Mahogany
Mustard (Kavli and Moseng, 1987)
Papain (Santucci et al., 1985)
Perfumes
Pickles (Edwards and Edwards, 1984a)
Rose (Kleinhans, 1985)
Rouge
Spices (Niinimäki, 1987)
Strawberry (Grattan and Harman, 1985)
Teak
Tobacco (Tosti et al., 1987)
Tulip (Lahti, 1986a)
Winged bean (Lovell and Rycroft, 1984)

Preservatives and disinfectants

Benzoic acid (Nethercott et al., 1984)
Benzyl alcohol
Butylated hydroxytoluene
Chlorhexidine (Bergqvist-Karlsson, 1988; Fisher, 1989; Nishioka et al., 1984)
Chloramine
Chlorocresol (Goncalo et al., 1987)
1,3-Diiodo-2-hydroxypropane (Löwenfeld, 1928)
Formaldehyde (Andersen and Maibach, 1984; Lindskov, 1982)
Gentian violet (Francois et al., 1970)
Hexantriol (Tachibana et al., 1977)
para-Hydroxybenzoic acid (Bottger et al., 1981)
Parabens (Henry et al., 1979)
Phenylmercuric propionate
ortho-Phenylphenate (Tuer et al., 1986)

TABLE 2.1 (continued)   Agents Producing Immunologic Contact Urticaria (ICU)

Polysorbates
Sodium hypochlorite
Sorbitan monolaurate
Tropicamide (Guill et al., 1979)

Enzymes

alpha-Amylase (Morren et al., 1993)
Cellulases (Tarvainen et al., 1991)
Xylanases (Tarvainen et al., 1991)

Miscellaneous

Acetyl acetone (Sterry and Schmoll, 1985)
Acrylic monomer
Alcohols (amyl, butyl, ethyl, isopropyl) (Rilliet et al., 1980)
Aliphatic polyamide
Ammonia
Ammonium persulfate
Aminothiazole
Benzophenone
Carbonless copy paper
Chlorothanil (Dannaker et al., 1993)
Cu(II)-acetyl acetonate (Sterry and Schmoll, 1985)
Denatonium benzoate
Diethyltoluamide
Epoxy resin (Jolanki et al., 1987)
Formaldehyde resin
Lanolin alcohols
Lindane
Methyl ethyl ketone (Varigos and Nurse, 1986)
Monoamylamine
Naphtha (Goodfield and Saihan, 1988)
Naphthylacetic acid (Camarasa, 1986)
Nylon (Dooms-Goossens et al., 1986b; Hatch and Maibach, 1985)
Oleylamide
Paraphenylenediamine (Edwards and Edwards, 1984b; Temesvari, 1984)
Patent blue dye
Perlon
Phosphorus sesquisulfide (Payero et al., 1985)
Plastic
Polypropylene (Tosti et al., 1986)
Polyethylene glycol
Potassium ferricyanide
Seminal fluid (Blair and Parish, 1985)
Sodium silicate
Sodium sulfide
Sulfur dioxide

TABLE 2.1 (continued)   Agents Producing Immunologic Contact Urticaria (ICU)

Terpinyl acetate
Textile finish (De Groot and Gerkens, 1989)
Vinyl pyridine
Zinc diethyldithiocarbamate

eruption indistinguishable from that seen in eczema (Hjorth and Roed-Petersen, 1976).

2.2.2   Tests for Immunologic Contact Urticaria

Open application as above is all that is required for most ICU agents. Prick testing is often the method of choice for testing patients with suspected allergic contact reactions when the open application method is negative.

The scratch test is a less standardized method than the prick test, but it is useful when nonstandardized allergens must be used (Paul, 1987). The allergen solutions in scratch testing are the same as those used in prick testing. Also, freeze-dried and other powdered allergens moistened with 0.1 N aqueous sodium hydroxide solution and fresh foods (e.g., potato, apple, carrot) can be used. When testing with poorly standardized or nonstandardized substances, control tests should be made on at least 20 people to avoid false interpretation of the test results.

The chamber scratch test was introduced for testing foods when commercial allergens with proven efficacy are not available (Hannuksela and Lahti, 1977). Potato, apple, and carrot lose their allergenicity when cooked, deep-frozen, or made into juice, and it is therefore best to use them fresh for skin testing.

In the chamber scratch test, the procedure is that of the ordinary scratch test, but the scratch and the foodstuff are covered with a small aluminum chamber (Finn Chamber, Epitest Ltd Oy, Hyryla, Finland) for 15 minutes. The result is read 5 minutes after the removal of the chamber according to the criteria of the scratch test. Reactions at least the size of a similarly produced histamine reaction are usually clinically significant. Histamine hydrochloride (10 mg/ml) is the positive reference and aqueous 0.1 N sodium hydroxide is the negative reference.

The Prausnitz-Kustner test or passive transfer test has been used in occupational dermatology for detecting immunologic contact urticaria to potato (Tuft and Blumstein, 1942) and to rubber (Kopman and Hannuksela, 1983). Today, because of concern regarding inadvertent transfer of infectous diseases among humans, this test is now generally limited to animal studies.

RAST is seldom needed for contact urticaria diagnosis, but RAST inhibition tests are used in investigating cross-allergenity (Halmepuro and Løvenstein, 1985). For this purpose, crossed radioimmunoelectrophoresis and its inhibition are also used. If there is a risk of anaphylaxis, a RAST may be performed before skin testing.

Nonsteroidal antiinflammatory drugs and antihistamines should not be taken by patients during tests for immediate contact reactions because these drugs may inhibit the reactions. Using the same test site repeatedly may result in the tachyphylaxis phenomenon and cause false negative results.

A positive open test (erythema alone or wheal and flare) is almost always of clinical significance in ICU, assuming that the same agent is not reactive in controls. With skin prick and scratch testing, great caution must be utilized to rule out nonspecific reactions. Also the need for more controls (>10) should be emphasized, since many substances produce positive reactions in a nonimmunologic manner. Normal saline or other appropriate diluents may be used for prick or scratch testing controls.

CAUTION: In testing for ICU when extracutaneous organs are also involved, it is extremely important to begin with very diluted allergen concentrations and use serial dilutions if required, in order to minimize allergen exposure and avoid reproducing systemic reactions (von Krogh and Maibach, 1982). Resuscitation facilities should also be immediately available.

When examining patients with a suspected allergic contact reaction, the prick, scratch, or scratch chamber tests may be done first because the test procedures are fast. The diagnosis should be based on the result of the open application test and interpreted by reviewing the clinical history and the background controls.

REFERENCES

Aaronson, C. M. 1969. Generalized urticaria from sensitivity to nifuroxime. *J. Am. Med. Assoc.* 210:557.

Adinoff, A. D., Tellez, P., and Clark, R. A. 1988. Atopic dermatitis and aeroallergen contact sensitivity. *J. Allergy Clin. Immunol.* 81:736-742.

Agrup, G. and Sjostedt, L. 1985. Contact urticaria in laboratory technicians working with animals. *Acta Derm. Venereol. (Stockh.)* 65:111-115.

Andersen, K. E. and Maibach, H. I. 1984. Multiple application delayed onset contact urticaria: possible relation to certain unusual formalin and textile reactions. *Contact Dermatitis* 10:227-234.

Apted, J. 1988a. Acute contact urticaria from *Grevillea juniperina. Contact Dermatitis* 18:126.

Apted, J. 1988b. Acute contact urticaria from *Hakea suaveolens. Contact Dermatitis* 18:126.

Assalve, D., Cicioni, P., Perno, P., and Lisi, P. 1988. Contact urticaria and anaphylactoid reaction from cornstarch surgical glove powder. *Contact Dermatitis* 19:61.

Axelsson, J. G. K., Johansson, S. G. O., and Wrangsjo, K. 1987. IgE-mediated anaphylactoid reactions to rubber. *Allergy* 42:46-50.

Axelsson, I. G., Ericksson, M., and Wrangsjo, K. 1989. Anaphylaxis and angioedema due to rubber allergy in children. *Acta Paediatr. Scand.* 77:314-316.

Baes, H. 1974. Allergic contact dermatitis to virginiamycin. *Dermatologica (Basel)* 149:231.

Barker, J. N. W. N., Alegre, V. A., and MacDonald, D. M. 1988. Surface-bound immunoglobulin E on antigenpresenting cells in cutaneous tissue of atopic dermatitis. *J. Invest. Dermatol.* 90:117-121.

Belsito, D.V. 1993. Contact urticaria from pentamidine isethionate. *Contact Dermatitis* 29:158.

Bergqvist-Karlsson, A. 1988. Delayed and immediate-type hypersensitivity to chlorhexidine. *Contact Dermatitis* 18:84-88.

Bernstein, D. I., Gallagher, J. S., and Bernstein, I. L. 1983. Mealworm asthma: clinical and immunological studies. *J. Allergy Clin. Immunol.* 72:475–480.

Blair, H. and Parish, W. E. 1985. Asthma and urticaria induced by seminal plasma in a woman with IgE antibody and T-lymphocyte responsiveness to a seminal plasma antigen. *Clinical Allergy* 15:117–130.

Boso, E. B. and Brestel, E. P. 1987. Contact urticaria to cow milk. *Allergy* 42:151–153.

Bottger, E. M., Mucke, C., and Tronnier, H. 1981. Kontaktdermatitis auf neuere Antikykotika and Kontakturtikaria. *Acta Derm. Venereol. Suppl. (Stockh.)* 7:70.

Bruynzeel-Koomen, C. 1986. IgE on Langerhans cells: new insights into the pathogenesis of atopic dermatitis. *Dermatologica* 172:181–183.

Bruynzeel-Koomen, C., van Wichen, D. F., Toonstra, J., Berrens, J., and Bruynzeel, P. L. B. 1986. The presence of IgE molecules on epidermal Langerhans cells in patients with atopic dermatitis. *Arch. Dermatol. Res.* 278:199-205.

Burns, D. A. 1987. Papular urticaria produced by the mite *Listrophorus gibbus*. *Clin. Exp. Dermatol.* 12:200-201.

Camarasa, J. G. 1986. Contact urticaria to naphthylacetic acid. *Contact Dermatitis* 14:113.

Capron, M., Capron, A., Dessaint, J., Johansson, S., and Prin, L. 1981. Fc-receptors for IgE on human and rat eosinophils. *J. Immunol.* 126:2087–2092.

Carrillo, T., Cuevas, M., Munoz, T., Hinojosa, M., and Moneo, I. 1986. Contact urticaria and rhinitis from latex surgical gloves. *Contact Dermatitis* 15:69-72.

Dannaker, C.J., Maibach, H.I., and O'Malley, M. 1993. Contact urticaria and anaphylaxis to the fungicide chlorothalonil. *Cutis* 52:312-315.

De Groot, A. C. and Gerkens, F. 1989. Contact urticaria from a chemical textile finish. *Contact Dermatitis* 20:63-64.

de Haan, P., von Blomberg-van der Flier, B. M., de Groot, J., Nieboer, C., and Bruynzeel, D. P. 1994. The risk of sensibilization and contact urticaria upon topical application of fumaric acid derivatives. *Dermatology* 188:126-130.

Dooms-Goossens, A., Deveylder, H., Duron, C., Dooms, M., and Degreef, H. 1986a. Airborne contact urticaria due to cinchona. *Contact Dermatitis* 15:258.

Dooms-Goossens, A., Duron, C., Loncke, J., and Degreef, H. 1986b. Contact urticaria due to nylon. *Contact Derrnatitis* 14:63.

Edwards, E. K. and Edwards, E. K. 1984a. Contact urticaria provoked by pickels. *Cutis* 33:230.

Edwards, E. K. and Edwards, E. K. 1984b. Contact urticaria and allergic contact dermatitis caused by paraphenylenediamine. *Cutis* 34:87–88.

El-Sayed, F., Manzur, F., Bayle, P., et al. 1995. Contact urticaria from abietic acid. *Contact Dermatitis* 32:361–362.

Estlander, T., Jolanki, R., and Kanerva, L. 1987. Contact urticaria from rubber gloves: a detailed description of four cases. *Acta Derm. Venereol. Suppl. (Stockh.)* 134:98–102.

Fisher, A. A. 1987. Contact urticaria and anaphylactoid reaction due to corn starch surgical glove powder. *Contact Dermatitis* 16:224-225.

Fisher, A. A. 1989. Contact urticaria from chlorhexidine. *Cutis* 43:17–18.

Francois, A., Henin, P., Carli Basset, C., and Ginies, G. 1970. Anaphylactic shock following applications of Milian's solution. *Bull. Soc. Fr. Dermatol. Syphiligr.* 77:834.

Frosch, P. J., Wahl, R., Bahmer, F. A., and Maasch, H. J. 1986. Contact urticaria to rubber gloves is IgE-mediated. *Contact Dermatitis* 14:241–245.

Gollhausen, R. and Kligman, A. M. 1985. Human assay for identifying substances which induce non-allergic contact urticaria: the NICU-test. *Contact Dermatitis* 13:98–106.

Goncalo, M., Gongalo, S., and Moreno, A. 1987. Immediate and delayed sensitity to chlorocresol. *Contact Dermatitis* 17:46–47.

Goodfield, M. J. D. and Saihan, E. M. 1988. Contact urticaria to naphtha present in a solvent. *Contact Dermatitis* 18:187.

Gottmann-Luckerath, I. 1982. Kontakturticaria nach DermoxinR. *Soc. Proc. Dermato sen* 30:124.

Grattan, C. E. H. and Harman, R. R. M. 1985. Contact urticaria to strawberry. *Contact Dermatitis* 13:191–192.

Grob, J. J., Pommier, G., Robaglia, A., Collet-Villette, A. M., and Bonerandi, J. J. 1987. Contact urticaria from rifamycin. *Contact Dermatitis* 16:284–285.

Guill, A., Goette, K., Knight, C. G., Peck, C. C., and Lupton, G. P. 1979. Erythema multiforme and urticaria. *Arch. Dermatol.* 115:742.

Halmepuro, L. and Løvenstein, H. 1985. Immunological investigation of possible structural similarities between pollen antigens and antigens in apple, carrot, and celery tuber. *Allergy* 40:264-272.

Halmepuro, L., Vuontela, K., Kalimo, K., and Bjorksten, F. 1984. Cross-reactivity of IgE antibodies with allergens in birch pollen, fruits, and vegetables. *Int. Arch. Allergy Appl. Immunol.* 74:235-240.

Hannuksela, M. 1986. Contact urticaria from foods. In *Nutrition and the Skin,* D. Roe, Ed., pp. 153-162. New York: Alan R. Liss.

Hannuksela, M. and Lahti, A. 1977. Immediate reactions to fruits and vegetables. *Contact Dermatitis* 3:79-84.

Hatch, K. L. and Maibach, H. I. 1985. Textile fiber dermatitis. *Contact Dermatitis* 12:1-11.

Henry, J. C., Tschen, E. H., and Becker, L. E. 1979. Contact urticaria to parabens. *Arch. Dermatol.* 115:1231.

Hjorth, N. and Roed-Petersen, J. 1976. Occupational protein contact dermatitis in foodhandlers. *Contact Dermatitis* 2:28-42.

Hostynek, J.J. 1997. Metals. In *Contact Urticaria Syndrome,* S. Amin, A. Lahti, and H.I. Maibach, Eds., Boca Raton: CRC Press.

Johansson, G. 1988. Contact urticaria from levomepromazine. *Contact Dermatitis* 19:304.

Jolanki, R., Estlander, T., and Kanerva, L. 1987. Occupational contact dermatitis and contact urticaria caused by epoxy resins. *Acta Derm. Venereol. Suppl. (Stockh.)* 134:90-94.

Joseph, M., Tonnel, A., Capron, A., and Voisin, C. 1980. Enzyme release and super oxide anion production by human alveolar macrophages stimulated with immunoglobulin E. *Clin. Exp. Immunol.* 40:416-422.

Joseph, M., Auriault, C., Capron, A., Vorng, H., and Viens, P. 1983. A new function for platelets: IgE-dependent killing of schistosomes. *Nature (Lond.)* 303:810-812.

Kalveram, K.-J., Kastner, H., and Frock, G. 1986. Detection of specific IgE antibodies in veterinarians suffering from contact urticaria. *Z. Hautkr.* 61:75-81.

Kassen, B. and Mitchell, J. C. 1974. Contact urticaria from a vitamin E preparation in two siblings. *Contact Derm. Newslett.* 16:482.

Kavli, G. and Moseng, D. 1987. Contact urticaria from mustard in fish stick production. *Contact Dermatitis* 17:153-155.

Keller, K. and Schwanitz, H. J. 1993. Combined immediate and delayed type hypersensitivity to Mezlocillin. *H + G* Band 68, Heft 3:178-180.

Kleinhans, D. 1985. Kontakt-Urtikaria. *Dermatosen* 33:198-203.

Kleinhans, D. and Zwissler, H. 1980. Anaphylaktischer Schock nach Anwendung einer Benzocainhaltigen Salbe. *Z. Hautkr.* 55:945.

Kopman, A. and Hannuksela, M. 1983. Contact urticaria to rubber. *Duodecim* 99:221-224.

Kremser, M. and Lindemayr, W. 1983. Celery allergy (celery contact urticaria syndrome) and relation to allergies to other plant antigens. *Wien. Klin. Wochenscher.* 95:838-843.

Lahti, A. 1986a. Contact urticaria and respiratory symptoms from tulips and lilies. *Contact Dermatitis* 14:317-319.

Lahti, A. 1986b. Contact urticaria to plants. *Dermatol. Clin.* 4:127-136.

Lahti, A. and Maibach, H. I. 1986. Immediate contact reactions (contact urticaria syndrome). In *Occupational and Industrial Dermatology,* 2nd ed., H. Maibach, Ed., pp. 32-44. Chicago: Year Book Medical.

Larkö, O., Lindstedt, G., Lundberg, P. A., and Mobacken, H. 1983. Biochemical and clinical studies in a case of contact urticaria to potato. *Contact Dermatitis* 9:108-114.

La Rosa, M., Crea, G. F., Di Francesco, S., Di Paola, M., and Castiglione, N. 1986. Fennel allergy: Case report. Abstr. *3rd Int. Symp. Immunological and Clinical Problems of Food Allergy,* Taormina, Giardini Naxos, Italy, October 1-4.

Leung, D. Y., Schneeberger, E. E., Siraganian, R. P., Geha, R. S., and Bhan, A. K. 1987. The presence of IgE on macrophages and dendritic cells infiltrating into the skin lesion of atopic dermatitis. *Clin. Immunol. Immunopathol.* 42:328-337.

Lewis-Jones, M. S. 1985. Papular urticaria caused by *Dermestes maculatus* Degeer. *Clin. Exp. Dermatol.* 10:181.

Lezaun, A., Igea, J.M., Quirce, S., Cuevas, M., Parra, F., Alonso, M.D., Martin, J.A., and Cano, M.S. 1994. Asthma and contact urticaria caused by rice in a housewife. *Allergy* 49:92-95.

Lindskov, R. 1982. Contact urticaria to formaldehyde. *Contact Dermatitis* 8:333.

Lombardi, P., Giorgini, S., and Achille, A. 1983. Contact urticaria from aminophenazone. *Contact Dermatitis* 9:428-429.

Lovell, C. R., Cronin, E., and Rhodes, E. L. 1986. Photocontact urticaria from chlorpromazine. *Contact Dermatitis* 14:290-291.

Lovell, C. R. and Rycroft, R. J. G. 1984. Contact urticaria from winged bean *(Psophocarpus tetragonolobus). Contact Dermatitis* 10:310-318.

Lowenfeld, W. 1928. Uberempfindlichkeit gegen lodthion mit gleichzeitiger urtikarieller reaction. *Derm. Wochenschr.* 78:502.

Maibach, H. I. 1986. Regional variation in elicitation of contact urticaria syndrome (immediate hypersensitivity syndrome): Shrimp. *Contact Dermatitis* 15:100.

Melewicz, F. and Spiegelberg, H. 1980. Fc-receptors for IgE on a subpopulation of human peripheral blood monocytes. *J. Immunol.* 125:1026-1031.

Melino, M., Toni, F., and Riguzzi, G. 1987. Immunologic contact urticaria to fish. *Contact Dermatitis* 17:182.

Mitchell, E. B., Crow, J., Williams, G., and Platts-Mills, T. A. E. 1986. Increase in skin mast cells following chronic house dust mite exposure. *Br. J . Dermatol.* 114:65-73.

Mittelbach, F. 1983. Urticaria and Quincke's edema caused by *Chironomidae (Chironomus thummi thummi)* as fishfood. *Z. Hautkr.* 58:1548-1555.

Mizutani, H., Ohyanagi, S., and Shimizu, M. 1994. Anaphylactic shock related to occupational handling of Cefotiam dihydrochloride [letter].*Clin. Exp. Dermatol.* 19(5):449.

Monk, B. E. 1988. Contact urticaria to locusts. *Br. J. Dermatol.* 118:707-708.

Morales, C., Basomba, A., Carreira, J., and Sastre, A. 1989. Anaphylaxis produced by rubber glove contact. Case reports and immunological identification of the antigens involved. *Clin. Exp. Allergy* 19:425-430.

Morren, M-A., Janssens, V., Dooms-Goosens, A., Van Hoeyveld, E., Cornelis, A., De Wolf-Peeters, C., and Heremans, A. 1993. Alpha-amylase, a flour additive: An important cause of protein contact dermatitis in bakers. *J. Am. Acad. Dermatol.* 29:723-728.

Muñoz, D., Leanizbarrutia, I., Lobera, T., and de Corres, F. 1985. Anaphylaxis from contact with carrot. *Contact Dermatitis* 13:345-346.

Nagano, T., Kanao, K., and Sugai, T. 1984. Allergic contact urticaria caused by raw prawns and shrimps: Three cases. *J. Allergy Clin. Immunol.* 74:489-493.

Najem, N. and Hull, D. 1989. Langerhans cells in delayed skin reactions to inhalant allergens in atopic dermatitis — An electron microscopic study. *Clin. Exp. Dermatol.* 14:218-222.

Nakayama, H. and Ichikawa, T. 1997. Occupational contact urticaria sundrome due to rhodium and platinum. In *Contact Urticaria Syndrome,* S. Amin, A. Lahti, and H.I. Maibach, Eds., Boca Raton: CRC Press.

Nethercott, J. R., Lawrence, M. J., Roy, A.-M., and Gibson, B. L. 1984. Airborne contact urticaria due to sodium benzoate in a pharmaceutical manufacturing plant. *J. Occup. Med.* 26:734-736.

Niinimäki, A. 1987. Scratch-chamber tests in food handler dermatitis. *Contact Dermatitis* 16:11 20.

Nishioka, K., Doi, T., and Katayama, I. 1984. Histamine release in contact urticaria. *Contact Dermatitis* 11:191.

Paul, E. 1987. Skin reactions to food and food constituents — Allergic and pseudoallergic reactions. *Z. Hautkr. Suppl.* 62:79-87.

Payero, M. L. P., Correcher, B. L., and Garcia-Perez, A. 1985. Contact urticaria and dermatitis from phosphorous sesquisulphide. *Contact Dermatitis* 13:126-127.

Pecquet, C. and Leynadier, F. 1993. IgE mediated allergy to natural rubber latex in 100 patients. *Clin. Rev. Allergy* 11:381-384.

Picardo, M., Rovina, R., Cristaudo, A., Cannistraci, C., and Santucci, B. 1988. Contact urticaria from *Tilia* (lime). *Contact Dermatitis* 19:72-73.

Pigatto, P. D., Riva, F., Altomare, G. F., and Parotelli, R. 1983. Short-term anaphylactic antibodies in contact urticaria and generalized anaphylaxis to apple. *Contact Dermatitis* 9:511.

Pinol, J. and Carapeto, F. J. 1984. Contact urticaria to etofenamate. *Contact Dermatitis* 11:132-133.

Quirce, S., Garcia-Figueroa, B., Olaguibel, J.M., Muro, M.D., and Tabar, A.I. 1993. Occupational asthma and contact urticaria from dried flowers of Limonium tataricum. *Allergy* 48:285-290.

Reitamo, S., Visa, K., Kahonen, K., Kayhko, K., Stubb, S., and Salo, O. P. 1986. Eczematous reactions in atopic patients caused by epicutaneous testing with inhalant allergens. *Br. J. Dermatol.* 114:303-309.

Reunala, T., Bjorksten, F., Forstrom, L., and Kanerva, L. 1983. IgE-mediated occupational allergy to a spider mite. *Clin. Allergy* 13:383-388.

Rilliet, A., Hunziker, N., and Brun, R. 1980. Alcohol contact urticaria syndrome (immediate type hypersensitivity). *Dermatologica (Basel)* 161:361.

Rivers, J. K. and Rycroft, R. J. G. 1987. Occupational allergic contact urticaria from colophony. *Contact Dermatitis* 17:181.

Rudzki, E. and Rebandel, P. 1985. Occupational contact urticaria from penicillin. *Contact Dermatitis* 13:192.

Salo, O. P., Makinen-Kiljunen, S., and Juntunen, K. 1986. Milk causes a rapid urticarial reaction on the skin of children with atopic dermatitis and milk allergy. *Acta Derm. Venereol. (Stockh.)* 66:438-442.

Santucci, B., Cristaudo, A., and Picardo, M. 1985. Contact urticaria from papain in a soft lens solution. *Contact Dermatitis* 12:233.

Seifert, H. U., Wahl, R., Vocks. E., Borelli, S., and Maasch, H. J. 1987. Immunoglobulin E-vermittelte Kontakturtikaria bzw. Asthma bronchiale durch Latexenthaltende Haushaltsgummihandschuhe. *Dermatosen* 35:137-139.

Schewach-Millet, M. and Shpiro, D. 1985. Urticaria and angioedema due to topically applied chloramphenicol ointment. *Arch. Dermatol.* 121:587.

Shelley, W. B., Shelley, E. D., and Ho, A. K. S. 1983. Cholinergic urticaria: Acetylcholine-receptor-dependent immediate-type hypersensitivity reaction to copper. *Lancet* i:843-846.

Spaner, D., Dolovich, J., Tarlo, S., Sussman, G., and Buttoo, K. 1989. Hypersensitivity to natural latex. *J. Allergy Clin. Immunol.* 83:1135-1137.

Steinman, H. K., Lovell, C. R., and Cronin, E. 1984. Immediate-type hypersensitivity to *Crataegus monogyna* (hawthorn). *Contact Dermatitis* 11:321.

Sterry, W. and Schmoll, M. 1985. Contact urticaria and dermatitis from self-adhesive pads. *Contact Dermatitis* 13:284-285.

Tachibana, S., Horio, T., and Hayakawa, M. 1977. Contact urticaria and dermatitis due to fluocinonide cream. *Acta Dermatol. (Kyoto)* 72:141.

Tanaka, T., Moriwaki, S., and Horio, T. 1987. Occupational dermatitis with simultaneous immediate and delayed allergy to *Chrysanthemum. Contact Dermatitis* 16:152-154.

Tarvainen, K., Kanerva, I., Tupasela, O., Grenquist-Norden, B., Jolanki, R., Estlander, T., and Keskinen, H. 1991. Allergy from cellulase and xylanase enzymes. *Clin. Exp. Dermatol.* 21:609-615

Tee, R. D., Gordon, D. J., Hawkins, E. R., Nunn, A. J., Lacey, J., Venables, K. M., Cooter, R. J., McCaffery, A. R., and Newman Taylor, A. J. 1988. Occupational allergy to locusts: An investigation of the sources of the allergen. *J. Allergy Clin. Immunol.* 81:517-525.

Temesvari, E. 1984. Contact urticaria from paraphenylenediamine. *Contact Dermatitis* 11:125.

Tigalonowa, M., Braathen, L. R., and Lea, T. 1988. IgE on Langerhans cells in the skin of patients with atopic dermatitis and birch allergy. *Allergy* 43:464-468.

Tosti, A., Bettoli, V., Iannini, G., and Forlani, L. 1986. Contact urticaria from polypropylene. *Contact Dermatitis* 15:51.

Tosti, A., Melino, M., and Veronesi, S. 1987. Contact urticaria to tobacco. *Contact Dermatitis* 16:225-226.

Trunell, T. N., Waisman, M., and Trunell, T. L. 1985. Contact dermatitis caused by *Brucella. Cutis* 35:379-381.

Tuer, W. F., James, W. D., and Summers, R. J. 1986. Contact urticaria to Ophenylphenate. *Ann. Allergy* 56:19-21.

Tuft, L. and Blumstein, G. I. 1942. Studies in food allergy II. Sensitization to fresh fruits: Clinical and experimental observations. *J. Allergy* 13:574-581.

Turjanmaa, K. 1987. Incidence of immediate allergy to latex gloves in hospital personnel. *Contact Dermatitis* 17:270-275.

Turjanmaa, K. and Reunala, T. 1988. Contact urticaria from rubber gloves. *Dermatol. Clin.* 6:47-51.

Turjanmaa, K. and Reunala, T. 1989. Condoms as a source of latex allergen and cause of contact urticaria. *Contact Dermatitis* 20:360-364.

Turjanmaa, K., Reunala, T., Tuimala, R., and Karkkainen, T. 1988a. Allergy to latex gloves: Unusual complication during delivery. *Br. J. Dermatol.* 297:1029.

Turjanmaa, K., Reunala, T., and Rasanen, L. 1988b. Comparison of diagnostic methods in latex surgical glove contact urticaria. *Contact Dermatitis* 19:241-247.

Turjanmaa, K., Laurila, K., Makinen-Kiljunen, S., and Reunala, T. 1988c. Rubber contact urticaria. Allergenic properties of 19 brands of latex gloves. *Contact Dermatitis* 19:362-367.

Turjanmaa, K., Rasanen, L., Lehto, M., Makinen-Kiljunen, S., and Reunala, T. 1989. Basophil histamine release and lymphocyte proliferation tests in latex contact urticaria. *Allergy* 44:181-186.

Valdivieso, R., Moneo, I., Pola, J., Munoz, T., Zapata, C., Hinojosa, M., and Losada, E. 1989. Occupational asthma and contact urticaria caused by buckwheat flour. *Ann. Allergy* 63:149-152.

Valsecchi, R. and Cainelli, T. 1987. Contact urticaria from nickel. *Contact Dermatitis* 17:187.

Valsecchi, R. and Cainelli, T. 1989. Contact urticaria from dog saliva. *Contact Dermatitis* 20:62.

Valsecchi, R., Foiadelli, L., Reseghetti, A., and Cainelli, T. 1986. Generalized urticaria from DNCB. *Contact Dermatitis* 14:254-255.

van der Meeren, H. L. M. and van Erp, P. E. J. 1986. Life-threatening contact urticaria from glove powder. *Contact Dermatitis* 14:190-191.

van Hecke, E. and Santosa, S. 1985. Contact urticaria to DNCB. *Contact Dermatitis* 12:282.

Varigos, G. A. and Nurse, D. S. 1986. Contact urticaria from methyl ethyl ketone. *Contact Dermatitis* 15:259-260.

von Krogh, G. and Maibach, H. I. 1982. The contact urticaria syndrome — 1982. *Semin. Dermatol.* 1:59-66.

Wahl, R. and Kleinhans, D. 1989. IgE-mediated allergic reactions to fruit gums and investigation of cross-reactivity between gelatine and modified gelatine-containing products. *Clin. Exp. Allergy* 19:77-80.

Weissenbach, T., Wutrich, B., and Weihe, W. H. 1988. Allergies to laboratory animals. An epidemiological, allergological study in persons exposed to laboratory animals. *Schweiz. Med. Wochenschr.* 118:930-938.

Wrangsjo, K., Wahlberg, J. E., and Axelsson, I. G. 1988. IgE-mediated allergy to natural rubber in 30 patients with contact urticaria. *Contact Dermatitis* 19:264-271.

Wuthrich, B. and Dietschi, R. 1985. The celery-carrot-mugwort-condiment syndrome: Skin test and RAST results. *Schweiz. Med. Wochenschr.* 115:258-264.

Yodoi, J. and Iskizaka, K. 1979. Lymphocytes bearing Fc-receptors for IgE. Presence of human and rat Iymphocytes with Fc-receptors. *J. Immunol.* 122:2577-2583.

Yoshikawa, M. 1985. Skin lesions of papular urticaria induced experimentally by *Chyletus malaccensis* and *Chelacaropsis sp. (Acari, Cheyletidae). J. Med. Entomol.* 22:115-117.

3

Model for Immunologic Contact Urticaria

Antti I. Lauerma and Howard I. Maibach

CONTENTS

3.1 INTRODUCTION

Immunologic contact urticaria (ICU) is not an uncommon problem; its importance has increased recently, especially in the face of natural rubber latex ICU epidemics. Therefore, a clear need for suitable animal models for screening medicaments for ICU exists. Although an animal model for nonimmunologic contact urticaria (NICU)[1] has been established, models for ICU are not readily available.

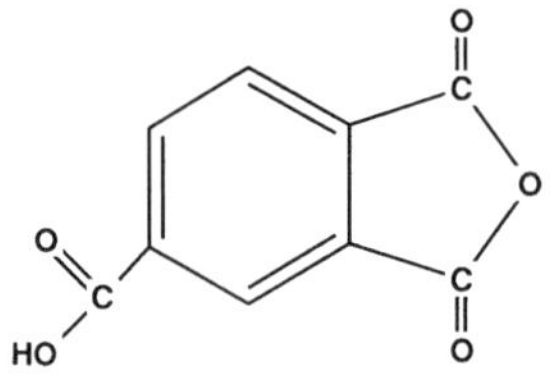

FIGURE 3.1 Chemical structure of TMA.

3.2 TRIMELLITIC ANHYDRIDE

3.2.1 Chemistry

Trimellitic anhydride (TMA) (Figure 3.1) is a hapten with a molecular weight of 192 Da. As a hapten, it has to bind to a carrier protein to become immunogenic. The nature of these carrier proteins is not clear; they could be membrane proteins on the surface of antigen-presenting cells (APC) or other cells, as has been suggested with some haptens participating in delayed-type hypersensitivity reactions. However, other proteins such as albumin can also act as carrier proteins.

3.2.2 Symptoms Caused by TMA

In the 1970s, it was observed that anhydrides such as TMA cause asthma-like symptoms in persons exposed to them.[2] The immunologic reactions seen in lungs of patients and experimental animals feature anaphylactic (Coombs-Gell Type I), complement-mediated (Coombs-Gell type II), antibody-complex-mediated (Coombs-Gell Type III), and cell-mediated (Coombs-Gell Type IV) reactions. Non-immunologic (irritant) reactions may participate,[3] possibly due to metabolization of trimellitic anhydride to trimellitic acid.

TMA causes skin reactions if sensitization is done through skin contact.[4] The skin reactions consist of two phases, immediate and delayed, possibly implying both immediate and delayed type hypersensitivity.[4,5]

3.3 TMA-SENSITIVE MOUSE AS A MODEL FOR ICU

3.3.1 Sensitization Procedures

Sensitization to TMA may be performed either through airways[6] or through skin. Cutaneous sensitization is done either intradermally[7] or topically.[4] Cutaneous sensitization seems to induce both immediate (1 h) and delayed (24 h) skin reactions when TMA is subsequently encountered.

Intradermal sensitization to TMA may be done with the free hapten. When guinea pigs have been sensitized, TMA has been suspended in corn oil at 30% and injected into skin at a 0.1 mL dose. Guinea pigs sensitized in this manner have been used for challenges 3 to 4 weeks after the injection.

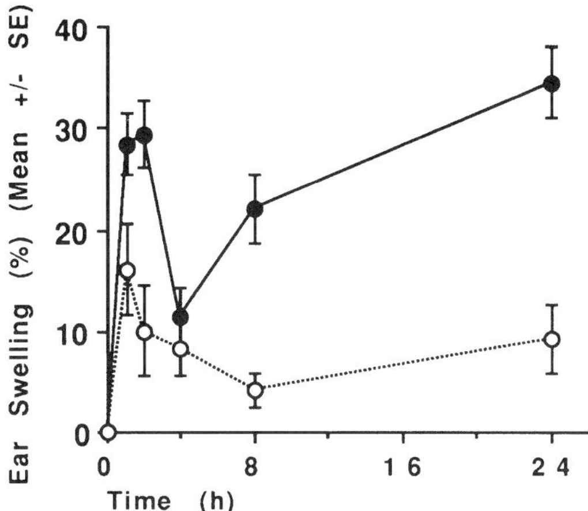

FIGURE 3.2   Reaction kinetics of ear swelling in mice exposed to topical TMA. Mice sensitized to TMA: Closed dots. Mice not sensitized to TMA: Open dots. Results are as mean +/– SE of percentage increase of ear pinnae thickness.

Immediate skin reactions to TMA have been studied using topical skin sensitization.[4,5] The study animal has been the BALB/C mouse and the animals have been sensitized topically on shaven skin on the trunk that has been tape-stripped prior to application. The dose used has been 100 μL TMA at 500 mg/mL. To enhance development of anti-TMA-IgE-antibodies, a second sensitization has been performed with 50 μL 250 mg/mL TMA at the same site. The animals have been used for elicitation one week after the second dosing.

3.3.2   Time-Course of Reaction

In mice sensitized to TMA, a two-phase reaction is seen after TMA application on ears; there is a first phase with swelling peaking at 1 h and a second phase peaking at 24 h.[4] However, a dose-dependent early swelling after TMA application is also observed in nonsensitized mice.[5] Nonimmunologic, possibly irritant reactions in lungs have been suggested to be caused by trimellitic acid, a hydrolization product of TMA.[3] The skin reactions in nonsensitized animals could possibly be considered a form of nonimmunologic contact urticaria (NICU). Reaction kinetics in sensitized and unsensitized mice are in Figure 3.2.

3.3.3   Effect of Topical Immunomodulatory Treatments

The effect of topical treatment with three immunomodulating chemicals, i.e., an antihistamine, diphenhydramine, a glucocorticosteroid, betamethasone dipropionate, and a nonsteroidal anti-inflammatory drug, indomethacin hydrochloride, on early ear swelling by TMA are shown in Figure 3.3. Treatment with diphenhydramine or betamethasone dipropionate suppresses the reaction, whereas indomethacin slightly increases swelling.[5]

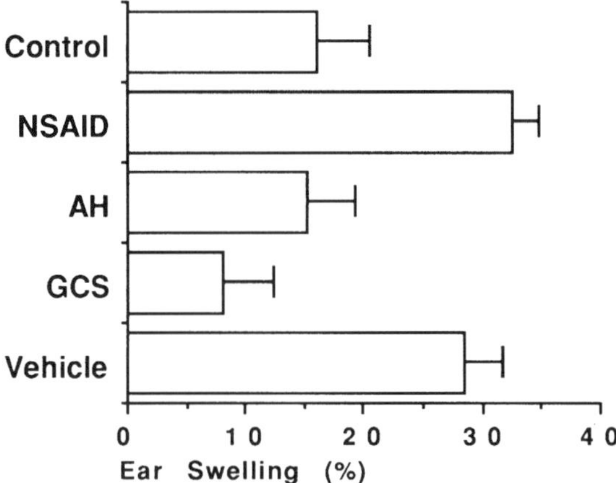

FIGURE 3.3   Effect of topical immunomodulatory treatments on TMA reactions. "Control" = A group of animals not sensitized with TMA and pretreated with vehicle. Other groups of animals were sensitized with TMA. Pretreatments prior to TMA elicitation: "Vehicle" = acetone:olive oil vehicle; "AH" = antihistamine diphenhydramine hydrochloride; "GCS" = glucocorticosteroid betamethasone valerate; "NSAID" = nonsteroidal anti-inflammatory drug indomethacin. Results are percentage increases of ear thickness from baseline with mean +/– SE.

3.4   OTHER POSSIBLE MODELS FOR ICU

3.4.1   Sensitization to Other Haptens Causing Respiratory Allergy

There are other also haptens capable of inducing respiratory allergy. Diphenyl-methane-4,4-diisocyanate (MDI) and phthalic anhydride are respiratory allergens that induce IgE antibody production in animals exposed by epicutaneous application.[8] These haptens could be used to establish a similar animal model for ICU as with TMA.

3.4.2   Sensitization to Protein Allergens

Rabbits sensitized through airways or through the skin with natural rubber latex (NRL) also have, in addition to respiratory symptoms, wheal-and-flare skin prick test reactions.[9] Therefore, it could be that such animals could possibly be used as models for ICU. However, it has to be determined whether percutaneous penetration of NRL proteins is sufficient to cause ICU reactions in this model. Additionally, mice exposed to NRL have elevated IgE levels and eosinophilia, and IgG antibodies against NRL antigens.[10] Similar models of immediate type hypersensitivity to other proteins may be worthwile to investigate.

3.4.3   Repeated Sensitization to Contact Allergens

In a recent study BALB/C mice repeatedly sensitized for up to 48 days with the contact allergen 2,4,6-trinitro-1-chlorobenzene (TNCB) had the time-course of

TNCB-specific hypersensitivity reactions shifted from delayed-type to an immediate-type response. The reaction kinetic shift coincided with an increase of mast cell number in the skin area used for sensitization and elicitation. These early reactions in mouse ears, also followed by a later phase, were dependent on the presence of skin mast cells on the application site as well as antigen-specific IgE.[11] Therefore, such reactions could resemble ICU.

3.5 CONCLUSIONS

It seems that animals sensitized through skin contact to TMA or possibly to other respiratory hapten allergens could be used as animal models for ICU. Such models would ease screening for topical drugs that may be used to treat ICU and other forms of skin diseases with immediate-type allergy. In addition, it could be that the topical sensitization method described here could be useful to screen for other contact urticants as well. In any case, further studies would still be needed to validate this model and to further characterize the reactions observed.

REFERENCES

1. Lahti, A. and Maibach, H. I., An animal model for nonimmunologic contact urticaria, *Toxicol. Appl. Pharmacol.*, 76, 219-224, 1984.
2. Zeiss, C.R., Patterson, R., Pruzansky, J. J., Miller, M. M., Rosenberg, M., and Levitz, D., Trimellitic anhydride-induced airway syndromes: clinical and immunologic studies, *J. Allergy Clin. Immunol.*, 60, 96-103, 1977.
3. Patterson, R., Zeiss, C.R., and Pruzansky, J. J., Immunology and immunopathology of trimellitic anhydride pulmonary reactions, *J. Allergy Clin. Immunol.*, 70, 19-23, 1982.
4. Dearman, R. J., Mitchell, J. A., Basketter, D. A., and Kimber, I., Differential ability of occupational chemical contact and respiratory allergens to cause immediate and delayed dermal hypersensitivity reactions in mice, *Int. Arch. Allergy Appl. Immunol.*, 97, 315-321, 1992.
5. Lauerma, A.I., Fenn B., and Maibach, H.I., Trimellitic anhydride sensitivity as an animal model for contact urticaria, *Joint Meeting of the International Association of Allergology and Clinical Immunology (ICACI XV) and European Academy of Allergology and Clinical Immunology (EAACI '94)*, Stockholm, Sweden, 1994.
6. Obata, H., Tao, Y., Kido, M., Nagata, N., Tanaka, I., and Kurowa, A., Guinea pig model of immunologic asthma induced by inhalation of trimellitic anhydride, *Am. Rev. Respir. Dis.*, 146, 1553-1558, 1992.
7. Hayes, J.P., Daniel, R., Tee, R.D., Barnes, P.J., Chung, K.F., and Newman Taylor, A.J., Specific immunological and bronchopulmonary responses following intradermal sensitization to free trimellitic anhydride in guinea pigs, *Clin. Exp. Allergy*, 22, 694-700, 1992.
8. Dearman, R.J., Basketter, D.A., and Kimber., I., Variable effects of chemical allergens on serum IgE concentration in mice. Preliminary evaluation of a novel approach to the identification of respiratory sensitizers, *J. Appl. Toxicol.*, 12, 317-323, 1992.
9. Reijula, K.E., Kelly, K.J., Kurup, V.P., Choi, H., Bongard, R.D., Dawson, C.A., and Fink, J.N., Latex-induced dermal and pulmonary hypersensitivity in rabbits, *J. Allergy Clin. Immunol.* 94: 891-902, 1994.

10. Kurup, V.P., Kumar, A., Choi, H., Murali, P.S., Resnick, A., Kelly, K.J., and Fink, J.N., Latex antigens induce IgE and eosinophils in mice, *Int. Arch. Allergy Immunol.,* 103: 370-377, 1994.
11. Kitagati, H., Fujisawa, S., Watanabe, K., Hayakawa, K., and Shiohara, T., Immediate-type hypersensitivity response followed by a late reaction is induced by repeated epicutaneous application of contact sensitizing agents in mice, *J. Invest. Dermatol.* 105, 749-755, 1995.

4

Skin Tests and Specific IgE Determinations in the Diagnostics of Contact Urticaria Caused by Low-Molecular-Weight Chemicals

Outi Tupasela and Lasse Kanerva

CONTENTS

4.1   INTRODUCTION

Allergic reactions may occur after exposure to low molecular weight chemicals (LMW). The frequency of such reactions will probably increase, because in today's environment people are increasingly exposed to a variety of chemicals both at home and at work. It has been estimated that more than 85,000 chemicals are currently used.[1]

Chemicals can cause delayed or cell-mediated hypersensitivity, e.g., allergic contact dermatitis, which develops in hours to days. On the other hand, immediate, IgE-mediated reactions develop in minutes. This article briefly reviews diagnostic methods to detect IgE-mediated allergies caused by LMW chemicals. Clinically, these reactions range from invisible contact urticaria,[2] and allergic rhinitis to dangerous, even fatal, anaphylactic shock.

Chemicals have not usually been regarded as potential inducers of immunoglobulin E (IgE) production because agents that can be recognized by the human immune system are usually of protein nature. Experience shows, however, that LMW chemicals may also induce allergic type I reactions. It is believed that the LMW chemical acts as a hapten and binds to a protein or other macromolecule *in vivo,* and that the resulting hapten-carrier conjugate acts as the allergen. A great number of LMW chemicals have been reported to cause contact urticaria (Table 4.1).[3-80] Nevertheless, appropriate methods to prove that contact urticaria has been IgE-mediated are in most cases lacking but have been documented in some cases.[6,53,63]

4.2 LOW MOLECULAR WEIGHT CHEMICALS

Proteins have molecular weights from approximately 10,000 to several hundred thousands, whereas the typical molecular weights of LMW chemicals are below 1000. Some examples of LMW chemicals that have elicited IgE-mediated responses are presented in Table 4.2. Diisocyanates are initial materials for polymers called polyurethanes. Polyurethanes are used, e.g., as foams, isolation materials, lacquers, and paints. Organic acid anhydrides are used in the production of unsaturated polyester resins and as hardeners for epoxy resins. Amines are also initial materials in the plastic industry. Acrylates, among other substances, are now widely used in fillings of teeth and in dentures. Ammonium persulphate is used, e.g., in hair bleaching.

Chemicals have the ability to react with nucleophiles, forming covalent linkages, predominantly with serum proteins. These chemical-protein conjugates are immunogenic. Other interactions of LMW chemicals with biomolecules also result in immunogenicity of the chemical hapten.[81] Nickel and platinum salts are examples of chemicals which seem to react through noncovalent bindings with host biomacromolecules. Evidence of the immunogenity of such conjugates has been obtained from detection of IgE antibodies in sensitized workers reactive to platinium-serum albumin complexes[82] and nickel-serum albumin complexes.[63]

4.3 PREPARATION AND CHARACTERIZATION OF HAPTEN-PROTEIN CONJUGATE ANTIGENS

Hapten-protein conjugates can be synthetised in the laboratory *in vitro.* Human serum albumin (HSA) has been considered as the best carrier for haptens.[83] HSA is a major respiratory tract protein, and practical experience shows that it is a stable protein and is therefore suitable as a carrier. The host response may be hapten-specific or directed against new antigenic determinants (NAD) formed on the protein carrier.[84]

Protein conjugates of reactive chemicals for use in immunoassays can be prepared by simply mixing the chemical and protein in a suitable buffer solution. The chemistry

TABLE 4.1 Low Molecular Weight Chemicals That Have Been Reported to Cause Contact Urticaria

Abietic acid	el Sayed, 1995[3]
Acetic acid	Lahti, 1980[4]
Acetylsalicylic acid	Odom and Maibach, 1976[5]
Acid anhydrides	Tarvainen, 1995[6]
Acrylic acid	Fowler, 1990[7]
	Daecke, 1993[8]
Acrylic monomer	Key, 1961[9]
Albendazole	Macedo,1991[10]
Aliphatic alcohols	Key, 1961[9]
	Lahti, 1980[4]
	Rilliet, 1980[11]
p-Aminodiphenylamine	von Liebe, 1979[12]
Aminophenazone	Camarasa, 1978[13]
	Lombardi, 1983[14]
Aminothiazole	Key, 1961[9]
Ammonium	Key, 1961[9]
Ammonium persulphate	Calnan and Shuster, 1963[15]
	Brubaker, 1972[16]
	Fisher and Dooms-Goossens, 1976[17]
Aziridine	Kanerva, 1995[18,19]
Bacitracin	Roupe and Strannegard, 1969[20]
	Palungwachira, 1991[21]
Benzaldehyde	Forsbeck and Skog, 1977[22]
	Seite-Bellezza, 1994[23]
Benzocaine	Ryan, 1980[24]
Benzoic acid	Forsbeck and Skog, 1977[22]
	Clemmensen and Hjorth, 1982[25]
Benzoyl peroxide	Tkach, 1982[26]
Butyric acid	Lahti, 1980[4]
Butylhydroxytoluol	Osmundsen, 1980[27]
Calcium hypochloride ($CaOCl_2$)	Neering, 1977[28]
Carbamates	Belsito, 1990[29]
Cefotiam hydrochloride	Miyahara, 1993[30]
Cephalosporin	Tuft, 1975[31]
Cetylalcohol	Gaul, 1969[32]
Chloramine	Dooms-Goossens, 1983[33]
Chlorhexidine	Okano, 1989[34]
	Fisher, 1988[35]
	Bergqvist-Karsson, 1988[36]
Chlorothalonil	Dannaker, 1993[37]
Chlorpromazine	Odom and Maibach, 1976[5]
Cinnamic acid	Forsbeck and Skog, 1977[22]
Cinnamic aldehyde	Forsbeck and Skog, 1977[22]
	Nater, 1977[38]
	Seite-Bellezza, 1994[23]

TABLE 4.1 (continued)   Low Molecular Weight Chemicals That Have Been Reported to Cause Contact Urticaria

Clioquinol	von Liebe, 1979[12]
Clobetasol-17-propionate	Gottmann-Lückerath, 1984[39]
Cobalt chloride	Smith, 1975[40]
Diethylfumarate	Lahti and Maibach, 1985[41]
Diethyltoluamide	Maibach and Johnson, 1975[42]
Dimethylsulfoxide	Odom and Maibach, 1976[5]
	Frosch, 1980[43]
Denatoniumbenzoate	Björkner, 1980[44]
Dimethylsulphoxide	Kanerva, 1991[45]
	Rilliet, 1980[11]
	Ophaswongse and Maibach, 1994[46]
Ethylaminobenzoate	Ryan, 1980[24]
Eugenol	Picardo, 1988[47]
Fluoride	Camarasa, 1993[48]
Formaldehyde	Key, 1961[9]
	Helander, 1977[49]
	McDaniel and Marks, 1979[50]
Fumaric acid	de Haan, 1994[51]
Iodine	Gronemeyer, 1967[52]
Iridium	Bergman, 1995[53]
Lindane	Key, 1961[9]
Mechloroethamine	Daughters, 1973[54]
Mercapto compounds	Belsito, 1990[29]
Mercury salts	Corrales Torres, 1985[55]
	Torresani, 1993[56]
Methylhexahydrophthalic anhydride	Jolanki, 1987[57]
	Jolanki, 1990[58]
	Tarvainen,1995[6]
Mexiletine hydrochloride	Yamazaki, 1994[59]
Monoamylamine	Tharp, 1973[60]
Neomycin	Goh, 1986[61]
Nickel sulphate	Osmundsen, 1980[27]
	Valsecchi and Cainelli, 1989[62]
	Estlander, 1993[63]
Nicotin acid ester	Lahti, 1980[4]
	Bandmann and Wahl, 1982[64]
Oleylamide	Osmundsen, 1980[27]
Parabens	Henry, 1979[65]
Pentamidine isethionate	Belsito, 1993[66]
p-Phenylene diamine (or mix)	Edwards Jr. and Edwards, 1984[67]
	Temesvári, 1984[68]
	Belsito, 1990[29]
Platinum salts	Key, 1961[9]
Polyethylene glycol	Fisher, 1978[69]
Polysorbic acid	Maibach and Conant, 1977[70]

TABLE 4.1 (continued)   Low Molecular Weight Chemicals That Have Been Reported to Cause Contact Urticaria

Propylene glycol	Funk and Maibach, 1994[71]
Reactive dyes	Estlander, 1990[72]
Rifamycin	Grob et al., 1987[73]
	Mancuso and Masara, 1992[74]
Salicylic acid	Odom and Maibach, 1976[5]
Sesquisulphide	White and Rycroft, 1983[75]
Sodium hypochloride(NaOCl)	Neering, 1977[28]
Sodium sulphide	Key, 1961[9]
Sorbitan monostearate	Maibach, 1977[70]
Sorbitan sesquioleate	Hardy and Maibach, 1995[76]
Streptomycin	Rudzki, 1981[77]
	Odom and Maibach, 1976[5]
Tartrazin	Rademaker and Forsyth, 1989[78]
Terpenylacetate	McDaniel and Marks, 1979[50]
Vinyl pyridine	Rudzki, 1981[77]
Xylene	Palmer, 1993[79]
Zinc diethyldithiocarbamate	Helander and Mäkelä, 1983[80]

TABLE 4.2 Low Molecular Weight Chemicals

Organic chemicals:	Diisocyanates
	2,4-TDI (2,4-Toluene diisocyanate)
	2,6-TDI (2,6-Toluene diisocyanate)
	HDI (1,6 Hexamethylene diisocyanate)
	MDI (4,4'-Diphenylmethane diisocyanate)
	Acid anhydrides
	PA (Phthalic anhydride)
	HHPA (Hexahydrophthalic anhydride)
	MHHPA (Methylhexahydrophthalic anhydride)
	MTHPA (Methyltetrahydrophthalic anhydride)
	TMA (Trimellitic anhydride)
	MA (Maleic anhydride)
	Amines
	Acrylates
	Reactive dyes
Inorganic chemicals:	Ammonium persulphate
	Nickel sulphate
	Platinum salts
Drugs:	Penicillin

of some haptens may be complex, and it is difficult to anticipate the factors that are important for preparation. For instance, time, temperature, concentration, and pH are factors that influence the structure of the hapten-protein conjugate.[83]

It is also possible to use some coupling agents for linking chemicals containing nucleophilic groups to protein carriers.[85] Welinder et al. have, for example, used carbodi-imide to couple heterocyclic amine piperazine to HSA.[86] Several methods have been used in the coupling of drugs to carbohydrate and protein carriers.[87]

In order to understand the nature of the *in vitro* synthesized HSA conjugates, they should be characterized immunochemically and physically. The ratio of chemical molecules bound per molecule of carrier protein (hapten density, HD) can be studied. Haptens with chromophores can be analyzed spectrophotometrically with the assumption that the absorbance of the conjugate is the sum of the absorbanses of the haptens and the protein. Haptens bound to amino groups in the protein can be quantified by analyzing the number of free amino groups before and after the conjugation. The change in electrophoretic mobility of the proteins after substitution can be studied. The conjugate can be hydrolyzed, and the released haptens can then be analyzed by conventional methods.[86] Wass and Belin have found that for diisocyanates HD at intervals of 6–10 mol/mol is optimal.[83] Welinder, on the other hand, has indicated that at synthesis 14–24 acid anhydride molecules could bind to an HSA molecule.

4.4   PRICK SKIN TEST AND SPECIFIC IgE DETERMINATIONS

Immediate allergic hypersensitivity can be diagnosed by *in vivo* or *in vitro* immunologic tests. The skin-prick test is the most general *in vivo* skin test, and radioallergosorbent tests (RAST) are widely used for *in vitro* detection of specific IgE antibodies.

Hapten-HSA-conjugate is used as the allergen in both tests.[45,63] The conjugate is synthesized by mixing a suitable quantity of hapten-chemical and human serum albumin.[83,86,88] After the incubation, the unconjugated, free hapten is dialyzed off, and the hapten-HSA-conjugate is concentrated namely for this purpose.

Skin prick tests with hapten-HSA-conjugates are performed as with common environmental allergens. A drop of hapten-HSA-conjugate solution is placed on the subject's arm. A lancet is placed in the solution, and the skin is gently pricked. After 15 minutes, a positive result is a wheal-and-flare response.

The RAST is the method used to detect specific IgE antibodies in serum. It was developed by Wide, Bennich, and Johansson in 1967,[89] and its principle is illustrated in Figure 4.1. Although the mechanism of RAST has been quite uniform, preparation of the hapten conjugates and analysis of assay results, including the establishment of criteria for ascertaining positivity, have been highly variable.[90] Usually the results are expressed as a percentage of the total activity added or as a RAST ratio, that is, the ratio between the binding to the hapten-HSA disc and to a disc onto which HSA had been coupled and run in the same experiment. False-negative values may result from high titres of other classes of specific IgE antibody in the sera . Such antibodies may block IgE from reacting with allergen on the disc. False-positive results may occur when sera contain large amounts of total IgE. This problem can be overcome by performing specific RAST inhibition tests.[81] The RAST inhibition test is also useful for studying the cross-reactivity of various hapten-allergens (Figure 4.2).

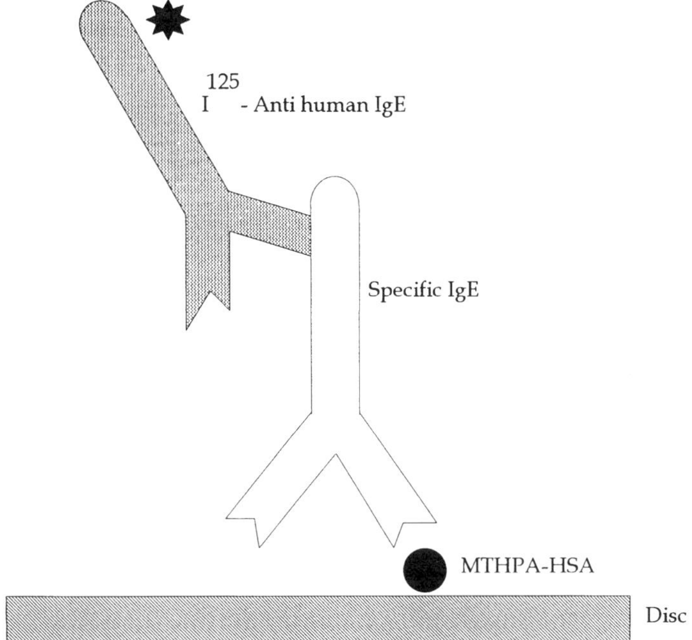

FIGURE 4.1 The principle of the RAST. Allergen, MTHPA-HSA, is coupled to a paper disc. IgE antibodies in a serum sample which are specific for MTHPA bind to MTHPA epitopes on the disc. Bound IgE is detected by I^{125}-labeled anti human IgE.

RAST inhibition studies were carried out by the method of Yman et al.[91] Serial dilutions of hapten-HSA-conjugates were allowed to react with patients' serum. The mixtures were then used for RAST determination. The degree of reduction of the serum RAST values after absorption was expressed as an inhibition percentage.

4.5 CONCLUDING REMARKS

It is uncertain whether the low amount of positive sera reflects the absence of IgE antibodies or the inadequate methods used for conjugation of hapten and HSA, including the selection of a protein carrier and the reactivity of a chemical. Interpretation of results produced with varied methods can also cause difficulties.[90]

Hapten-prick tests and hapten RAST are not the prime methods to diagnose contact urticaria and other immediate allergies. However, in order to diagnose an IgE-mediated allergy, including contact urticaria, caused by LMW chemicals, the above methods need to be used. Therefore, dermatologists should be familiar with these methods.[93–95]

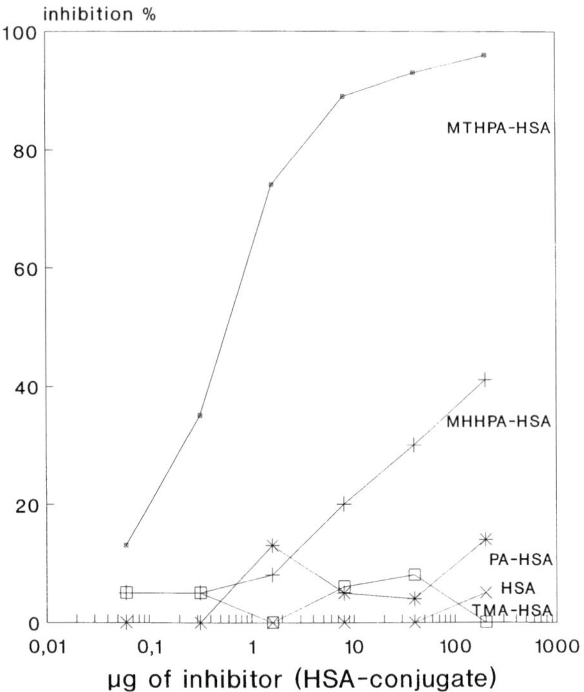

FIGURE 4.2　The inhibition of MTHPA-RAST by MTHPA-HSA and other acid anhydride-HSA-conjugates. 200 µg of MTHPA-HSA-conjugate inhibit the RAST reaction by 96%, which indicates specificity of RAST. The cross-reactivity with other acid anhydride conjugates is minor.

REFERENCES

1. Drake, L.A., Dorner, W., Goltz, R.W. et al., Guidelines of care for contact dermatitis, *J. Am. Acad. Dermatol.*, 32, 109, 1995.
2. Kligman, A.M., The spectrum of contact urticaria. Wheals, erythema and pruritus, *Dermatol. Clin.*, 8(1), 57, 1990.
3. el Sayed, F., Manzur, F., Bayle, P., Marquery, M.S., and Bazek, J., Contact urticaria from abietic acid, *Cont. Derm.*, 32, 361, 1995.
4. Lahti, A., Nonimmunologic contact urticaria, *Acta. derm. Venereol. (Stockh.)*, Suppl. 91, 1, 1980.
5. Odom, R.B. and Maibach, H.I., Kontakt-Urtikaria (KU) eine besondere Form der Kontaktdermatitis, *Z. Hautkr.*, 51, 815, 1976.
6. Tarvainen, K., Jolanki, R., Estlander, T., Tupasela, O., Pfäffli, P., and Kanerva, L., Immunologic contact urticaria due to airborne methylhexahydrophthalic and methyltetrahydrophthalic anhydrides, *Cont. Derm.*, 32, 204. 1995.
7. Fowler, J.F., Immediate contact hypersensitivity to acrylic acid, *Dermatol. Clinics*, 8, 193, 1990.

8. Daecke, C., Schaller, S., Schaller, S., and Goos, M., Contact urticaria from acrylic acid in Fixomull tape, *Cont. Derm.,* 29, 216, 1993.

9. Key, M.M., Some unusual reactions in industry. *Arch. Dermatol.,* 83, 3, 1961.

10. Macedo, N.A., Pineiro, M.I., and Carmona, C., Contact urticaria and contact dermatitis from albendazole, *Cont. Derm.,* 25, 73, 1991.

11. Rilliet, A., Hunziker, N., and Brun, R., Alcohol contact urticaria syndrome (immediate-type hypersensitivity), *Dermatologica,* 161, 361, 1980.

12. von Liebe, V., Karge, H.-J., and Burg, G., Kontakturtikaria, *Hautarzt* 30, 544, 1979.

13. Camarasa, J.M. et al., Contact urticaria and anaphylaxis from aminophenazone, *Cont. Derm.,* 4, 243, 1978.

14. Lombardi, P., Giorgini, S., and Achille, A., Contact urticaria from aminophenazone, *Cont. Derm.,* 9, 428, 1983.

15. Calnan, C.D. and Shuster, S., Reactions to ammonium persulfate, *Arch. Dermatol.,* 88, 812, 1963.

16. Brubaker, M.M., Urticarical reactions to ammonium persulfate, *Arch. Dermatol.,* 106, 413, 1972.

17. Fisher, A.A. and Dooms-Goossens, A., Persulfate hair bleach reactions, *Arch. Dermatol.,* 112, 1407, 1976.

18. Kanerva, L., Keskinen, H., Autio, P., Estlander, T., Tuppurainen, M., and Jolanki, R., Occupational respiratory and skin sensitization caused by polyfunctional aziridine hardener, *Clin. Exp. Allergy,* 25, 432, 1995.

19. Kanerva, L., Estlander, T., Jolanki, R., and Tarvainen, K., Occupational allergic contact dermatitis and contact urticaria caused by polyfunctional aziridine hardener, *Cont. Derm.,* 33, 304, 1995.

20. Roupe, G. and Strannegard, Ö., Anaphylactic shock elicited by topical administration of bacitracin, *Arch. Dermatol.,* 100, 450, 1969.

21. Palungwachira, P., Contact urticaria syndrome and anaphylatoid reaction from topical clioquinol and bacitracin (Banocin): a case repot, *J. Med. Assoc. Thai.,* 74(1), 43, 1991.

22. Forsbeck, M. and Skog, E., Immediate reactions to patch tests with balsam of Peru, *Cont. Derm.,* 3, 201, 1977.

23. Seite-Bellezza, D., el-Sayed, F., and Bazek, J., Contact urticaria from cinnamic aldehyde and benzaldehyde in a confectioner, *Cont. Derm.,* 31, 272, 1994.

24. Ryan, M.E., Brian, M.D., and Marks, J.G., Contact urticaria and allergic contact dermatitis to benzocaine gel, *J. Am. Acad. Dermatol.,* 2, 221, 1980.

25. Clemmensen, O. and Hjorth, N., Perioral contact urticaria from sorbic acid and benzoic acid in a salad dressing, *Cont. Derm.,* 8, 1, 1982.

26. Tkach, J.R., Allergic contact urticaria to benzoyl peroxide, *Cutis,* 29, 187, 1882.

27. Osmundsen, P.E., Contact urticaria from nickel and plastic additives (butylhydroxytoluene, oleylamide), *Cont. Derm.,* 6, 452, 1980.

28. Neering, H., Contact urticaria from chlorinated swimmingpool water, *Cont. Derm.,* 3 279, 1977.

29. Belsito, D.V., Contact urticaria caused by rubber. Analysis of seven cases, *Dermatol. Clin.,* 8(1) 61, 1990.

30. Miyahara, H., Koga, T., Imayama, S., and Hori, Y., Occupational contact urticaria syndrome from cefotiam hydrochloride, *Cont. Derm.,* 29 210, 1993.

31. Tuft, L., Contact urticaria from cephalosporins, *Arch. Dermatol.,* 111, 1609, 1975.

32. Gaul, L.E., Dermatisis from cetyl and stearyl alcohol, *Arch. Dermatol.,* 99, 593, 1969.

33. Dooms-Goossens, A., Gevers, D., Mertens, A., and Vanderheyden, D., Allergic contact urticaria due to chloramine, *Cont. Derm.,* 9, 319, 1983.
34. Okano, M., Nomura M., Hata, S., Okado, N., Sato, K., Kitan, Y., Tashiro, M., Yoshimoto, Y., Hama, R., and Aoki, T., Anaphylactic symptoms due to chlorhexidine gluconate, *Arch. Dermatol.,* 125, 50, 1989.
35. Fisher, A.A., Contact urticaria from chlorhexidine, *Cutis,* 43(1), 17, 1988.
36. Bergqvist-Karlsson, A., Delayed and immediate-type hypersensitivity to chlorhexidine, *Cont. Derm.,* 18(2), 84, 1988.
37. Dannaker, C.J., Maibach, H.I., and O'Malley, M., Contact urticaria and anaphylaxis to the fungicide chlorothalonil, *Cutis,* 52, 312, 1993.
38. Nater, J.P., de John, J.M., Baar, A.J.M. et al., Contact urticarial skin responses to cinnamaldehyde, *Cont. Derm.,* 3:151, 1977.
39. Gottmann-Lückerath, I., Kontakturtikaria nach Dermoxin, *Allergologie,* 7, 344, 1984.
40. Smith, J.D., Odom, R.B., and Maibach, H.I., Contact urticaria from cobalt chloride, *Arch. Dermatol.,* 111, 1610, 1975.
41. Lahti, A. and Maibach, H.I., Contact urticaria from diethyl fumarate, *Cont. Derm.,* 12, 130, 1985.
42. Maibach, H.I. and Johnson, H.L., Contact urticaria syndrome, *Arch. Dermatol.,* 111, 726, 1975.
43. Frosch, P.J., Duncan, S., and Kligman, A.M., Cutaneous biometrics I. The response of human skin to dimethyl sulphoxide, *Br. J. Dermatol.,* 102, 263, 1980.
44. Björkner, B., Contact urticaria and asthma from denotonium benzoate (Bitrex), *Cont. Derm.,* 6, 466, 1980.
45. Kanerva, L., Jolanki, R., Tupasela, O., Halmepuro, L., Keskinen, H., Estlander, T., and Sysilampi, M.-L., Immediate and delayed allergy from epoxy resins besed on diglycidyl ether of bisphenol A, *Scand. J. Work Environ. Health,* 17, 208, 1991.
46. Ophaswongse, S. and Maibach, H.I., Alcohol dermatitis: allergic contact dermatitis and contact urticaria syndrome. A review. *Cont. Derm.,* 30, 1, 1994.
47. Picardo, M., Rovina, R., Christando, A., Cannistraci, C., and Santucci, B., Contact urticaria from Tilia (lime), *Cont. Derm.,* 19(1), 72, 1988.
48. Camarasa J.G., Serra-Baldrich, E., Lluch, M., and Malet, A., Contact urticaria from sodium fluoride, *Cont. Derm.,* 28, 294, 1993.
49. Helander, I., Contact urticaria from leather containing formaldehyde, *Arch. Dermatol.,* 113, 1443, 1977.
50. McDaniel, W.H. and Marks, J.G., Jr., Contact urticaria due to sensitivity to spray starch, Arch. Dermatol., 115:628, 1979.
51. de Haan, P., von Blomberg-van-der-Flier, B.M., de Groot, J., and Nieboer, C., The risk of sensibilization and contact urticaria upon topical application of fumaric acid derivatives, *Dermatology,* 188, 126, 1994.
52. Gronemeyer, W., Urtikaria, Quincke-ödem und verwandte Zustände, in *Lehrbuch der klinischen Allergie,* Hansen, K. and Werner, M., Eds., Thieme, Stuttgart, 1967.
53. Bergman, A., Svedberg, U., and Nilsson, E., Contact urticaria with anaphylactic reactions caused by occupational exposure to iridium salt, *Cont. Derm.,* 32, 14, 1995.
54. Daughters, D., Zackenheim, H., and Mailbach, H. I., Urticaria and anaphylactoid reactions after topical application of mechlorethamine, *Arch. Dermatol.,* 107, 429, 1973.
55. Corrales Torres, J.L. and de Corres, F., Anaphylactic hypersensitivity to mercurochrome (merbromin), *Ann. Allergy,* 54, 230, 1985.

56. Torresani, C., Caprari, E., and Manara, G.C., Contact urticaria syndrome due to phenylmercuric acetate, *Cont. Derm.*, 29, 282, 1993.

57. Jolanki, R., Estlander, T., and Kanerva, L., Occupational contact dermatitis and contact urticaria caused by epoxy resins, *Acta. derm. Venerol. Suppl. (Stockh.)*, 134, 90, 1987.

58. Jolanki, R., Kanerva, L., Estlander, T., Tarvainen, K., and Henriks-Eckerman, M.-L., Occupational dermatoses from epoxy resin compounds, *Cont. Derm.*, 23, 172, 1990.

59. Yamazaki, S., Katayama, I., Kurumaji, Y., Yokozeki, H., and Nishioka, K., Contact urticaria induced by mexiletine hydrochloride in a patient receiving iontophoresis, *Br. J. Dermatol.*, 130, 538, 1994.

60. Tharp, C.V., Contact urticaria (monoamylamine), *Arch. Dermatol.*, 108, 135, 1973.

61. Goh, C.L., Anaphylaxis from topical neomycin and bacitracin, *Aust. J. Derm.*, 27, 125, 1986.

62. Valsecchi, R. and Cainelli, T., Contact urticaria from dog saliva, *Cont. Derm.*, 17(3), 182, 1989.

63. Estlander, T., Kanerva L., Tupasela O., Keskinen H., and Jolanki, R., Immediate and delayed allergy to nickel with contact urticaia, rhinitis, asthma and contact dermatitis, *Clin. Exp. Allergy*, 23, 306, 1993.

64. Bandmann, H.-J. and Wahl, B., Contact urticaria artefacta (witchcraft syndrome), *Cont. Derm.*, 8, 145, 1982.

65. Henry, H.C., Tschen, E.H., and Becker, L.E., Contact urticaria to parabens, *Arch. Dermatol.*, 115, 1231, 1979.

66. Belsito, D.V., Contact urticaria from pentamidine isethionate, *Cont. Derm.*, 29, 158, 1993.

67. Edwards, E.K., Jr. and Edwards, E.K., Contact urticaria and allergic contact dermatitis caused by paraphenylendiamine, *Cutis*, 34, 87, 1984.

68. Temesvári, E., Contact urticaria from parapheylendiamine, *Cont. Derm.*, 11, 125, 1984.

69. Fisher, A.A., Immediate and delayed allergic contact reactions to polyethylene glycol, *Cont. Derm.*, 4, 135, 1978.

70. Maibach, H.I. and Conant, M., Contact urticaria to a corticosteroid cream: polysorbate 60, *Cont. Derm.*, 3, 350, 1977.

71. Funk, J.O. and Maibach, H.I., Propylene glycol dermatitis: re-evaluation of an old problem, *Cont. Derm.*, 31, 236, 1994.

72. Estlander, T., Kanerva, L., and Jolanki, R., Occupational allergic dermatoses from textile, leather, and fur dyes, *Am. J. Cont. Derm.*, 1, 13, 1990.

73. Grob, J.J., Pommier, G., Robaglia, A., Collet-Villette, A.M., and Bonerendi, J.J., Contact urticaria from rifamycin, *Cont. Derm.*, 16(5), 284, 1987.

74. Mancuso, G. and Masara, N., Contact urticaria and severe anaphylaxis from rifamycin SV, *Cont. Derm.*, 27, 125, 1992.

75. White, I.R. and Rycroft, R.J., Contact urticaria from phosphorus sesquisulphide, *Cont. Derm.*, 9, 162, 1983.

76. Hardy, M.P. and Maibach, H.I., Contact urticaria syndrome from sorbitan sesquioleate in a corticoisteroid ointment, *Cont. Derm.*, 32, 114, 1995.

77. Rudzki, E., Rebandel, P., and Rogozinski, T., Contact urticaria from rat tail, guinea pig, streptomycin, and vinyl pyridine, *Cont. Derm.*, 7, 186, 1981.

78. Rademaker, M. and Forsyth, A., Contact urticaria in children, *Cont. Derm.*, 20(2), 104, 1989.

79. Palmer, K.T. and Rycroft, R.J., Occupational airborne contact urticaria due to xylene, *Cont. Derm.*, 28, 44, 1993.

80. Helander, I. and Mäkelä, A., Contact urticaria to zinc diethyldithiocarbamate (ZDC), *Con. Derm*, 9, 327, 1983.
81. Karol, M.H., Occupational asthma and allergic reactions to inhaled compounds, in *Principles and Practice of Immunotoxicology*, Miller, K., Turk, J., and Nicklin, S., Eds., Blackwell Scientific, London, 1992, 228.
82. Cromwell, O., Pepys, J., Parish, W.E., and Hughes, E.G., Specific IgE antibodies to platinum salts in sensitized workers, *Clin. Allergy*, 9, 109, 1979.
83. Wass, U., Studies on IgE antibodies induced by low-molecular weight chemicals, University of Gothenburg, Gothenburg, Sweden, 1989 (Dissertation).
84. Bernstein, D.I. and Zeiss R.C., Guidelines for preparation and characterization of chemical-protein conjugate antigens. Report of the subcommittee on preparatiom and characterization of low molecular weight antigens, *J. Allergy Clin. Immunol.*, 84, 820, 1989.
85. Welinder, H., Hagmar, L., and Gustavsson, C., IgE antibodies against piperazine and N- methyl piperazine in two asthmatic subjects. *Int. Archs. Allergy Appl. Immun.*, 79, 259, 1986.
86. Welinder, H., Occupational airways hypersensitivity to some small organic molecules. Exposure, response and pathomechanism, Lund University, Lund, Sweden, 1991 (Dissertation).
87. Balbo, A.B. and Pham, N.H., Structure-activity studies on drug-induced anaphylactic reactions, *Chem. Res. Toxicol.*, 7 (6), 703, 1994.
88. Howe, W., Venables, K.M., Topping, M.D., Dally M.B., Hawkins, R., Laws, J.S., and Newman Taylor, A.J., Tetrachlorophthalic anhydride asthma: evidence for specific IgE antibody. *J. Allergy Clin. Immunol.*, 71, 5, 1983.
89. Wide, L., Bennich, H., and Johansson, S.G.O., Diagnosis of allergy by an *in vitro* test for allergen antibodies, *The Lancet*, 2, 1105, 1967.
90. Karol, M.H., Kramarik, J.A., and Ferguson, J., Methods to assess RAST results in patients exposed to chemical allergens, *Allergy*, 50, 48, 1995.
91. Yman, L., Ponterius, G., and Brandt, R., RAST-based allergen assay methods. International WHO-IABS Symposium on Standardization and Control of Allergens Administered to Man, Geneva 1974, *Develop. Biol. Standard*, Karger, Basel, 29, 151, 1975.
92. Kanerva, L., Tupasela, O., Jolanki, R., Tarvainen, K., and Estlander, T., Histopathology and electron microscopy of long-lasting IgE-mediated skin prick test reaction caused by methyltetrahydrophthalic anhydride (MTHPA)and methylhexahydrophthalic andydride (MHHPA), in: *Immunological and Pharmacological Aspects of Atopic and Contact Eczema*, Czernielewski, J.M., Eds., Pharmacol. skin, Karger Basel, 4(4), 106, 1991.
93. Keskinen, H., Tupasela, O., Tiikkainen, U., and Nordman, H., Experiences of Specific IgE in Asthma Due to Diisocyanates. *Clin. Allergy*, 18, 597, 1988.
94. Jolanki, R., Estlander, T., and Kanerva, L., Occupational contact dermatitis and contact urticaria caused by epoxy resins, *Acta. Derm. Venerel.*, Suppl. 134, 90, 1987.
95. Tupasela, O., Kanerva, L., and Mölsä, K., Prick-ja RAST-tekniikat pienimolekyylisten kemikaalien aiheuttamien välittömien allergioiden tutkimuksissa (Prick tests and RASTs in the study of immediate allergy caused by low molecular weight chemicals), *Suomen Lääkärilehti*, 46(Suppl. 29), 2721, 1991.

5

Chemical Respiratory Allergens and the Contact Urticaria Syndrome

Ian Kimber and Rebecca J. Dearman

CONTENTS

5.1   INTRODUCTION

The contact urticaria syndrome was described first by Maibach and Johnson in 1975.[1] Since then, an increasing number of food, plant and animal products, medicaments, metals, and chemicals has been shown to cause the characteristic symptoms of an immediate local wheal-and-flare reaction.[2] The term *contact urticaria* describes the clinical picture resulting from topical exposure to the causative agent. It is clear, however, that several mechanisms may operate to provoke symptoms that are indistinguishable clinically. Three broad categories are recognized: immunologic contact

TABLE 5.1 Examples of Chemical Respiratory Allergens

Chemical	References
Acid anhydrides	
Phthalic anhydride	6–9
Trimellitic anhydride	10–13
Tetrachlorophthalic anhydride	14–17
Hexahydrophthalic anhydride	18,19
Maleic anhydride	13,20
Isocyanates	
Toluene diisocyanate	21–24
Diphenylmethane diisocyanate	25–28
Hexamethylene diisocyanate	29–31
Reactive dyes	32–35
Platinum salts	36–40
Carmine	20,41
Plicatic acid	42–45
Chloramine T	46–49

urticaria, nonimmunologic contact urticaria, and contact urticaria where the pathogenetic mechanisms are unknown and/or may comprise both immunological and nonimmunologic processes. In this chapter, the possible relationship between chemical respiratory allergens and immunologic contact urticaria is explored.

5.2 CHEMICAL RESPIRATORY ALLERGENS

Many chemicals are allergenic. There is a long list of chemicals that are able in susceptible individuals to cause skin sensitization and allergic contact dermatitis.[3] It is also clear that some chemicals, fewer in number, may induce sensitization of the respiratory tract resulting in occupational asthma and rhinitis.[4] Among the chemical agents known or suspected to cause respiratory allergy in humans are isocyanates, acid anhydrides, reactive dyes, metals, and other miscellaneous materials that find industrial application. Comprehensive details are available elsewhere,[5] and a list of some of the more common or better characterized chemical respiratory allergens is shown in Table 5.1.

Naturally, not all cases of occupational asthma associated with exposure to chemicals have an immunological basis. Nevertheless, for many chemicals there is evidence for an allergic mechanism characterized by the presence of specific homocytotropic (IgE or IgG4) antibodies. There is, however, some debate regarding whether there exists a universal obligatory role for IgE-related mechanisms in all cases of chemical respiratory sensitization.[50,51] This uncertainty arises in part from the fact that in some instances, particularly with respect to isocyanate-induced occupational asthma, it has proven difficult to detect specific IgE antibodies in symptomatic patients. It is possible, of course, that allergic sensitization of the respiratory tract may proceed via mechanisms that are independent of IgE antibody. Alternatively, the failure to identify IgE anti-hapten antibody in the serum of patients might be attributable to the use of inappropriate or insufficiently sensitive detection methods. Moreover, it is possible that in the absence of IgE, allergic inflammatory reactions could be effected by IgG4 antibody. Irrespective of an absolute requirement for IgE antibody in the pathogenesis of chemical respiratory allergy, it is likely that in many cases IgE- and/or IgG4-associated mechanisms play a prominent pathogenetic role.[52-54]

5.3　CHARACTERIZATION OF IMMUNE RESPONSES INDUCED IN MICE BY CHEMICAL RESPIRATORY ALLERGENS

The assumption is, therefore, that in many instances chemical respiratory allergens induce IgE (or IgG4) antibody production and that this antibody distributes systemically and associates with mast cells, including mast cells in the respiratory tract. If the now-sensitized individual subsequently inhales the inducing allergen, then mast cell degranulation will initiate a respiratory hypersensitivity reaction which may manifest itself as asthma or rhinitis. Such is consistent with what is known of immune responses provoked in mice by chemical respiratory allergens.

5.3.1　Cellular and Humoral Immune Responses to Chemical Respiratory Allergens

Chemical allergens of different types provoke in mice qualitatively divergent immune responses. In initial investigations, the characteristics of immune responses induced in mice by trimellitic anhydride (TMA) and by 2,4-dinitrochlorobenzene (DNCB) were examined. The former is a known human respiratory allergen,[10-13] while DNCB, a potent contact sensitizer, is considered not to cause respiratory hypersensitivity.[55] Groups of BALB/c strain mice were exposed topically to concentrations of these chemicals that stimulated equivalent levels of cellular proliferation in draining lymph nodes and comparable total IgG anti-hapten antibody responses. Under these conditions of equivalent overall immunogenicity, exposure only to TMA caused an increase in the serum concentration of IgE. In contrast, DNCB failed to influence the level of IgE found in serum, but induced a more vigorous production of specific IgG2a antibody than did TMA.[56] Further evidence for the stimulation by these chemicals of divergent immune responses derived from an examination of antibody production following inhalation exposure. Although exposure of mice to atmospheres of TMA or DNCB each induced the production of IgG anti-hapten antibody, only TMA provoked the synthesis of specific IgE antibody.[57]

In subsequent experiments, it was found that similar qualitative differences were observed following treatment of mice with other contact and respiratory chemical allergens.[58-62] On the basis of these investigations, the conclusion drawn was that chemical allergens of different types induce in mice divergent immune responses consistent with the selective stimulation of discrete T lymphocyte responses. It has been recognized for some time that T helper (Th) lymphocytes, characterized by the possession of the CD4 membrane determinant, display functional heterogeneity in mice and in other species.[63,64] Two main populations have been identified and these are designated Th_1 and Th_2 cells. These subpopulations of Th cells differ with respect to the pattern of cytokines they secrete. While some cytokines are produced by both cell types, only Th_1 cells secrete interleukin 2 (IL-2), interferon γ (IFN-γ) and tumor necrosis factor β (TNF-β) and only Th_2 cells produce interleukins 4, 5, 6 and 10 (IL-4, IL-5, IL-6, and IL-10).[65,66] The existence of functional subpopulations of Th cells is of some relevance for the development of allergic disease. The generation and maintenance of IgE responses are dependent upon the availability of IL-4, while IFN-γ antagonizes IgE production.[67,68] The implication from the experimental studies in mice described above was that chemical respiratory allergens provoke preferential Th_2-type immune responses resulting in the production of sufficient IL-4 to drive the production of specific IgE responses. Conversely, contact allergens are believed to elicit in mice selective Th_1-type responses in which the production of IFN-γ prohibits the generation of IgE antibody. The activation of Th_1 cells and their production of IFN-γ is, however, consistent with the induction of contact hypersensitivity.[69,70] Recently it has been shown that the other major class of T lymphocytes, $CD8^+$ cytotoxic T cells (Tc), also exhibit some degree of heterogeneity, again with two main subpopulations, Tc_1 and Tc_2, being recognized.[71] There is some evidence that these cells may contribute in important ways to the development of immune responses induced by allergenic chemicals.[72] However, the cytokine secretion patterns of Tc_1 and Tc_2 cells are similar to those of Th_1 and Th_2 cells, respectively, and the role of $CD8^+$ T lymphocytes in the development of responses to chemical respiratory allergens will not be considered further here.

The stimulation in mice of discrete Th cell responses by different classes of chemical allergens is consistent with the cytokine secretion patterns that are elicited. Exposure of mice to chemical respiratory allergens induces the development of Th_2-type cytokine production profiles by draining lymph node cells, with high levels of IL-4 and IL-10, but little IFN-γ. The converse is seen following treatment with contact allergens where lymph node cells produce IFN-γ, but little or no IL-4 or IL-10.[73-75] It is apparent therefore that chemical respiratory allergens provoke the class of response, and the pattern of cytokine production, necessary for the induction of IgE antibody responses. The role of such IgE responses in cutaneous reactions to respiratory allergens is considered below.

5.3.2   IgE Antibody, Mast Cells, and Cutaneous Reactions to Chemical Respiratory Allergens

The assumption that hapten-specific IgE antibody stimulated by exposure of mice to chemical respiratory allergens associates systemically with tissue mast cells is borne out by experimentation. Treatment of mice with TMA was shown to result in the specific sensitization of peritoneal mast cells *in situ,* as measured by the TMA-protein conjugate-induced release of serotonin *in vitro*. Exposure of mice under the same conditions to DNCB failed to result in mast cell sensitization.[76] In parallel experiments, the characteristics of cutaneous hypersensitivity reactions elicited in mice by chemical allergens were investigated. In animals sensitized previously to

TMA or DNCB, subsequent challenge to the ears with the same chemical was found in each case to result in a delayed (24 hour) edematous reaction. However, only in TMA-sensitized mice did such challenge result also in an immediate (1 hour) ear swelling response.[77] It was shown in addition that immediate, but not delayed, cutaneous hypersensitivity reactions could be transferred to naive recipients with serum from TMA-sensitized mice; an observation consistent with such immediate responses being effected by hapten-specific IgE antibody.[77] Recently, the ability of TMA to induce and elicit immediate-type dermal hypersensitivity reactions in mice has been confirmed in an independent investigation.[78]

With respect to TMA at least, it is clear that conventional topical sensitization provokes the quality of immune response necessary for the production of IgE antibody such that subsequent challenge causes an immediate (and delayed) dermal hypersensitivity reaction. The stimulation of Th_2-type immune responses by chemical respiratory sensitizers will facilitate the elicitation of immediate allergic reactions in ways other than, and in addition to, the generation of IgE antibody. The cytokine products of Th_2 cells are able to influence the development, differentiation, tissue distribution, and function of cells involved in allergic reactions. Interleukins 3, 4, and 10, all of which are Th_2 cell cytokines, are recognized as mast cell growth factors.[79,80] Moreover, IL-4 is known to augment the secretory potential of mast cells and will stimulate the increased release of inflammatory mediators following stimulation, a response inhibited by IFN-γ.[81-85] Interleukin 5 is a growth and differentiation factor for eosinophils, cells that are associated with immediate-type allergic responses.[86]

The integrated view is that many, at least of the known chemical respiratory allergens, have the ability to induce the class of immune response necessary for induction of homocytotropic antibody and for the subsequent elicitation of immediate-type allergic reactions.

5.4 CHEMICAL RESPIRATORY ALLERGENS AND THE CONTACT URTICARIA SYNDROME

Despite the controversy regarding an obligatory role for IgE antibody in the pathogenesis of occupational asthma, there is evidence that chemical respiratory allergens are able to induce in humans IgE and/or IgG4 antibody responses. Certainly this is true for the acid anhydrides,[7,13,14,18,19,87,88] isocyanates,[26,29,30,89] and reactive dyes.[32-35] If such antibody is produced in sufficient quantity and distributes systemically, then there is no reason to suppose that cutaneous sensitization will not occur. Indeed, skin prick tests remain important for the diagnosis of IgE-mediated allergic disease, including allergy induced by chemicals such as, for instance, the acid anhydrides.[88] Assuming, therefore, that exposure to chemical allergens, via whatever route, has resulted in the sensitization of cutaneous mast cells, and if the inducing chemical is able to gain access to the viable skin through the stratum corneum, then conditions exist for the provocation of an immediate-type dermal reaction. The stimulation of mast cell degranulation is dependent upon the association of the chemical allergen with proteins such as to effect cross-linking of IgE borne by mast cells.

The extent to which chemical respiratory allergens are associated with contact urticaria is presently unclear, although there is evidence that acid anhydrides are active.[90-92] It has been reported recently, for instance, that two individuals who worked with epoxy resins developed contact urticaria following airborne exposure to methylhexahydrophthalic and methyltetrahydrophthalic anhydrides. In both cases, specific IgE antibody was found.[92] There are also indications that platinum salts and chloramine T are associated with immunologic contact urticaria.[2]

In the context of the ability of chemical respiratory allergens to provoke contact urticaria, it is worth reflecting on latex allergy. Latex products are known to cause IgE-mediated hypersensitivity, including contact urticaria.[93-97] It has been found that latex proteins induce immune responses in mice comparable with those provoked by chemical respiratory allergens. Animals exposed to latex proteins by either intranasal or intraperitoneal administration displayed an increased serum concentration of IgE and elevated expression of the Th_2 cell cytokine products IL-4 and IL-5.[98] The assumption is that contact urticaria induced by chemical allergens results from similar immunobiological processes.

5.5 CONCLUDING COMMENTS

In theory, chemical respiratory allergens have a clear potential to induce in susceptible individuals the class of immune response necessary for the induction and elicitation of contact urticaria. The extent to which this intrinsic hazard translates into an important risk for man is unknown, although some chemicals, notably the anhydrides, have been associated with contact urticaria. The likelihood that contact urticaria will result from exposure to certain chemical allergens will be determined by the route, duration, and extent of that exposure; the inherent sensitizing properties of the chemical; and the genetic and/or acquired susceptibility of the individual. More detailed analyses of the associations between exposure to chemical respiratory allergens and contact urticaria would be of value.

REFERENCES

1. Maibach, H.I. and Johnson, H.L., Contact urticaria syndrome to diethyltoluamide (immediate-type hypersensitivity), *Arch. Dermatol.*, 112, 1289, 1975.
2. Amin, S., Lahti, A., and Maibach, H.I., Contact urticaria and the contact urticaria syndrome (immediate contact reactions), in *Dermatotoxicology*, 5th ed., Marzulli, F.N. and Maibach, H.I., Eds., Taylor and Francis, Washington, D.C., 1996, Chap. 38.
3. Cronin, E., *Contact Dermatitis*, Churchill Livingstone, London, 1990.
4. Bernstein, I.L., Chan-Yeung, M., Malo, J-L., and Bernstein, D.I., *Asthma in the Workplace*, Marcel Dekker, New York, 1993.
5. Chan-Yeung, M. and Malo, J-L., Compendium 1. Table of major inducers of occupational asthma, in *Asthma in the Workplace*, Bernstein, I.L., Chan-Yeung, M., Malo, J-L., and Bernstein, D.I., Eds., Marcel Dekker, New York, 1996, p. 595.
6. Kern, R.A., Asthma and allergic rhinitis due to sensitization to phthalic anhydride: report of a case, *J. Allergy*, 10, 164, 1939.

7. Maccia, C.A., Bernstein, I.L., Emmett, E.A., and Brooks, S.M., *In vitro* demonstration of specific IgE in phthalic anhydride hypersensitivity, *Am. Rev. Respir. Dis.*, 113, 701, 1976.
8. Wernfors, M., Nielsen, J., Schutz, A., and Skerfving, S., Phthalic anhydride-induced occupational asthma, *Int. Arch. Allergy Appl. Immunol.*, 79, 77, 1986.
9. Nielsen, J., Welinder, H., Schutz, A., and Skerfving, S., Specific serum antibodies against phthalic anhydride in occupationally exposed subjects, *J. Allergy Clin. Immunol.*, 82, 126, 1988.
10. Zeiss, C.R., Patterson, R., Pruzansky, J.J., Miller, M., Rosenberg, M., and Levitz, D., Trimellitic anhydride-induced airway syndromes: clinical and immunologic studies, *J. Allergy Clin. Immunol.*, 60, 96, 1977.
11. Bernstein, D.I., Patterson, R., and Zeiss, C.R., Clinical and immunological evaluation of trimellitic anhydride- and phthalic anhydride-exposed workers using a questionnaire and comparative analysis of enzyme-linked immunosorbent and radioimmunoassay studies, *J. Allergy Clin. Immunol.*, 69, 311, 1982.
12. Zeiss, C.R., Wolkonsky, P., Chacon, R., Tuntland, R.N., Levitz, D., Pruzansky, J.J., and Patterson, R., Syndromes in workers exposed to trimellitic anhydride. A longitudinal clinical and immunologic study, *Ann. Int. Med.*, 98, 8, 1983.
13. Topping, M.D., Venables, K.M., Luczynska, C.M., Howe, W., and Newman Taylor, A.J., Specificity of the human IgE response to inhaled acid anhydrides, *J. Allergy Clin. Immunol.*, 77, 834, 1986.
14. Howe, W., Venables, K.M., Topping, M.D., Dally, M.B., Hawkins, R., Law, S.J., and Newman Taylor, A.J., Tetrachlorophthalic anhydride asthma: evidence for specific IgE antibody, *J. Allergy Clin. Immunol.*, 71, 5, 1983.
15. Grammer, L.C., Harris, K.E., Chandler, M.J., Flaherty, D., and Patterson, R., Establishing clinical and immunologic criteria for diagnosis of occupational immunologic lung disease with phthalic anhydride and tetrachlorophthalic anhydride exposures as a model, *J. Occ. Med.*, 29, 806, 1987.
16. Venables, K.M., Topping, M.D., Nunn, A.J., Howe, W., and Newman Taylor, A.J., Immunologic and functional consequences of chemical (tetrachlorophthalic anhydride)-induced asthma after four years of avoidance of exposure, *J. Allergy Clin. Immunol.*, 80, 212, 1987.
17. Liss, G.M., Bernstein, D., Genesove, L., Roos, J.O., and Lim, J., Assessment of risk factors for IgE-mediated sensitization to tetrachlorophthalic anhydride, *J. Allergy Clin. Immunol.*, 92, 237, 1993.
18. Moller, D.R., Gallagher, J.S., Bernstein, D.I., Wilcox, T.G., Burroughs, H.E., and Bernstein, I.L., Detection of IgE-mediated respiratory sensitization in workers exposed to hexahydrophthalic anhydride, *J. Allergy Clin. Immunol.*, 75, 663, 1985.
19. Nielsen, J., Welinder, H., Ottoson, H., Bensryd, I., Venge, P., and Skerfving, S., Nasal challenge shows pathogenetic relevance of specific IgE serum antibodies for nasal symptoms caused by hexahydrophthalic anhydride, *Clin. Exp. Allergy*, 24, 440, 1994.
20. Durham, S.R., Graneek, B.J., Hawkins, R., and Newman Taylor, A.J., The temporal relationship between increases in airway responsiveness to histamine and late asthmatic responses induced by occupational agents, *J. Allergy Clin. Immunol.*, 79, 398, 1987.
21. Butcher, B.T., Salvaggio, J.E., Weill, H., and Ziskind, M.M., Toluene diisocyanate (TDI) pulmonary disease: immunologic and inhalation challenge studies, *J. Allergy Clin. Immunol.*, 58, 89, 1976.

22. O'Brien, I.M., Harries, M.G., Burge, P.S., and Pepys, J., Toluene di-isocyanate-induced asthma. 1. Reactions to TDI, MDI, HDI and histamine, *Clin. Allergy*, 9, 1, 1979.
23. Banks, D.E., Butcher, B.T., and Salvaggio, J.E., Isocyanate-induced respiratory disease, *Ann. Allergy*, 57, 389, 1986.
24. Karol, M.H., Tollerud, D.J., Campbell, T.P., Fabbri, L., Maestrelli, P., Saetta, M., and Mapp, C.E., Predictive value of airways hyperresponsiveness and circulating IgE for identifying types of responses to toluene diisocyanate inhalation challenge, *Am. J. Respir. Crit. Care Med.*, 149, 611, 1994.
25. Tansar, A.R., Bourke, M.P., and Blandford, A.G., Isocyanate asthma: respiratory symptoms caused by diphenylmethane diisocyanate, *Thorax*, 28, 596, 1973.
26. Zeiss, C.R., Kanellakes, T.M., Bellone, J.D., Levitz, D., Pruzansky, J.J., and Patterson, R., Immunoglobulin E-mediated asthma and hypersensitivity pneumonitis with precipitating anti-hapten antibodies due to diphenylmethane diisocyanate (MDI) exposure, *J. Allergy Clin. Immunol.*, 65, 346, 1980.
27. Zammit-Tabona, M., Sherkin, M., Kijek, K., Chan, H., and Chan-Yeung, M., Asthma caused by diphenylmethane diisocyanate in foundry workers. Clinical, bronchial provocation and immunologic studies, *Am. Rev. Respir. Dis.*, 128, 226, 1983.
28. Nemery, B. and Lenaerts, L., Exposure to methylene diphenyl diisocyanate in coal mines, *The Lancet*, 341, 318, 1993.
29. Keskinen, H., Tupasela, O., Tiikkainen, U., and Nordman, H., Experience of specific IgE in asthma, *Clin. Allergy*, 18, 597, 1988.
30. Cartier, A., Grammer, L.C., Malo, J-L., Lagier, F., Ghezzo, H., Harris, K., and Patterson, R., Specific serum antibodies against isocyanates. Association with occupational asthma, *J. Allergy Clin. Immunol.*, 84, 507, 1989.
31. Vandenplas, O., Cartier, A., Lesage, J., Cloutier, Y., Perreault, G., Grammer, L.C., Shaughnessy, M.A., and Malo, J-L., Prepolymers of hexamethylene diisocyanate as a cause of occupational asthma, *J. Allergy Clin. Immunol.*, 91, 850, 1993.
32. Docker, A., Wattie, J.M., Topping, M.D., Luczynska, C.M., Newman Taylor, A.J., Pickering, C.A.C., Thomas, P., and Gompertz, D., Clinical and immunological investigation of respiratory disease in workers using reactive dyes, *Br. J. Ind. Med.*, 44, 534, 1987.
33. Topping, M.D., Forster, H.W., Ide, C.W., Kennedy, F.M., Leach, A.M., and Sorkin, S., Respiratory allergy and specific immunoglobulin E and immunoglobulin G antibodies to reactive dyes used in the wool industry, *J. Occ. Med.*, 31, 857, 1989.
34. Park, H.S. and Hong, C-S., The significance of specific IgG and IgG4 antibodies to a reactive dye in exposed workers, *Clin. Exp. Allergy*, 21, 357, 1991.
35. Hong, C-S. and Park, H.S., Heterogeneity of IgE antibody response to reactive dye in sera from four different sensitized workers, *Clin. Exp. Allergy*, 22, 606, 1992.
36. Pepys, J., Pickering, C.A.C., and Hughes, E.G., Asthma due to inhaled chemical agents: complex salts of platinum, *Clin. Allergy*, 2, 391, 1972.
37. Cromwell, O., Pepys, J., Parish, W.J., and Hughes, E.G., Specific IgE antibodies to platinum salts in sensitized workers, *Clin. Allergy*, 9, 109, 1979.
38. Biagini, R.E., Bernstein, I.L., Gallagher, J.S., Moorman, W.J., Brooks, S., and Gann, P.H., The diversity of reaginic immune responses to platinum and palladium salts, *J. Allergy Clin. Immunol.*, 79, 794, 1985.
39. Murdoch, R.D., Pepys, J., and Hughes, E.G. IgE antibody responses to platinum group metals: a large scale refinery survey, *Br. J. Ind. Med.*, 43, 37, 1986.

40. Brooks, S.M., Baker, D.B., Gann, P.H., Jarabek, A.M., Hertzberg, V., Gallagher, J., Biagini, R.E., and Bernstein, I.L., Cold air challenge and platinum skin reactivity in platinum refinery workers, *Chest*, 97, 1041, 1990.

41. Quirce, S., Cuevas, M., Olaguibel, J.M., and Tabar, A.I., Occupational asthma and immunologic responses induced by inhaled carmine among employees at a factory making natural dyes, *J. Allergy Clin. Immunol.*, 93, 44, 1994.

42. Chan-Yeung, M., Barton, G., MacLean, L., and Grzybowski, S., Occupational asthma and rhinitis due to western red cedar (*Thuja plicata*), *Am. Rev. Respir. Dis.*, 108, 1094, 1973.

43. Chan-Yeung, M., Immunologic and nonimmunologic mechanisms in asthma due to western red cedar (*Thuja plicata*), *J. Allergy Clin. Immunol.*, 70, 32, 1982.

44. Cartier, A., Chan, H., Malo, J-L., Pineau, L., Tse, K.S., and Chan-Yeung, M., Occupational asthma caused by eastern white cedar (*Thuja occidentalis*) with demonstration that plicatic acid is present in this wood dust and is the causal agent, *J. Allergy Clin. Immunol.*, 77, 639, 1986.

45. Frew, A., Chan, H., Dryden, P., Salari, H., Lam, S., and Chan-Yeung, M., Immunologic studies of the mechanisms of occupational asthma caused by western red cedar, *J. Allergy Clin. Immunol.*, 92, 466, 1993.

46. Feinberg, S.M. and Watrous, R.M., Atopy to simple chemical compounds: sulphonechloramides, *J. Allergy,* 16, 109, 1945.

47. Bourne, M.S., Flindt, M.L.H., and Walker, J.M., Asthma due to industrial use of chloramine, *Br. Med. J.*, 2, 10, 1979.

48. Dijkman, J.H., Vooren, P.H., and Kramps, J.A., Occupational asthma due to inhalation of chloramine T. 1. Clinical observations and inhalation provocation studies, *Int. Arch. Allergy Appl. Immunol.*, 64, 422, 1981.

49. Wass, U., Belin, L., and Eriksson, N.E., Immunological specificity of chloramine-T-induced IgE antibodies in serum from a sensitized worker, *Clin. Allergy,* 19, 463, 1989.

50. Chan-Yeung, M., Occupational asthma, *Chest*, 98, 148S, 1990.

51. Chan-Yeung, M., Occupational asthma, *Environ. Health Perspect.*, 106, 249, 1995.

52. Kimber, I., Mechanisms of pulmonary sensitization, in *Toxicology of Industrial Compounds*, Thomas, H., Hess, R., and Waechter, F., Eds., Taylor and Francis, London, 1995, p. 141.

53. Kimber, I., Mechanisms of chemical respiratory allergy, in *Allergic Hypersensitivities Induced by Chemicals. Recommendations for Prevention,* Vos, J.G., Younes, M., and Smith, E., Eds., CRC Press, Boca Raton, 1996, Chap. 3.

54. Kimber, I. and Dearman, R.J., Immunobiology of chemical respiratory sensitization, in *Toxicology of Chemical Respiratory Hypersensitivity,* Kimber, I. and Dearman, R.J., Eds., Taylor and Francis, London, 1997, Chap. 5.

55. Botham, P.A., Rattray, N.J., Woodcock, D.R., Walsh, S.T., and Hext, P.M., The induction of respiratory allergy in guinea-pigs following intradermal injection of trimellitic anhydride: a comparison with the response to 2,4-dinitrochlorobenzene, *Toxicol. Lett.*, 47, 25, 1989.

56. Dearman, R.J. and Kimber, I., Differential stimulation of immune function by respiratory and contact chemical allergens, *Immunology*, 72, 563, 1991.

57. Dearman, R.J., Hegarty, J.M., and Kimber, I., Inhalation exposure of mice to trimellitic anhydride induces both IgG and IgE anti-hapten antibody, *Int. Arch. Allergy Appl. Immunol.*, 95, 70, 1991.

58. Dearman, R.J. and Kimber, I., Divergent immune responses to respiratory and contact chemical allergens: antibody elicited by phthalic anhydride and oxazolone, *Clin. Exp. Allergy*, 22, 241, 1992.

59. Dearman, R.J., Spence, L.M., and Kimber, I., Characterization of murine immune responses to allergenic diisocyanates, *Toxicol. Appl. Pharmacol.*, 112, 190, 1992.

60. Dearman, R.J., Basketter, D.A., Coleman, J.W., and Kimber, I., The cellular and molecular basis for divergent allergic responses to chemicals, *Chem. Biol. Interactions*, 84, 1, 1992.

61. Kimber, I. and Dearman, R.J., Immune responses to contact and respiratory allergens, in *Immunotoxicology and Immunopharmacology*, 2nd. ed., Dean, J.H., Luster, M.I., Munson, A.E., and Kimber, I., Eds., Raven Press, New York, 1994, Chap. 38.

62. Kimber, I., Chemical-induced hypersensitivity, in *Experimental Immunotoxicology*, Smialowicz, R.J. and Holsapple, M.P., Eds., CRC Press, Boca Raton, 1996, Chap. 19.

63. Mosmann, T.R., Cherwinski, H., Bond, M.W., Giedlin, M.A., and Coffman, R.L., Two types of murine helper T cell clone. 1. Definition according to profiles of lymphokine activities and secreted proteins, *J. Immunol.*, 136, 2348, 1986.

64. Romagnani, S., Human T_{H1} and T_{H2} subsets: doubt no more, *Immunol. Today*, 12, 256, 1991.

65. Mosmann, T.R. and Coffman, R.L., Heterogeneity of cytokine secretion patterns and functions of helper T cells, *Adv. Immunol.*, 46, 111, 1989.

66. Mosmann, T.R., Schumacher, J.H., Street, N.F., Budd, R., O'Garra, A., Fong, T.A.T., Bond, M.W., Moore, K.W.M., Sher, A., and Fiorentino, D.F., Diversity of cytokine synthesis and function of mouse CD4+ T cells, *Immunol. Rev.*, 123, 209, 1991.

67. Finkelman, F.D., Katona, I.M., Urban, J.F.Jr., Holmes, J., Ohara, J., Tung, A.S., Sample, J.G., and Paul, W.E., IL-4 is required to generate and sustain *in vivo* IgE responses, *J. Immunol.*, 141, 2335, 1988.

68. Finkelman, F.D., Katona, I.M., Mosmann, T.R., and Coffman, R.L., IFN-γ regulates the isotypes of Ig secreted during *in vivo* humoral immune responses, *J. Immunol.*, 140, 1022, 1988.

69. Cher, D. and Mosmann, T.R., Two types of murine helper T clones. II. Delayed type hypersensitivity is mediated by Th_1 clones, *J. Immunol.*, 138, 3688, 1987.

70. Fong, T.A.T. and Mosmann, T.R., The role of IFN-γ in delayed-type hypersensitivity mediated by Th_1 clones, *J. Immunol.*, 143, 2887, 1989.

71. Croft, M., Carter, L., Swain, S.L., and Dutton, R.W., Generation of polarized antigen-specific CD8 effector populations: reciprocal action of interleukin (IL)-4 and IL-12 in promoting type 2 versus type 1 cytokine profiles, *J. Exp. Med.*, 180, 1715, 1994.

72. Xu, H., DiIulio, N.A., and Fairchild, R.L., T cell populations primed by hapten sensitization in contact sensitivity are distinguished by polarized patterns of cytokine production. Interferon-γ-producing (Tc_1) effector CD8+ T cells and interleukin (IL)4/IL-10-producing (Th_2) negative regulatory CD4+ T cells, *J. Exp. Med.*, 183, 1001, 1996.

73. Dearman, R.J., Ramdin, L.S.P., Basketter, D.A., and Kimber, I., Inducible interleukin-4-secreting cells provoked in mice during chemical sensitization, *Immunology*, 81, 551, 1994.

74. Dearman, R.J., Basketter, D.A., and Kimber I., Differential cytokine production following chronic exposure of mice to chemical respiratory and contact allergens, *Immunology*, 86, 545, 1995.

75. Dearman, R.J., Basketter, D.A., and Kimber, I., Characterization of chemical allergens as a function of divergent cytokine secretion profiles induced in mice, *Toxicol. Appl. Pharmacol.*, 138, 308, 1996.

76. Holliday, M.R., Coleman, J.W., Dearman, R.J., and Kimber, I., Induction of mast cell sensitization by chemical allergens: a comparative study, *J. Appl. Toxicol.*, 13, 137, 1993.

77. Dearman, R.J., Mitchell, J.A., Basketter, D.A., and Kimber, I., Differential ability of occupational chemical contact and respiratory allergens to cause immediate and delayed dermal hypersensitivity reactions in mice, *Int. Arch. Allergy Immunol.*, 97, 315, 1992.

78. Lauerma, A.I., Aioi, A., and Maibach, H.I., Topical cis-urocanic acid suppresses both induction and elicitation of contact hypersensitivity in BALB/c mice, *Acta Derm. Venereol. (Stockh.)*, 75, 272, 1995.

79. Smith, C.A. and Rennick, D.M., Characterization of a murine lymphokine distinct from interleukin 3 (IL-3) possessing a T-cell growth factor activity and a mast cell growth factor activity that synergizes with IL-3, *Proc. Natl. Acad. Sci. U.S.A.*, 83, 1857, 1986.

80. Thompson-Snipes, L., Dhar, V., Bond, M.W., Mosmann, T.R., Moore, K.W., and Rennick, D.M., Interleukin-10: a novel stimulatory factor for mast cells and their progenitors, *J. Exp. Med.*, 173, 507, 1991.

81. Coleman, J.W., Buckley, M.G., Holliday, M.R., and Morris, A.G., Interferon-γ inhibits serotonin release from mouse peritoneal mast cells, *Eur. J. Immunol.*, 21, 2559, 1991.

82. Coleman, J.W., Holliday, M.R., and Buckley, M.G., Regulation of the secretory function of mouse peritoneal mast cells by IL-3, IL-4 and IFN-γ, *Int. Arch. Allergy Immunol.*, 99, 408, 1992.

83. Coleman, J.W., Holliday, M.R., Kimber, I., Zsebo, K.M., and Galli, S.J., Regulation of mouse peritoneal mast cell secretory function by stem cell factor, IL-3 or IL-4, *J. Immunol.*, 150, 556, 1993.

84. Holliday, M.R., Banks, E.M.S., Dearman, R.J., Kimber, I., and Coleman, J.W., Interactions of IFN-γ with IL-3 and IL-4 in the regulation of serotonin and arachidonate release from mouse peritoneal mast cells, *Immunology*, 82, 70, 1994.

85. Coleman, J.W., Holliday, M.R., Dearman, R.J., and Kimber, I., Cytokine-mast cell interactions: relevance to IgE-mediated chemical allergy, *Toxicology*, 88, 225, 1994.

86. Yokota, T., Coffman, R.L., Hagiwara, H., Rennick, D.M., Takebe, Y., Yokota, K., Gemmell, L., Schrader, B., Yang, G., Meyerson, P., Luh, J., Hoy, P., Pene, J., Briere, F., Spits, H., Banchereau, J., de Vries, J., Lee, F.D., Arai, N., and Arai, K-I., Isolation and characterization of lymphokine cDNA clones encoding mouse and human IgA-enhancing and eosinophil-colony stimulating factor activities. Relationship to interleukin 5, *Proc. Natl. Acad. Sci. U.S.A.*, 84, 7388, 1987.

87. Newman Taylor, A.J., Venables, K.M., Durham, S.R., Graneek, B.J., and Topping, M.D., Acid anhydrides and asthma, *Int. Arch. Allergy Appl. Immunol.*, 82, 435, 1987.

88. Drexler, H., Schaller, K-H., Weber, A., Letzel, S., and Lehnert, G., Skin prick tests with solutions of acid anhydrides in acetone, *Int. Arch. Allergy Immunol.*, 100, 251, 1993.

89. Wass, U. And Belin, L., Immunologic specificity of isocyanate-induced IgE antibodies in serum from 10 sensitized workers, *J. Allergy Clin. Immunol.*, 83, 126, 1989.

90. Jolanki, R., Estlander, T., and Kanerva, L., Occupational contact dermatitis and contact urticaria caused by epoxy resins, *Acta. Dermatol. Venereol. Suppl. (Stockh.)*, 134, 90, 1987.

91. Jolanki, R., Kanerva, L., Estlander, T., Tarvainen, K., Keskinen, H., and Henricks-Eckerman, M-L., Occupational dermatoses from epoxy resin compounds, *Contact Derm.*, 23, 172, 1990.

92. Tarvainen, K., Jolanki, R., Estlander, T., Tupasela, O., Pfaffli, P., and Kanerva, L., Immunologic contact urticaria due to airborne methylhexahydrophthalic and methyltetrahydrophthalic anhydrides, *Contact Derm.*, 32, 204, 1995.

93. Wrangsjo, K., Wahlberg, J.E., and Axelsson, I.G.K., IgE-mediated allergy to natural rubber in 30 patients with contact urticaria, *Contact Derm.*, 19, 264, 1988.

94. Turjanmaa, I., Laurila K., Makinen-Kiljunen, S., and Reunala, T., Rubber contact urticaria. Allergenic properties of 19 brands of latex gloves, *Contact Derm.*, 19, 362, 1988.

95. Turjanmaa, K. and Reunala, T., Condoms as a source of latex allergen and cause of contact urticaria, *Contact Derm.*, 20, 360, 1989.

96. Belsito, D.V., Contact urticaria caused by rubber. Analysis of seven cases, *Dermatol. Clin.*, 8, 61, 1990.

97. Fernandez de Corres, L., Moneo, I., Munoz, D., Bernaola, G., Fernandez, E., Audicana, M., and Urrutia, I., Sensitization from chestnuts and bananas in patients with urticaria and anaphylaxis from contact with latex, *Ann. Allergy*, 70, 35, 1993.

98. Kurup, V.P., Kumar, A., Choi, H., Murali, P.S., Resnick, A., Kelly, K.J., and Fink, J.N., Latex antigens induce IgE and eosinophils in mice, *Int. Arch. Allergy Immunol.*, 103, 370, 1994.

6

Statistics on Occupational Contact Urticaria

Lasse Kanerva, Riitta Jolanki, Jouni Toikkanen, and Tuula Estlander

CONTENTS

6.1 INTRODUCTION

Statistics are available on occupational contact urticaria caused by natural rubber latex,[1] but otherwise very little is known.[2,3] In Finland, occupational contact urticaria has been classified as a separate occupational skin disease since 1989. Earlier, all allergic contact dermatoses, i.e., allergic contact dermatitis and contact urticaria, were grouped together. The number of cases of occupational contact urticaria has

"

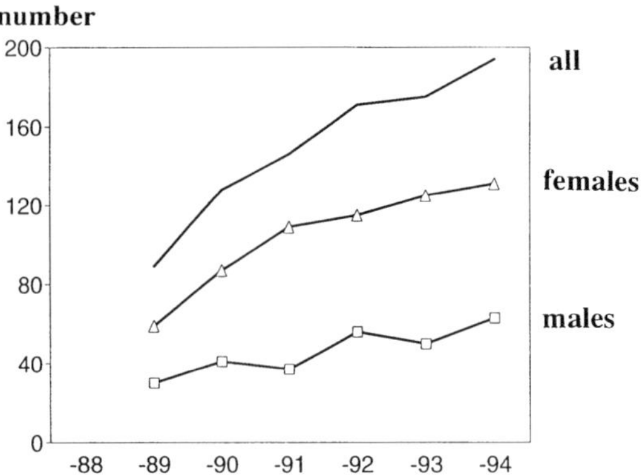

FIGURE 6.1   Number of occupational cases of contact urticaria (protein contact dermatitis included) by gender during 1989–1994.

more than doubled during the observation period: 89 cases were reported in 1989 and 194 cases in 1994 (Figure 6.1). In this article, we have compiled data from a 5-year period, namely 1990–1994.

6.2   COMPILING STATISTICS ON OCCUPATIONAL DISEASES IN FINLAND

The Department of Social Research of the Ministry of Social Affairs and Health started compiling statistics on occupational diseases in Finland in 1926. Since 1974, the Act on the Supervision of Labor Protection has obligated physicians to report every case of occupational disease. In 1975, the Finnish Institute of Occupational Health assumed the responsibility for compiling these statistics. The collection of data is illustrated in Figure 6.2. All the occupational disease cases have been diagnosed by a physician. The insurance companies provide the Register with data on every case reported to them, irrespective of the final decision with regard to compensation. Statistics on new cases of occupational diseases are published annually in Finnish.[4] An English edition is published every 3–4 years.[5]

Only the main cause is considered as the source of an occupational dermatosis. If the disease is diagnosed as an occupational allergic disease, it is recorded as an occupational allergic disease despite the fact that irritant factors have probably also been involved. A patient's occupational skin disease is registered only once. Contact urticaria (CU) and protein contact dermatitis (PCD) are dealt with together under the heading of contact urticaria.

6.3   CLASSIFICATION OF OCCUPATIONS

The currently used classification of occupations was published in 1987, and is based on work done by the Central Statistical Office of Finland in collaboration with the Ministry of Labor of Finland. The classifications used in employment service and

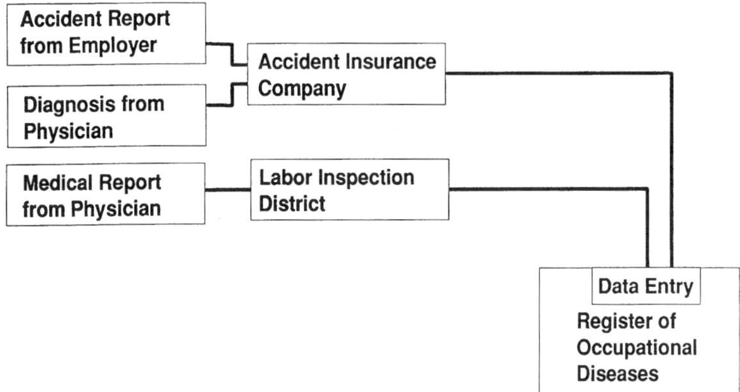

FIGURE 6.2   Flow chart outlining data collection routes for the Register of Occupational Diseases in Finland.

the official statistics are nearly identical down to the 3-digit level. Both classifications are based on the Nordic Classification of Occupations (NYK 1982)[6] which, in principle, is based on the International Standard Classification of Occupations (ISCO) published in 1958 and revised in 1986.[7] Furthermore, national needs and institutional circumstances have been given preference in compiling the Finnish standard. The basic classification criterion in the grouping of occupations has been the type of work performed irrespective of education, status in employment, or industry.

The identification code of the Finnish standard consists of four digits and uses a decimal system of coding. There are eight major groups (e.g., ISCO has nine groups).[8] The structure of the Finnish classification system is as follows:

8 major groups (1-digit level)
85 groups in the 2-digit level
362 groups in the 3-digit level
231 groups in the 4-digit level
about 7800 title words (occupations) altogether

The structure of the coding scheme is illustrated in Table 6.1. In the present statistics, occupational contact urticaria of occupations has been analyzed at the 3-digit level (Table 6.2).

6.4   PREVALENCE OF OCCUPATIONAL CONTACT URTICARIA

The prevalence of occupational contact urticaria during 1990–1994 per 100,000 employed workers is given in Table 6.2, both for women and men. Table 6.3 shows a prevalence ranking list, indicating that bakers, preparers of processed food, and dental assistants have the highest risk to develop occupational contact urticaria.

TABLE 6.1 The Major Occupational Groups (1-digit level) and an Example of the Structure of the Coding Scheme (1-digit, 2-digit, 3-digit and 4-digit level) of the Finnish Classification of Occupations

	Number of Cases
0. Technical, scientific, juridical, humanistic, and artistic work	
1. Health care and social work (1-digit level)	NG
10. Medical and nursing work (2-digit level)	127
101 Physicians (3-digit level)	20
102 Chief nurses	0
103 Nurses	42
1031 Ward nurses (4-digit level)	NG
1032 Specialized nurses	NG
1033 Nurses (general)	NG
1034 Midwives	NG
1035 Public health nurses	NG
104 Laboratory technologists, radiology technologists	9
105 Psychiatric attendants	1
106 Assistant nurses, medical orderlies	14
1061 Assistant nurses, practical nurses	NG
1062 Orderlies, ambulance attendants	NG
107 Children's nurses	0
108 Technical nursing assistants	5
1081 Hospital maids	NG
1082 Ward assistants, patient receptionists	NG
1083 Instrument keepers, technical assistants	NG
1083 Examinations assistants (in hospitals, etc.)	NG
109 Other medical and nursing work	0
1091 Podiatrists	NG (=0)
1092 Chiropractors, naprapaths, etc.	NG (=0)
11. Therapeutical work (2-digit level)	0
12. Dental work	33
121 Dentists	5
122 Dental nurses	28
etc.	
2. Managerial, administrative, and clerical work	
3. Commerical work	
4. Agricultural, forestry, and fishing work	
5. Transport and communication work	
6/7/8. Manufacturing, machinery operation, and related work	
9. Service work, etc.	

Note: The number of cases of contact urticaria during 1990–1994 are given in the health care and social work-group (= 1-digit level) at the 2-digit and the 3-digit level; for details see Table 4.2.

NG = not given.

TABLE 6.2 Occupational Contact Urticaria by Occupation per 100,000 Employed Persons in Finland during 1990–1994 (815 cases), According to the Finnish Register of Occupational Diseases. Classification of the Occupations at the 3-digit level (see Table 6.1).

		Men		Women		Total	
Code	Occupation	Number	Per 100,000 employed persons	Number	Per 100,000 employed persons	Number	Per 100,000 employed persons
001	Construction engineers and technicians	1	0.9	0	0.0	1	0.8
005	Chemical engineers and technicians	1	2.2	0	0.0	1	1.9
010	Chemists	1	10.8	1	14.1	2	12.3
012	Laboratory assistants	0	0.0	15	34.9	15	24.6
021	Biologists	1	30.1	0	0.0	1	19.7
031	Teachers at universities and other institutions of higher education	1	3.4	0	0.0	1	2.3
032	Secondary school teachers	0	0.0	2	1.3	2	0.9
081	Librarians, etc.	0	0.0	1	3.2	1	2.7
101	Physicians	6	18.1	14	50.8	20	33.0
103	Nurses	2	31.1	40	20.8	42	21.2
104	Laboratory technicians, radiographers	0	0.0	9	37.4	9	35.6
105	Psychiatric attendants	0	0.0	1	6.3	1	3.7
106	Assistant nurses, hospital attendants	3	27.6	11	8.7	14	10.2
108	Technical nursing assistants	0	0.0	5	4.3	5	4.2
121	Dentists	2	32.1	3	19.8	5	23.4
122	Dental assistants	0	0.0	28	95.7	28	95.5
141	Veterinary surgeons	2	83.5	1	57.4	3	72.5
155	Homemakers, home helps (municipal)	0	0.0	5	6.3	5	6.2
211	Managers of business enterprises	0	0.0	1	1.1	1	0.2
231	Financial planners and cost estimation officers	0	0.0	1	7.7	1	4.4
311	Real estate and personal property agents	1	13.9	0	0.0	1	7.7
342	Shop managers, etc.	0	0.0	2	5.5	2	3.3
343	Shop assistants, shop cashiers	2	1.8	7	2.2	9	2.1

TABLE 6.2 (continued) Occupational Contact Urticaria by Occupation per l00,000 Employed Persons in Finland during 1990–1994 (815 cases), According to the Finnish Register of Occupational Diseases. Classification of the Occupations at the 3-digit level (see Table 6.1).

		Men		Women		Total	
Code	Occupation	Number	Per 100,000 employed persons	Number	Per 100,000 employed persons	Number	Per 100,000 employed persons
400	Farmers, silviculturalists	124	33.3	217	99.2	341	57.7
401	Agricultural supervisors	1	42.7	0	0.0	1	33.7
406	Domestic animal attendants	27	65.5	34	72.2	61	69.1
409	Others belonging to group 40	0	0.0	2	63.9	2	46.3
410	Commercial gardeners	1	16.1	0	0.0	1	8.8
411	Horticultural supervisors	1	11.6	5	68.7	6	37.8
412	Horticultural workers	0	0.0	5	19.8	5	10.7
541	Lorry and articulated vehicle drivers	1	0.4	0	0.0	1	0.4
542	Goods shippers	0	0.0	1	420.7	1	101.1
705	Textile finishers, dyers	1	52.4	0	0.0	1	16.7
709	Others belonging to group 70	1	207.5	0	0.0	1	79.7
716	Industrial sewers, etc.	0	0.0	4	9.3	4	9.1
741	Precision instrument mechanics	1	6.9	0	0.0	1	5.7
751	Turners, machinists, and toolmakers	1	1.3	0	0.0	1	1.3
752	Machine fitters, etc.	1	1.2	0	0.0	1	1.2
753	Machine and engine mechanics, etc.	7	4.0	0	0.0	7	3.9
756	Welders, flame cutters, etc.	1	1.7	0	0.0	1	1.6
757	Machine and metal product assemblers	1	11.5	0	0.0	1	6.0
765	Electrical and teletechnical equipment assemblers	1	8.2	2	6.0	3	6.6

Code	Occupation						
772	Sawyers	1	2.9	0	0.0	1	2.4
773	Plywood and fibreboard workers	1	15.4	1	16.1	2	15.7
777	Woodworking machine operators	1	2.6	0	0.0	1	2.3
782	Other painters and lacquerers	1	6.6	0	0.0	1	5.8
801	Printing foremen and typesetters, etc.	1	4.7	0	0.0	1	2.6
822	Bakers	26	157.2	27	127.4	53	140.5
823	Chocolate and confectionery workers	1	94.8	0	0.0	1	27.8
826	Butchers and sausage makers	4	21.7	3	51.4	7	28.9
827	Dairy workers	2	42.7	3	35.3	5	37.9
828	Processed food preparers	0	0.0	4	117.0	4	101.8
829	Others belonging to minor group 82	1	17.5	1	14.7	2	16.0
839	Others belonging to group 83	0	0.0	3	68.1	3	27.3
862	Tanners, fellmongers, and pelt dressers	1	96.5	1	119.1	2	106.6
881	Packers	1	4.3	7	14.5	8	11.2
911	Housekeeping managers, snack bar managers, etc.	0	0.0	9	13.9	9	11.5
912	Chefs, cooks, cold buffet managers	9	47.0	31	36.5	40	38.5
913	Kitchen assistants, restaurant workers, etc.	1	13.4	15	13.7	16	13.6
921	Headwaiters, restaurant waiters, etc.	1	6.3	0	0.0	1	1.3
922	Waiters in cafes and snack bars, etc.	0	0.0	9	16.1	9	15.1
941	Building caretakers, etc.	2	1.8	0	0.0	2	1.4
942	Cleaners, etc.	0	0.0	21	7.3	21	6.7
951	Hairdressers, beauticians, bath attendants, etc.	0	0.0	9	12.2	9	11.8
961	Laundry workers	0	0.0	1	6.9	1	6.0
992	Burial service personnel	0	0.0	1	112.0	1	42.6
999	Others belonging to group 99	2		4		6	
	Total	248	2.2	567	5.3	815	3.7

TABLE 6.3 The Ranking List of Occupations with Occupational Contact Urticaria in Finland During 1990–1994 (n = 815)

Occupation	Number per 100,000 workers	Total number
1. Bakers	140.5	53
2. Preparers of processed food	101.8	4
3. Dental assistants	95.5	28
4. Veterinary surgeons	72.5	3
5. Domestic animal attendants	69.1	61
6. Farmers, silviculturalists	57.7	341
7. Chefs, cooks, cold buffet managers	38.5	40
8. Dairy workers	37.9	5
9. Horticultural supervisors	37.8	6
10. Laboratory technicians, radiographers	35.6	9
11. Physicians	33.0	20
12. Butchers and sausage makers	28.9	7
13. Laboratory assistants	24.6	15
14. Dentists	23.4	5
15. Nurses	21.2	42
16. Waiters in cafes and snack bars, etc.	15.1	9
17. Kitchen assistants, restaurant workers, etc.	13.6	16
18. Hairdressers, beauticians, bath attendants, etc.	11.8	9
19. Housekeeping managers, snack bar managers, etc.	11.5	9
20. Packers	11.2	8
21. Horticultural workers	10.7	5
22. Assistant nurses, hospital attendants	10.2	14
23. Industrial sewers, etc.	9.1	4
24. Cleaners, etc.	6.7	21
25. Electrical and teletechnical equipment assemblers	6.6	3
26. Homemakers, home helps (municipal)	6.2	5
27. Technical nursing assistants	4.2	5
28. Machine and engine mechanics, etc.	3.9	7
29. Shop assistants, shop cashiers	2.1	9
Total	3.7	815

Note: Only occupations in which at least three persons had an occupational urticaria were included.

Occupations with less than three cases of occupational contact urticaria during 1990–1994 have been omitted.

6.5 THE MOST COMMON CAUSES OF OCCUPATIONAL CONTACT URTICARIA

Table 6.4 gives a ranking list of the most common causes of occupational contact urticaria. The three most common causes are first, cow dander, second, natural rubber latex, and third, flour, grains, and feed. These three groups (n = 647) comprise 79% of all cases of occupational contact urticaria (n = 815). Contact urticaria from cow

TABLE 6.4 The Causes of Occupational Contact Urticaria and Protein Contact Dermatitis During 1990–1994 (815 cases) According to the Finnish Register of Occupational Diseases

Cause	Number of Cases		Men/Women
1. Cow dander	362		132/230
2. Natural rubber latex	193		22/171
3. Flour, grains, and feed	92		
4. Handling of foodstuffs	25		9/16
5. Enzymes	14		
cellulase		8	
alfa-amylase		2	
6. Decorative plants	13		1/12
7. Roots	10		2/8
8. Spices	9		1/8
9. Pork	8		4/4
Vegetables	8		
11. Storage mites	6		5/1
12. Ethylhexyl acrylate	5		0/5
13. Onions	4		1/3
Egg	4		1/3
14. Fish, fish meal	3		0/3
Poultry, chicken, other birds	3		1/3
Total	815		248/567

dander and natural rubber latex, as well as the total number of cases of contact urticaria, is much more common in women than in men (Table 6.3).

6.6 OCCUPATIONAL CONTACT URTICARIA CAUSED BY LOW MOLECULAR WEIGHT CHEMICALS

We have reported cases of contact urticaria caused by low molecular weight chemicals, but the prevalence is very low, and only occasional cases were detected during 1990–1994 (Table 6.5). The most common low molecular chemical was ethylhexyl acrylate, but we have no additional data on these cases, as they have not been diagnosed at our institute.

6.7 REMARKS ON THE MOST COMMON CAUSES OF OCCUPATIONAL CONTACT URTICARIA

Cow dander has only rarely been reported to cause occupational skin diseases,[9] although both immediate and delayed contact allergy to cow dander was described already in 1948 by Epstein.[10] Van Ketel and Dieggelen[11] reported in 1982 a farmer with hand eczema, positive immediate skin tests, and RASTs to cow hair and dander.

**TABLE 6.5 Occupational Contact Urticaria
Caused by Low Molecular Weight
Chemicals During 1990–1994**

2-ethylhexyl acrylate	5
Methylhexahydrophthalic anhydride	2
Acetic acid	1
Furfuryl aldehyde	1
Ammonium persulfate	1
Potassium persulfate	1
Epoxy resin	1

Recently, Susitaival[12] showed that hand eczema is common in Finnish dairy farmers, partly due to immediate and delayed allergy to cow dander.[13]

Finland is geographically located above the 60th degree of northern lattitude, and is thus the most northern country with dairy farming. Accordingly, cows are kept in cowhouses during most of the year, generally from September to May or June. For example, in neighboring Sweden, most dairy farming takes place further south, and to our knowledge, cow dander has not been considered an occupational skin hazard in Sweden. In a Danish farmer population with one third having dairy cattle, 3.2% had a positive skin prick test reaction to cow dander,[14] but skin symptoms were not monitored in that report.

It is common in Finland that farmers brush the cows to keep them tidy, and as this also is performed inside the cowhouses, the exposure to cow dander may be exceptionally high. Accordingly, hand eczema is common in Finnish farmers,[12] and cow dander is also the most common cause of occupational rhinitis and asthma in Finland.[2,15] Contact urticaria caused by cow dander is IgE-mediated, and recently major bovine allergens have been characterized by immunoassays.[16,17] Allergy to cow dander is well known in Finland, but may elsewhere not be recognized and looked for.[18]

Contact urticaria caused by natural rubber latex has been extensively reviewed in the literature,[1] including this book (Turjanmaa), whereas flour, grains, and feed have received much less attention in the dermatological literature. Both bakers (Table 6.2) and farmers, as well as workers in various food industries, are at risk. It is emphasized that flour contains two groups of allergens, the protein flour itself, and natural enzymes[19] in the flours. Enzymes were the fourth most common cause of occupational contact urticaria. Contact urticaria from enzymes have been dealt with elsewhere in this book.[19] The relatively high number of cases caused by enzymes in Finland is due to a relatively large enzyme industry, as well as the recent research interest in allergy caused by enzymes in Finland.

Decorative plants, roots, spices,[20,21] pork,[22] and vegetables[23] are well known causes of contact urticaria, whereas storage mites are less well known, although they are relatively well known as respiratory allergens.[24,25] We routinely prick test farmers and other exposed workers with three storage mites, namely *Acarus siro, Lepidoglyphus destructor,* and *Tyrophagus putrescentiae* (ALK, Copenhagen, Denmark). It seems evident that if prick tests or alternatively radioallergosorbent tests (RAST) to storage mites are not performed, it is not possible to investigate storage mites as a possible cause of contact urticaria.

Low molecular weight chemicals are a rare cause of contact urticaria. We have had cases caused by, e.g., methylhexahydrophthalic and methyltetrahydrophthalic anhydride,[26] diglycidyl ether of bisphenol A epoxy resin,[27] polyfunctional aziridines,[28,29] nickel,[30] and reactive dyes.[31] The low molecular weight chemicals that have caused contact urticaria have been summarized in this book.[32]

6.8 CONCLUDING REMARKS

Data on 815 occupational cases of contact urticaria, based on a recent report,[33] are presented. As the clinical picture ranges from an invisible skin disease[34] to anaphylactic shock and death, the clinician needs to have great skill and knowledge to be able to make the diagnosis. It is probable that a high number of cases of contact urticaria remain undetected.

REFERENCES

1. Turjanmaa, K., Mäkinen-Kiljunen, S., Reunala, T., Alenius, H., and Palosuo, T., Natural rubber latex allergy. The European experience, *Immunol. Allergy Clinics North America,* 15, 71-88, 1995.
2. Kanerva, L., Jolanki, R., and Toikkanen, J., Frequencies of occupational allergic diseases and gender differences in Finland, *Int. Arch. Occ. Environ. Health,* 66, 111-116, 1994.
3. Kanerva, L., Jolanki, R., Toikkanen, J., Tarvainen, K., and Estlander, T., Statistics on occupational dermatoses in Finland, *Curr. Probl. Dermatol.,* Basel, Karger, 23, 28-40, 1995.
4. Kauppinen, T., Vaaranen, V., Vasama, M., Toikkanen, J., and Jolanki, R., Ammattitaudit 1993, Katsauksia 130, Työterveyslaitos, Helsinki 1994 (in Finnish).
5. Toikkanen, J., Kauppinen, T., Vaaranen, V., Vasama, M., and Jolanki, R., Occupational diseases in Finland in 1993. New cases of occupational diseases reported to the Finnish Register of Occupational Diseases, Finnish Institute of Occupational Health, Reviews 21, Helsinki, Finland, 1994.
6. Nordisk Yrkesklassifiering, NYK-82, Rapport till Nordiska Ministerrådet, Sept., 1982, NAUT-rapport, 10, 1982 (in Swedish).
7. International Standard Classification of Occupations, Revised edition 1968, International Labour Office, Geneva, Third Impression, 1978.
8. Classificaton of Occupations 1980, Handbooks No. 14, Helsinki, 1981.
9. Kanerva, L. and Susitaival, P., Cow dander — the most common cause of occupational contact urticaria in Finland, *Contact Dermatitis,* 35, 309–310, 1996.
10. Epstein, S., Milker's eczema, *J. Allergy,* 19, 333-341, 1948.
11. van Ketel, W.G. and van Diggelen, M. W., A farmer with allergy to cows, *Contact Dermatitis,* 8, 269, 1982.
12. Susitaival, P., Epidemiological study of hand dermatoses and other skin diseases in a cohort of Finnish farmers, Kuopio University Publications D. Medical Sciences (Thesis), 93, 1-104, 1996.

13. Susitaival, P., Husman, L., Hollmen, A., Horsmanheimo, M., Husman, K., and Hannuksela, M., Hand eczema in Finnish farmers. A questionnaire-based clinical study, *Contact Dermatitis,* 32, 150-155, 1995.

14. Iversen, M. and Pedersen, B., The prevalence of allergy in Danish farmers, *Allergy,* 45, 347-353, 1990.

15. Kanerva, L. and Vaheri, E., Occupational rhinitis in Finland, *Int. Arch. Occ. Environ. Health,* 64, 565-568, 1993.

16. Ylönen, J., Mäntyjärvi, R., Taivainen, A., and Virtanen, T., IgG and IgE antibody responses to cow dander and urine in farmers with cow-induced asthma, *Clin. Exp. Allergy,* 22, 83-90, 1992.

17. Ylönen, J., Virtanen, T., Horsmanheimo, L., Parkkinen, S., Pelkonen, J., and Mäntyjärvi, R., Affinity purification of the major bovine allergen by a novel monoclonal antibody, *J. Allergy Clin. Immunol.,* 93, 851-858, 1994.

18. Janssens, J., Morren, M., Dooms-Goossens, A., and Degreef, H., Protein contact dermatitis: myth or reality, *Br. J. Dermatol.,* 132, 1-6, 1995.

19. Kanerva, L. and Brisman, J., Contact urticaria, dermatitis, and respiratory allergy caused by enzymes, In: *Contact Urticaria Syndrome,* Amin, S., Lahti, A., and Maibach, H. I., Eds., CRC Press Inc, Boca Raton, FL, 1997.

20. Niinimäki, A., Spice allergy. Investigations on the prevalence of positive skin test reactions and the appearance of clinical symptoms (Thesis), Acta Univ Oul D 357, Oulun Yliopisto, Oulu, 1-81, 1995.

21. Kanerva, L., Estlander, T., and Jolanki, R., Occupational allergic contact dermatitis from spices, *Contact Dermatitis,* 35, 157–162, 1996.

22. Kanerva, L., Occupational IgE-mediated protein contact dermatitis from pork in a slaughterman, *Contact Dermatitis,* 34, 301–302, 1996.

23. Hjorth, N. and Roed-Petersen, J., Occupational protein contact dermatitis in food handlers, *Contact Dermatitis,* 2, 28-42, 1976.

24. Terho, E.O., Husman, K., Vohlonen, I., Rautalahti, M., and Tukiainen, H., Allergy to storage mites or cow dander as a cause of rhinitis among Finnish farmers, *Allergy,* 40, 23-26, 1985.

25. Cuthbert, O. D., Storage mite allergy, *Clin. Rev. Allergy,* 8, 69-86, 1990.

26. Tarvainen, K., Jolanki, R., Estlander, T., Tupasela, O., Pfäffli, P., and Kanerva, L., Immunologic contact urticaria due to airborne methylhexahydrophthalic and methyltetrahydrophthalic anhydrides, *Contact Dermatitis,* 32, 204-209, 1995.

27. Kanerva, L., Jolanki, R., Tupasela, O., Halmepuro, L., Keskinen, H., Estlander, T., and Sysilampi, M-L., Immediate and delayed allergy from epoxy resins based on diglycidyl ether of bisphenol A. *Scand. J. Work Environ. Health,* 17, 208-215, 1991.

28. Kanerva, L., Keskinen, H., Autio, P., Estlander, T., Tuppurainen, M., and Jolanki, R., Occupational respiratory and skin sensitization caused by polyfunctional aziridine hardener, *Clin. Exp. Allergy,* 25, 432-439, 1995.

29. Kanerva, L., Estlander, T., Jolanki, R., and Tarvainen, K., Occupational allergic contact dermatitis and contact urticaria caused by polyfunctional aziridine hardener, *Contact Dermatitis,* 33, 304-309, 1995.

30. Estlander, T., Kanerva, L., Tupasela, O., Keskinen, H., and Jolanki, R., Immediate and delayed allergy to nickel with contact urticaria, rhinitis, asthma, and contact dermatitis, *Clin. Exp. Allergy,* 23, 306-310, 1993.

31. Estlander, T., Occupational allergic dermatoses and respiratory diseases from reactive dyes, *Contact Dermatitis,* 18, 290-297, 1988.

32. Tupasela, O. and Kanerva L., Skin tests and specific IgE determinations in the diagnostics of contact urticaria caused by low-molecular-weight chemicals. In: *Contact Urticaria Syndrome,* Amin, S., Lahti, A., and Maibach H. I., Eds., CRC Press Inc, Boca Raton, FL, 1997.

33. Kanera, L., Toikkanen, J., Jolanki, R., and Estlander, T., Statistical data on occupational contact urticaria, *Contact Dermatitis,* 35, 229–233, 1996.

34. Kligman, A., The spectrum of contact urticaria: wheals, erythema, and pruritus, *Derm. Clin.,* 8, 57-60, 1990.

7

Substance P in Contact Urticaria

Joanna Wallengren

Contact urticaria is associated with flare and wheal and accompanied by burning, stinging, or itching. These symptoms are part of the triple response[1] and can be mimicked by intradermal injection of histamine. Not surprisingly, therefore, histamine is thought to be involved in contact urticaria. The histamine-evoked reactions, in particular the flare and itch, are dependent on an intact nervous network in the skin.[2] Nonimmunologic contact urticaria (NICU) arises without previous sensitization. It is due to the release of vasoactive substances without the involvement of immunological processes.[3] It is exemplified by the reaction to nettles. Immunologic contact urticaria (ICU) requires previous exposition to an allergen which elicits either IgE-mediated degranulation of mast cells and basophils or IgG/IgM-mediated activation of the complement cascade.[3] There is a morphological relationship between nerves and the immune system, and it is conceivable that the nervous system can modulate immune responses.[4]

The innervation of human skin is necessary for the response to external stimuli. The sensory outflow to the skin runs in nerves that are gradually segregated to form cutaneous nerve fibers. These nerves contain a high proportion of unmyelinated fibers, C-fibers.[5]

Dermal nerve fibers have been analyzed by means of immunocytochemical methods. A large proportion of the free nerve endings located in the papillary dermis and epidermis contain neuropeptides, such as substance P (SP), neurokinin A (NKA), and calcitonin gene-related peptide (CGRP).[6] Substance P, NKA, and CGRP seem to coexist in the same (nociceptive) nerve fibers (C-fibers),[6] although fibers that only contain CGRP can be detected as well. These neuropeptides are released in response to physical and chemical irritants.[7] The C-fiber peptides have effects on microvascular tone and permeability, on the contractile activity of smooth muscle (intestines and airways), and on the secretory activity of epithelial cells and glands.[8] The intradermal injection of SP induces flare, wheal, and itch.[4,9] These responses resemble the urticarial reaction in appearence and time course (the flare is maximal after 5 minutes, and the wheal after 15 minutes). Substance P is 100 to 400 times more potent than histamine.[2,9] The flare appears to be highly dependent upon histamine released from dermal mast cells since depletion of histamine by compound 48/80 reduces the response to SP.[2,10,11] The flare is also dependent upon axon reflexes, as local anesthesia greatly depresses the response. Also, drugs that inhibit prostaglandin synthesis will suppress the SP- induced flare.[12] The SP- evoked wheal is unaffected by these pretreatments, and seems to reflect a direct effect of the peptide on vascular permeability. There is evidence that ICU and NICU are influenced by sensory nerves. Prick test reactions to house dust (ICU)[13] and NICU[14] can be suppressed by local anesthesia.

The critical involvement of neuropeptides in the mediation of hypersensitivity reactions has been suggested by findings in recent experiments, one involving SP inhibitors and another involving capsaicin. Capsaicin, the pungent agent of pepper, is a useful tool in exploring the function of nociceptive nerves. An acute challenge with capsaicin excites the C-fibers.[15] Upon repeated topical applications, it depletes the skin of C-fiber neuropeptides.[15] Capsaicin has been used to treat localized pain and itch in postherpetic neuralgia[16] and notalgia paresthetica.[17-19] Capsaicin pretreatment has been shown to suppress symptoms of cold and heat urticaria,[20] and to abolish the flare but not the wheal response to prick tests in human subjects.[21] Interestingly, the symptoms of NICU induced by benzoic acid, sorbic acid, and cinnamic acid were intensified by capsaicin pretreatment.[22] Capsaicin pretreatment thus seems to influence immunologic and nonimmunologic immediate hypersensitivity reactions differently. Alternatively, the explanation of the apparent paradox lies in the different time course of the two reactions: ICU being elicited within 15 minutes and NICU within 45 minutes. Perhaps the early phase of the immediate hypersensitivity reaction is inhibited, whereas the later phase is enhanced.

We have explored the involvement of SP in ICU and NICU using spantide, an antagonist to SP.[23] Spantide, injected at a dose of 800 pmol/0.05 ml in itself induced a modest triple response.[24] The itch subsided after a few minutes and the flare and wheal after 75–90 minutes. A dermal response to spantide could still be produced following three consecutive injections of the drug at 1-hour intervals, indicating that spantide did not totally deplete the mast cell-derived histamine.[25] A single 800 pmol dose of spantide was used prior to induction of NICU (benzoic acid) and ICU (scratch test in patients sensitized to tomato, beef, shrimp, fish, egg, flour, or latex). Of eleven patients (all atopic), seven manifested reduced ICU reactions after pretreatment with spantide, as compared to controls, whereas NICU reactions were unchanged.[24] The results suggest that SP is involved in allergic but not in nonallergic immediate hypersensitivity reactions.

Patients with atopic disease are characterized by increased wheal and flare responses to intracutaneous SP.[13] Conceivably, mast cells in such individuals release their mediators more readily, or are more numerous than in normal individuals. According to a review of reported cases of ICU, 22 of 67 patients developed a positive delayed test response after the initial wheal and flare reaction to an antigen.[26] These reports indicate that both immediate and delayed hypersensitivity to a substance may occur simultaneously in the same individual. For such cases, the term "contact dermatitis of the immediate and delayed type" has been suggested.[26] Substance P is in fact a good candidate as a stimulatory mediator in this reaction.

Substance P has been shown to enhance the proliferation of T-lymphocytes[27-31] and to promote elicitation of allergic contact dermatitis in mice.[32] The delayed hypersensitivity responses to nickel and tuberculin in humans were suppressed by spantide, whereas the UVB reaction and the irritant delayed reaction to benzalconium chloride were unaffected.[24,33] This supports the view that SP is involved in immunologic rather than in nonimmunologic delayed hypersensitivity reactions.

Suprisingly, capsaicin has been shown to augment the elicitation phase of allergic contact dermatitis in man,[22] mouse,[34] and guinea pig,[35] and in the latter case even the sensitization phase of contact allergy. CGRP has been shown to inhibit the antigen presenting capacity of the Langerhans cell.[36] The consequence is a suppression of the delayed allergic reaction, which is opposite to the effect of SP. The net result of the capsaicin-evoked depletion of CGRP and SP (CGRP being most abundant in the skin) may result in potentiation of the inflammatory reaction.

Substance P is released from C-fibers in response to physical or chemical irritants. Substance P is capable of releasing histamine from local mast cells, and hence may contribute to contact urticaria (stage 1).[26] Mobilized histamine will excite C-fibers, not only locally but also antidromically to release more SP (together with NKA and CGRP). This sequence of events will then repeat itself, possibly until all ramifications of the nerve are engaged in axon reflexes. When adjacent nerves become engaged, the contact urticaria becomes generalized (stage 2).[26] Subsequent to skin contact with an eliciting substance, symptoms from the airways, gastrointestinal tract, or vascular system may develop, representing more advanced stages (stages 3 and 4)[26] in the contact urticaria syndrome. These symptoms occur only in ICU and may originate from an Ig-E mediated hypersensitivity. Such reactions may be elicited by specific IgE-mediated degranulation of mast cells. Sudden activation of IgE may cause "arousal" of mast cell-dependent defense mechanisms.

Another hypothetical route for "cross talk" between different organs, elicited by percutaneous absorbtion of an allergen, would be a nervous pathway initiated by C-fiber dependent reflexes originating in the skin. Such a nerve-mediated reflex may result in efferent nerve stimulation in a number of organs. Substance P may induce bronchoconstriction,[13,37] for instance, and vasodilatation of blood vessels (flushing and tachycardia).[38] Anti-inflammatory drugs may act at many steps along the line to modulate mediator release or to inhibit the effects of mediators. Even if the effect of spantide may in part reflect depletion of mast-cell histamine, SP antagonists may prove useful in the treatment of allergic reactions. Pretreatment with topical capsaicin, which depletes mediators from C-fibers, may yield at least partial symptom relief in ICU but none in NICU.

REFERENCES

1. Lewis T., The nocifensor system of nerves and its reactions, *Br. Med. J.*, 3973, 1937.
2. Wallengren J. and Håkanson R., Effects of substance P, neurokinin A and calcitonin gene-related peptide in human skin and their involvement in sensory nerve-mediated responses, *Eur. J. Pharmacol.*, 143, 267, 1987.

3. Lahti A., Krogh G., and Maibach H. I., Contact urticaria syndrome, in *Dermatologic Immunology and Allergy*, Stone J., Ed., C. V. Mosby Company, St. Louis, 1985, Chap 28.

4. Blalock J., The immune system as a sensory organ, *J. Immunol.*, 132, 3,1067, 1984.

5. Winkelmann R. K., Cutaneous Sensory Nerves, *Sem. Derm.*, 7, 4, 236, 1988.

6. Wallengren J., Ekman R., and Sundler F., Occurrence and distribution of neuropeptides in the human skin, *Acta Derm. Venereol. (Stockh.)*, 67,185, 1987.

7. Wallengren J., Pathophysiology of itch, *Eur. J. Derm.*, 3, 643, 1993.

8. Goetzl E. J., Chernov T., Renold F., and Payan D. G., Neuropeptide regulation of the expression of immediate hypersensitivity, *J. Immunol.*, 135, 2, 802s, 1985.

9. Hägermark Ö., Hökfelt T., and Pernow B., Flare and itch induced by substance P in human skin, *J. Invest. Dermatol.*, 71, 233, 1978.

10. Fjellner B. and Hägermark Ö., Studies on pruritogenic and histamine-releasing effects of some putative neurotransmitters, *Acta Derm. Venereol. (Stockh.)*, 61, 245, 1981.

11. Barnes P. J., Brown M. J., Dollery C. T., Fuller R. W., Heavy D. J., and Ind P. W., Histamine is released from skin by substance P but does not act as the final vasodilator in the axon reflex, *Br. J. Pharmacol.*, 88, 741, 1986.

12. Ståhle M. and Hägermark Ö., Separate effects of topical indomethacin on the itch response and on the flare reaction induced by histamine in human skin. *Acta Derm. Venereol. (Stockh.)*, 85, 340, 1985.

13. Nakai S., Iikura Y., Akimoto K., and Shiraki K., Substance P-induced cutaneous and bronchial reactions in children with bronchial asthma, *Ann. Allergy*, 66, 155, 1991.

14. Lahti A., Non-immunol contact urticaria, *Acta Derm. Venereol. (Stockh.)*, 60, suppl 91, 1980.

15. Fitzgerald M., Capsaicin and sensory neurons-a review. *Pain*, 15, 109, 1983.

16. Bernstein J. E., Korman N. J., Bickers D. R., Dahl M. V., and Milikan L. E., Topical capsaicin treatment of chronic post-herpetic neuralgia. *J. Am. Acad. Derm.*, 15, 504, 1986.

17. Wallengren J.,Treatment of notalgia paresthetica with topical capsaicin, *J. Am. Acad. Derm.*, 24, 286, 1991.

18. Leibsohn E., Treatment of notalgia paresthetica with capsaicin. *Cutis,* 49, 335, 1992.

19. Wallengren J. and Klinker M., Successful treatment of notalgia paresthetica with topical capsaicin. Vehicle controlled, double-blind, cross-over study. *J. Am. Acad. Dermatol.*, 32, 287, 1995.

20. Toth-Kasa J., Jancso G., Obal F., Husz S., and Simon N., Involvement of sensory nerve endings in cold and heat urticaria, *J. Invest. Dermatol.*, 80, 34, 1983.

21. Lundblad L., Lundberg J. M., Änggård A., and Zetterström O., Capsaicin sensitive nerves and the cutaneous allergy reaction in man, *Allergy*, 42, 20, 1987.

22. Wallengren J. and Möller H.,The effect of capsaicin on some experimental inflammations in human skin, *Acta Derm. Venereol. (Stockh.)*, 66, 375, 1986.

23. Folkers K., Håkanson R., Hörig J., Jie-Cheng X., and Leander S., Biological evaluation of substance P antagonist, *Br. J. Pharmacol.*, 83, 449, 1984.

24. Wallengren J., Substance P antagonist inhibits immediate and delayed type cutaneous hypersensitivity reactions, *Br. J. Dermatol.*, 124, 324, 1991.

25. Wallengren J., Substance P antagonist and immune hypersensitivity reactions, Reply, *Br. J. Derm.*, 125, 605, 1992.

26. Krogh G. and Maibach H. I., The contact urticaria syndrome, in *Dermatotoxocology,* Marzulli F. N. and Maibach H. I., Eds., Hemisphere Publishing Corporation, Washington, 1987, Chap. 15.

27. Payan D. D., Brewster D. R., Missirian-Bastian A., and Goetzl E. J., Substance P recognition by a subset of human T lymphocytes. *J. Clin. Invest.*, 74, 1532, 1984.
28. Payan D. D., Brewster D. R., and Goetzl E. J., Specific stimulation of human T lymphocytes by substance P. *J. Immunol.*, 131,1613, 1983.
29. Bienenstock J., Denburg J., Scicchitano R. et al., Role of neuropeptides, nerves and mast cells in intestinal immunity and physiology. *Monogr. Allergy*, 24, 134, 1988.
30. Nordlind K. and Mutt V., Modulating effect of beta-endorphin, somatostatin, substance P and vasoactive intestinal peptide on the proliferative response of peripheral blood T lymphocytes of nickel-allergic patients to nickel sulfate, *Int. Arch. Allergy Appl. Immun.*, 81, 368, 1986.
31. Ek L. and Theodorsson E., Tachykinins and Calcitonin Gene-Related peptide in Oxazolone-Induced Allergic Contact dermatitis in Mice, *J. Invest. Dermatol.*, 94, 761, 1990.
32. Gutwald J., Goebler M., and Sorg C., Neuropeptides enhance irritant and allergic dermatitis, *J. Invest. Dermatol.*, 96, 695, 1991.
33. Wallengren J. and Möller H., Some neuropeptides as modulators of experimental contact allergy. *Contact Dermatitis*, 19, 35, 1988.
34. Girolomoni G. and Tigelaar R. E., Peptidergic neurons and vasoactive intestinal peptide modulate experimental delayed-type hypersensitivity reactions. *Ann. N.Y. Acad. Sci.*, 650, 9, 1992.
35. Wallengren J., Ekman R., and Möller H., Capsaicin enhances allergic contact dermatitis in guinea pig. *Contact Dermatitis*, 24, 30 1991.
36. Hosoi J., Murphy G. F., Egan C. L., Lerner E. A., Grabbe S., Asahina A., and Granstein R. D., Regulation of Langerhans cell function by nerves containing calcitonin gene related peptide, *Lett. Nature, 363,159, 1993.*
37. Barnes P. J., Asthma as an axon reflex, *Lancet*, 242, 1986.
38. Eklund B., Jogestrand T., and Pernow B., Effect of substance P on resistance and capacitance vessels in the human forearm, *Substance P*, Euler U. S. and Pernow B., Eds., Raven Press, New York, 275, 1977.

8

Prostaglandin D$_2$ Mediates Contact Urticaria Caused by Sorbic Acid, Benzoic Acid, and Esters of Nicotinic Acid

L. Jackson Roberts II and Jason D. Morrow

CONTENTS

8.1 INTRODUCTION

Benzoic acid and sorbic acid are commonly used as preservatives in cosmetics, foods, and drug formulations.[1-3] Although these agents are generally considered non-toxic and safe, they induce cutaneous erythema, urticaria, and stinging when applied topically at concentrations used in creams and ointments, etc., in a large percentage of people. For example, Fryklof reported the development of erythema in nearly 50% of patients who had creams or ointments containing sorbic acid applied to their cheeks.[4] Clemmensen and Hjorth reported contact urticaria in 18 of 20 playful kindergarten children who applied salad dressing containing sorbic acid and benzoic acid to their face during an unsupervised lunch period.[5] In another study, application of 1% sorbic acid to the face, back, and forearms of normal volunteers induced erythema, edema, and flare in 100% of the subjects and the intensity of the reaction was dose-dependent over the range of concentrations tested (0.05–1%).[6] Contact cheilitis has also been reported in association with the use of a toothpaste containing benzoic acid.[7] Transient episodes of urticaria have also occurred in workers exposed to airborne sodium benzoate at a pharmaceutical manufacturing plant.[8]

Although contact reactions from sorbic acid and benzoic acid are well known to occur, the underlying mechanism of these reactions to these agents has been very poorly understood.[9,10] A role for mast cell derived histamine was implicated in one study because of a partial suppression of the response with the use of topical antihistamine.[5] However, in other studies, pretreatment of individuals with oral antihistamines was found to have no effect on inhibiting these cutaneous reactions.[6,11] Further, no evidence of significant mast cell degranulation was seen in skin in which contact urticaria was induced by sorbic acid and was examined histologically.[6] A role for prostaglandins in mediating the contact urticaria induced by these agents has been suggested by the findings that administration of cyclooxygenase inhibitors greatly suppresses these reactions.[6,12] However, Lahti, et al. found no differences in the concentrations of prostaglandin (PG) $F_{2\alpha}$, PGI_2 (prostacyclin), and thromboxane B_2 in suction blisters raised on forearm skin of volunteers treated with topical benzoic acid compared to untreated skin.[13] Thus, if a prostaglandin(s) plays an important role as a mediator of these reactions, its identity remained unclear.

Our interest in pursuing the potential role of prostaglandins as mediators of sorbic acid and benzoic acid induced contact urticaria evolved from our previous studies in which we explored the role of prostaglandins in mediating the cutaneous vasodilation which occurs following ingestion of pharmacologic doses of niacin (nicotinic acid) to lower levels of serum cholesterol. We found that ingestion of niacin induced a profound release of the vasodilatory prostaglandin, PGD_2. Further, the prostaglandin release induced by niacin was selective in that niacin did not induce a release of the other vasodilatory prostaglandins, PGI_2 (prostacyclin) and PGE_2. In addition, we found that the niacin-induced release of PGD_2 was not accompanied by a release of histamine, suggesting that niacin did not cause degranulation of mast cells.[14] Further studies demonstrated that the skin was a major site of PGD_2 release following ingestion of niacin and that topical application of the methyl ester of niacin (methyl-nicotinate) causes intense cutaneous erythema which is accompanied by a dramatic release of PGD_2 from a cell that resides in the skin.[15] Spurred by the striking similarities of the cutaneous reactions which occur following topical application of methylnicotinate with that of sorbic acid and benzoic acid, we explored the possibility that PGD$_2$ may also mediate the contact urticarial reactions induced by the latter two commonly used preservatives.

8.2 THE ROLE OF PROSTAGLANDIN D$_2$ IN SORBIC ACID INDUCED CONTACT URTICARIAL REACTIONS

Four normal volunteers were studied to explore the role of PGD$_2$ in sorbic acid induced contact urticarial reactions.[16] In all subjects, topical application of a 15 cm-wide patch of filter paper saturated with 1% sorbic acid (prepared in isopropyl alcohol:water, 50:50) on a forearm for 20 min. induced intense cutaneous erythema limited to the site of application. The erythema was also accompanied by a feeling of warmth, stinging, and urticaria. The intensity of the erythema was maximal between 20–30 min and began to subside after 45–60 min, similar to previous observations.[6] To assess the role of prostaglandins and histamine in this reaction, blood was sampled serially from the antecubital vein draining the treated site and analyzed for PGD$_2$, the initial metabolite of PGD$_2$ (9α,11β-PGF$_2$),[17] PGE$_2$, the stable hydrolysis product of PGI$_2$ (6-keto-PGF$_{1\alpha}$), and histamine using highly accurate mass spectrometric assays.[18,19]

As shown in Figure 8.1, levels of both PGD$_2$ and its metabolite, 9α,11β-PGF$_2$, increased dramatically, 250–620-fold and 15–58-fold above baseline, respectively, in blood draining the site of skin treated with 1% sorbic acid. The time course of these increases correlated temporally with the peak intensity and disappearance of cutaneous vasodilation observed. Levels of PGE$_2$ and 6-keto-PGF$_{1\alpha}$ were undetectable (<5 pg/ml) in all blood samples, suggesting that the release of vasodilatory prostaglandins induced by sorbic acid was selective for PGD$_2$. The major cyclooxygenase product produced by human mast cells is PGD$_2$.[20] However, levels of histamine measured at the time of peak erythema were not different than pretreatment levels (277–455 pg/ml pretreatment compared to 233–544 pg/ml at peak erythema). This not only suggests that histamine does not participate in sorbic acid contact urticarial reactions, but also that the mast cell is not the primary cellular source of sorbic acid induced release of PGD$_2$.

Because of the fact that the cutaneous erythema that occurs following topical application of sorbic acid to the skin is limited to the site of application, it is unlikely that the levels of PGD$_2$ measured in blood draining the site of application arose from systemic absorption of sorbic acid and subsequent release of PGD$_2$ from distal sites. Nonetheless, we assessed this possibility by measuring levels of PGD$_2$ and 9α,11β-PGF$_2$ in blood simultaneously drawn from the antecubital vein of the contralateral untreated arm in three individuals (Table 8.1). A very small amount of PGD$_2$ was detected in one individual only, and in all subjects levels of 9α,11β-PGF$_2$ remained below the limits of detection. The small amount of PGD$_2$ detected in the one individual may have arisen either from the release of PGD$_2$ into the circulation at the site of sorbic acid application or artifactual generation of PGD$_2$ from formed elements of blood during blood sampling and plasma isolation.

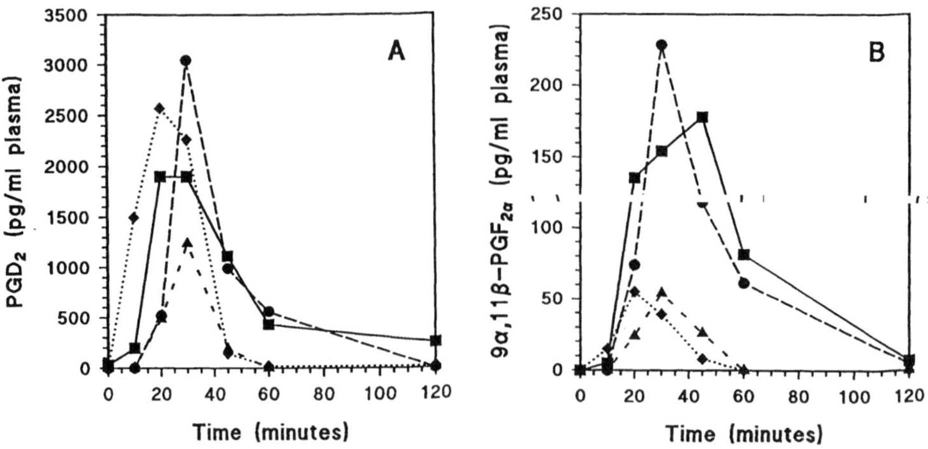

FIGURE 8.1 Time course of the increase in levels of PGD_2 (A) and its metabolite, $9\alpha,11\beta\text{-}PGF_2$, (B) measured in plasma obtained from the antecubital vein following topical application of 1% sorbic acid to the forearm for 20 minutes. Results obtained in each volunteer are represented by a different symbol. Pretreatment levels were below the assay limits of detection (<4 pg/ml). (From Morrow, J. D., *Arch. Dermatol.*, 130, 1408, 1994. With permission.)

TABLE 8.1 Levels of PGD_2 and $9\alpha,11\beta\text{-}PGF_2$ in Plasma Obtained Simultaneously from the Antecubital Vein of an Arm Treated with Topical Sorbic Acid and from the Contralateral Area of an Untreated Arm[a]

Subject No.	Treated Skin		Untreated Skin	
	PGD_2	$9\alpha,11\beta\text{-}PGF_2$	PGD_2	$9a11\beta\text{-}PGF_2$
1	546	37	29	<4
2	2017	162	<4	<4
3	398	62	<4	<4

[a] Prostaglandin levels are expressed as pg/ml. Detection limits of the assays are 4 pg/ml for PGD_2 and $9\alpha,11\beta\text{-}PGF_2$.

From Morrow, J. D., *Arch. Dermatol.*, 130, 1408, 1994. With permission.

The concentration-dependent effects of sorbic acid induced erythema and release of PGD_2 were also examined in three volunteers (Figure 8.2). The threshold concentration of sorbic acid which induced slight erythema in the subjects was 0.1%. This was also the lowest concentration in which a release of PGD_2 was detected. Concentrations greater than 0.1% induced more intense erythema and a higher dose-dependent release of PGD_2. The increase in release of PGD_2 plateaued between 1–3% sorbic acid. Importantly, cutaneous erythema accompanied by a significant release of PGD_2 occurred following application of sorbic acid at the concentration that is most commonly used in topically applied vehicles and cosmetics (0.2%).[21]

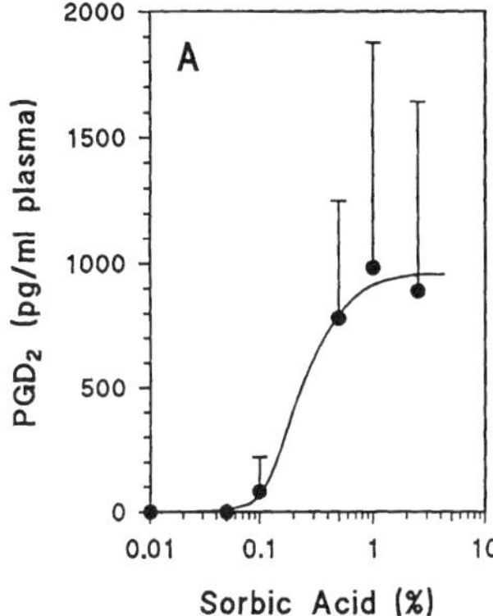
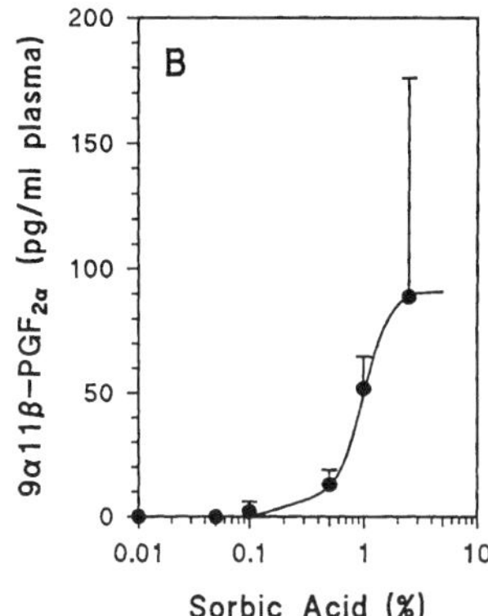

FIGURE 8.2 Concentration-dependent effects of sorbic acid applied to a forearm of three volunteers on plasma levels of PGD_2 (A) and $9\alpha,11\beta\text{-}PGF_2$ (B) measured in antecubital venous blood draining the treated site. Each value given is the mean ± SD. (From Morrow, J. D., *Arch. Dermatol.*, 130, 1408, 1994. With permission.)

TABLE 8.2 Levels of PGD_2 and $9\alpha,11\beta\text{-}PGF_2$ in Plasma Obtained from the Antecubital Vein of an Arm Treated with Sorbic Acid in Three Subjects with and without Pretreatment with Aspirin[a]

Subject No.		PGD_2	$9\alpha,11\beta\text{-}PGF_2$
1	Without aspirin	1908	155
	With aspirin	<4	<4
2	Without aspirin	3052	229
	With aspirin	<4	<4
3	Without aspirin	2270	39
	With aspirin	<4	<4

[a] Prostaglandin levels are expressed as pg/ml. Detection limits of the assays are 4 pg/ml for PGD_2 and $9\alpha,11\beta\text{-}PGF_2$. Aspirin (325 mg) was administered twice daily for 3 days and sorbic acid was applied 1 hour following the last dose of aspirin.

From Morrow, J. D., *Arch. Dermatol.*, 130, 1408, 1994. With permission.

It had been previously reported that pretreatment of individuals with aspirin markedly attenuates the cutaneous erythema induced by sorbic acid.[6] Thus, we assessed the effect of aspirin to inhibit the release of PGD_2 and the cutaneous erythema induced by sorbic acid in three normal volunteers. The subjects were given 325 mg of aspirin orally twice daily for 3 days and sorbic acid (1%) was applied 1 h following the last dose of aspirin. Aspirin pretreatment markedly attenuated the cutaneous vasodilation and profoundly inhibited sorbic acid induced release of PGD_2 and $9\alpha,11\beta\text{-}PGF_2$ in all three subjects (Table 8.2).

TABLE 8.3 Levels (mean ± SD) of Prostaglandins and Histamine
in Plasma Obtained From the Antecubital Vein
Draining Skin Before and After Treatment With 10%
Benzoic Acid Solution for 60 Minutes
(n = 4 volunteers)[a]

Mediator	Baseline	After Treatment
PGD_2 (pg/ml)	<4	11,508 ± 13,380
$9\alpha11\beta$-PGF_2 (pg/ml)	<4	523 ± 576
PGE_2	<5	<5
6-keto-$PGF_{1\alpha}$ (pg/ml)	<5	<5
Histamine (ng/ml)	0.67 ± 0.42	0.74 ± 0.51

[a] Limits of detections of the assays are 4 pg/ml for PGD_2 and $9\alpha,11\beta$-PGF_2 and 5 pg/ml for PGE_2 and 6-keto-$PGF_{1\alpha}$.

From Downard, C. D., *Clin. Pharmacol. Ther.*, 57, 441, 1995. With permission.

8.3 THE ROLE OF PROSTAGLANDIN D_2 IN BENZOIC ACID INDUCED CONTACT URTICARIAL REACTIONS

The role of PGD_2 in benzoic acid induced contact urticarial reactions was investigated using an almost identical protocol used above for the sorbic acid studies.[22] Varying concentrations of benzoic acid (0.01–15%) in petrolatum were applied to a forearm of four volunteers and covered with plastic wrap for 60 min. The cutaneous vasodilation induced by benzoic acid was limited to the site of application and was accompanied by sensations of stinging and pruritis. The erythema became maximal after 60 min. and gradually resolved over a 3–4 h period.

Application of a 10% concentration of benzoic acid for 60 min. in four volunteers was accompanied by a dramatic increase in plasma concentrations of PGD_2 and its metabolite, $9\alpha,11\beta$-PGF_2, in blood obtained from the antecubital vein draining the site of application. As was found in the sorbic acid studies, the release of PGD_2 was not associated with a release of PGE_2, 6-keto-$PGF_{1\alpha}$, or histamine (Table 8.3). The time course of the increase in plasma concentrations of $9\alpha,11\beta$-PGF_2 following application of a 10% concentration of benzoic acid is shown in Figure 8.3. The time course of the release of PGD_2 closely correlated temporally with the appearance and disappearance of the cutaneous erythema. Plasma concentrations of $9\alpha,11\beta$-PGF_2 drawn simultaneously from the contralateral untreated arm did not increase above baseline (≤4 pg/ml).

The concentration dependent effect of varying concentrations of benzoic acid to induce a release of PGD_2 is shown in Figure 8.4. No cutaneous erythema or release of PGD_2 occurred at concentrations of benzoic acid below 1%. A 1% concentration caused a detectable increase in plasma concentrations of $9\alpha,11\beta$-PGF_2 and slight patchy erythema. Higher concentrations produced more intense erythema and a release of much larger quantities of PGD_2. Pretreatment with aspirin using the same protocol as was used in the sorbic acid studies (325 mg aspirin twice daily for three days) markedly attenuated the erythema that occurred following application of 10% benzoic acid and prevented the release of PGD_2 (Table 8.4).

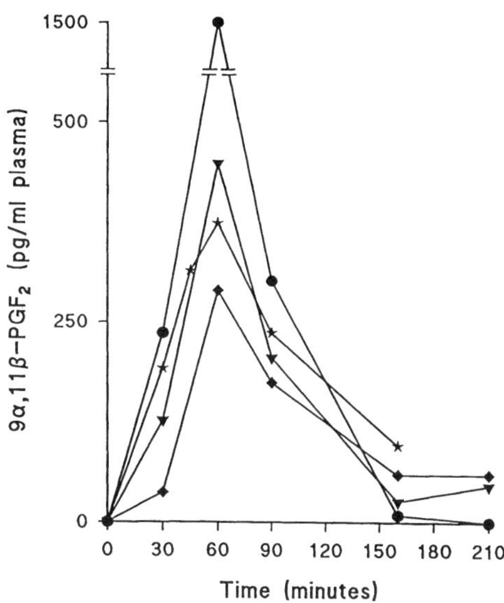

FIGURE 8.3 Time course of the increase in levels of the PGD$_2$ metabolite, 9α,β-PGF$_2$, measured in plasma obtained from the antecubital vein following topical application of 10% benzoic acid for 60 minutes. Results obtained in each volunteer are represented by a different symbol. Pretreatment levels were below the assay limits of detection (<4 pg/ml). (From Downard, C. D., *Clin. Pharmacol. Ther.*, 57, 441, 1995. With permission.)

8.4   THE ROLE OF PROSTAGLANDIN D$_2$ IN NICOTINIC ACID ESTER INDUCED CONTACT URTICARIAL REACTIONS

Trifuril (Ciba-Geigy, Basel, Switzerland) is a tetrahydrofurfuryl ester of nicotinic acid which is not available in the U.S. but is used in Europe as a rubefacient in inflammatory joint diseases and mild disorders of the circulation of the hands and feet.[23-25] Application of Trifuril causes intense cutaneous erythema in the vast majority of individuals. The erythema persists for 1–3 h. but may be evident for as long as 24 h. in some individuals. Although the role of PGD$_2$ in mediating the cutaneous vasodilation induced by Trifuril has not been directly evaluated, we previously reported that the methyl ester of nicotinic acid when applied to the skin evokes intense erythema which is associated with a selective release of PGD$_2$ and is not accompanied by a release of histamine,[15] analogous to what we found with the topical application of sorbic acid and benzoic acid. An ester of nicotinic acid is used for topical application to enhance its absorption through the skin. In this context, the type of ester used is unlikely to alter the pharmacological properties of nicotinic acid and thus, it is reasonable to assume that the contact erythema that occurs following application of the tetrahydrofurfuryl ester of nicotinic acid (Trifuril) to the skin, like methylnicotinate, is mediated primarily by a release of PGD$_2$. This notion is greatly supported by the fact that treatment with aspirin also attenuates the erythema induced by Trifuil.[26]

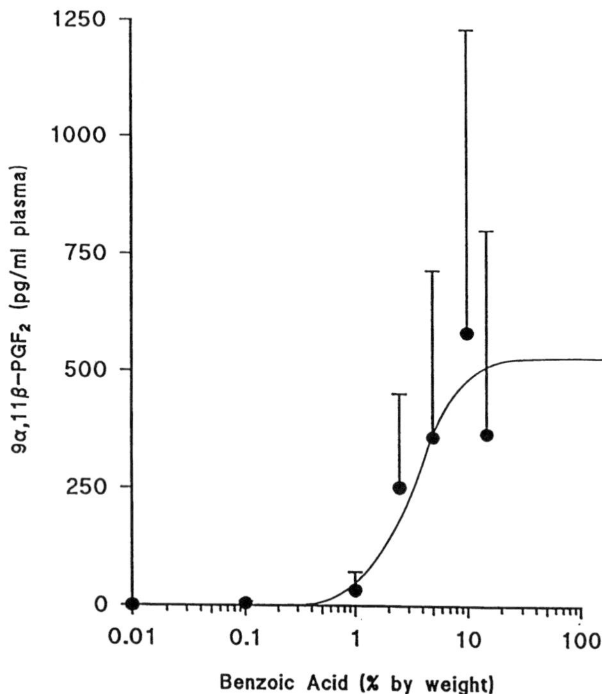

FIGURE 8.4 Concentration-dependent effects of benzoic acid applied to a forearm of three volunteers on plasma levels of the PGD_2 metabolite, $9\alpha,11\beta$-PGF_2, measured in antecubital venous blood draining the treated site. Each value given is the mean ± SD. (From Downard, C. D., *Clin. Pharmacol. Ther.*, 57, 441, 1995. With permission.)

TABLE 8.4 Levels of $9\alpha,11\beta$-PGF_2 in Plasma of Four Volunteers Obtained From the Antecubital Veins Draining the Skin After Treatment With 10% Benzoic Acid Solution for 60 Minutes With or Without Pretreatment With Aspirin[a]

Volunteer	Without aspirin	With aspirin
1	1509	<4
2	373	<4
3	448	<4
4	289	<4

[a] Levels are expressed as pg/ml. The limits of detection of the assay is 4 pg/ml. Aspirin (325 mg) was administered twice daily for 3 days and benzoic acid was applied 1 hour following the last dose of aspirin.

From Downard, C. D., *Clin. Pharmacol. Ther.*, 57, 441, 1995. With permission.

8.5 DISCUSSION

These data provide compelling evidence that the primary mediator of the contact urticarial reactions induced by sorbic acid, benzoic acid, and Trifuril is PGD_2. This is consistent with the findings that intradermal injection of PGD_2 into human skin causes long-lasting erythema and wheal formation.[27,28] Further, neutrophil infiltration, which characterizes some forms of contact dermatitis,[29] is a potential source of leukotriene B_4 production and PGD_2 markedly potentiates leukocyte infiltration and induration caused by leukotriene B_4 in human skin.[27] Interestingly, in rabbit skin, PGD_2 has been shown to be an intermediate in agonist-stimulated nitric oxide release and the cutaneous vasodilation induced by PGD_2 can be abroggated by N^G-nitro-L-arginine methyl ester (L-NAME), a nitric oxide synthase inhibitor.[30] This suggests that the vasodilation induced by PGD_2 is mediated by nitric oxide. Whether the mechanism by which PGD_2 causes vasodilation in human skin is similar to that in rabbit skin, however, remains unknown.

There are two questions of considerable interest in regards to the release of PGD_2 by these agents: (1) what is the identity of the cell(s) that resides in the skin that is activated by these agents to release PGD_2, and (2) what is the mechanism by which these agents induce the release PGD_2? Unfortunately, neither of these questions can be definitely answered at the present time. The skin has a large capacity to produce prostaglandins and PGD_2 is the predominant prostanoid formed by both the epidermis and dermis.[31] Data obtained by Urade et al. suggests that the cell in the skin that is activated by these agents to release PGD_2 may be the dermal macrophage and/or epidermal Langerhans cell.[32] The basis for this suggestion is that in the skin of rats, it was found that dermal macrophages and Langerhans cells contain the highest level of PGD-synthase and, thus, have the highest capacity to produce PGD_2. This is further supported by the finding that large quantities of PGD_2 are produced by guinea pig Langerhans cells whereas only very small quantities of other prostaglandins are produced.[33] We have also obtained evidence which supports the notion that mononuclear cells/macrophages are activated by these agents by demonstrating that incubation of normal circulating human monocytes and human cultured THP-1 macrophages with nicotinic acid induces a dose-dependent release of prostanoids whereas incubation of other cells with nicotinic acid, e.g., human neutrophils, does not induce the production of prostanoids.[34] Further, as described above, we have demonstrated that cutaneous mast cells are unlikely to be the cellular source of the release of PGD_2 since the release of PGD_2 is not accompanied by a release of histamine. Although certain agents, e.g., neuropeptides, have been found to selectively release histamine from mast cells but not PGD_2, no agents have been identified which selectively induce a release PGD_2 from mast cells without a concomitant release of histamine.[19] Important information that is currently lacking that would greatly support the notion that sorbic acid, benzoic acid, and nicotinic acid activate dermal macrophages and/or Langerhans cells would be the demonstration that incubation of purified populations of these cells but not other cells in the skin with these agents induces a release of PGD_2.

Although there are some insights regarding the potential cell(s) in the skin that is activated by esters of nicotinic acid, sorbic acid, and benzoic acid to release PGD_2, almost nothing is known about the mechanism by which these agents induce arachidonic acid metabolism and PGD_2 release. It is interesting that all three of these agents, which are structurally unrelated, induce the same biochemical response and thus, are likely activating the same cell(s) in the skin. Some evidence has been previously obtained suggesting that there may be a receptor for nicotinic acid on adipocytes which is not present on human platelets and rabbit myocardium.[35,36] The possibility that there may be receptors for nicotinic acid on cells that reside in the skin, however, has not been investigated. Understanding the mechanism by which these agents activate arachidonic acid metabolism could lead to ways to prevent the contact urticarial reactions associated with the use of these agents, other than pretreatment with cyclooxygenase inhibitors. Another interesting question is why do these agents, which are not endogenously produced in humans, activate arachidonic acid metabolism in these cells? Although quite speculative, this raises the possibility that an endogenously produced substance may also activate these cells via the same mechanism. Thus, information regarding the mechanism by which these agents activate the responsive cells may advance our understanding of the normal cellular biology of these cells *in vivo*.

ACKNOWLEDGMENTS

This work was supported in part by grants GM15431, ES00267, DK07383, HL02499, and GM07569 from the National Institutes of Health.

REFERENCES

1. Kolly, M., Pecoud, A., and Frei, P. C., Additives contained in drug formulations most frequently prescribed in Switzerland, *Ann. Allergy*, 62, 21, 1989.
2. Kumar, A., Rawlings, R. D., and Beaman, D. C., The mystery ingredients: sweetners, flavorings, dyes, and preservatives in analgesic/antipyretic, antihistamine/decongestants, cough and cold, antidiarrheal, and liquid theophylline preparations, *Pediatrics*, 91, 927, 1993.
3. Moneret-Vautrin, D. A., Food antigens and additives, *J. Allergy Clin. Immunol.*, 78, 1039, 1986.
4. Juhlin, L., Recurrent urticaria: clinical investigations of 330 patients, *Br. J. Dermatol.*, 104, 369, 1981.
5. Clemmensen, O. and Hjorth, N., Perioral contact urticaria from sorbic acid and benzoic acid in a salad dressing, *Contact Dermatitis*, 8, 1, 1982.
6. Soschin, D. and Leyden, J. J., Sorbic acid-induced erythema and edema, *J. Am. Acad. Dermatol.*, 14, 234, 1986.
7. Aguirre, A., Izu, R., Gardeazabal, J., and Diaz-Perez, J. L., Edematous anergic contact cheilitis from a toothpaste, *Contact Dermatitis*, 28, 42, 1993.
8. Nethercott, J. R., Lawrence, M. J., Roy, A. M., and Gibson, B. L., Airborne contact urticaria due to sodium benzoate in a pharmaceutical plant, *J. Occup. Med.*, 26, 734, 1984.

9. Safford, R. J. and Leyden, J. J., Immediate contact reactions to chemicals in the fragrance mix and a study of the quenching action of eugenol, *Br. J. Dermatol.*, 123, 595, 1990.

10. Kligman, A. M., The spectrum of contact urticaria, *Dermatol. Clinics*, 8, 57, 1990.

11. Lahti, A., Terfenadine does not inhibit nonimmunologic contact urticaria, *Contact Dermatitis*, 16, 220, 1990.

12. Lahti, A., Vaananen, A., Kokkonen, E. L., and Hannuksela, M., Acetylsalicylic acid inhibits nonimmunologic contact urticaria, *Contact Dermatitis*, 16, 133, 1987.

13. Lahti, A., Oikarinen, A., Viinikka, L., Ylikorkala, O., and Hannuksela, M., Prostaglandins in contact urticaria induced by benzoic acid, *Acta Derm. Venereol.*, 63, 425, 1983.

14. Morrow, J. D., Parsons, W. G., III, and Roberts, L. J., II, Release of markedly increased quantities of prostaglandin D_2 *in vivo* in humans following the adminstration of nicotinic acid, *Prostaglandins*, 38, 263, 1989.

15. Morrow, J. D., Awad J. A., Oates, J. A., and Roberts, L. J., II, Identification of skin as a major site of prostaglandin D_2 release following oral administration of niacin in humans, *J. Invest. Dermatol.*, 98, 812, 1992.

16. Morrow, J. D., Minton, T. A., Awad, J. A., and Roberts, L. J., II, Release of markedly increased quantities of prostaglandin D_2 from the skin *in vivo* in humans following the application of sorbic acid, *Arch. Dermatol.*, 130, 1408, 1994.

17. Liston, T. E. and Roberts, L. J., II, Transformation of prostaglandin D_2 to 9a,11β,15(S)-trihydroxy-5(Z),13(E)-dien-1-oic acid: A unique biologically active prostaglandin produced enzymatically *in vivo* in humans, *Proc. Natl. Acad. Sci. U.S.A.*, 82, 6030, 1985.

18. Parsons, W. G., III and Roberts, L. J., II, Transformation of prostaglandin D_2 to isomeric prostaglandin F_2 compounds by human eosinophils, *J. Immunol.*, 141, 2413, 1988.

19. Arzubiaga, C., Morrow, J. D., Roberts, L. J., II, and Biaggioni, I., Neuropeptide Y, a putative cotransmitter in noradrenergic neurons, induces mast cell degranulation but not prostaglandin D_2 release, *J. Allergy Clin. Immunol.*, 87, 88, 1991.

20. Lewis, R. A., Soter, N. A., Diamond, P. T., Austen, K. F., Oates, J. A., and Roberts, L. J., II, Prostaglandin D_2 generation after activation of rat and human mast cells with anti-IgE, *J. Immunol.*, 129, 1627, 1982.

21. Fischer, A. A., Contact dermatitis from food additives and dyes, in *Fischer's Contact Dermatitis*, 4th edition, Rietschel, R. L. and Fowler, J. F., Jr., Eds., Williams and Wilkins, Baltimore, 1995, 275.

22. Downard, C. D., Roberts, L. J., II, and Morrow, J. D., Topical benzoic acid induces the increased synthesis of prostaglandin D_2 in human skin *in vivo*, *Clin. Pharmacol. Ther.*, 57, 441, 1995.

23. McCabe, R. J., Studies with the local use of the furfuryl ester of nicotinic acid, *Arch. Dermatol.*, 74, 283, 1956.

24. Fischer, A. A., Contact Urticaria, in *Fischer's Contact Dermatitis*, 4th ed., Rietschel, R. L. and Fowler, J. F., Jr., Eds., Williams and Wilkins, Baltimore, 1995, 780.

25. Fischer, A. A., Four flusher's: topical agents producing facial flushing simulating systemic variety, *Cutis*, 51, 225, 1993.

26. Juhlin, L. and Michaelsson, G., Abnormal cutaneous reactions to a nicotinic acid ester, *Acta Dermatol.*, 51, 448, 1971.

27. Soter, N. A., Lewis, R. A., Corey, E. J., and Austen, K. F., Local effects of synthetic leukotrienes (LTC_4, LTD_4, LTE_4, and LTB_4) in human skin, *J. Invest. Dermatol.*, 80, 115, 1983.

28. Flower, R. J., Harvey, E. A., and Kingston, W. P., Inflammatory effects of prostaglandin D_2 in rat and human skin, *Br. J. Pharmacol.*, 56, 229, 1976.

29. Willis, C. M., Stephens, C. J., and Wilkinson, J. D., Differential patterns of epidermal leukocyte infiltration in patch test reactions to structurally unrelated chemical irritants, *J. Invest. Dermatol.*, 101, 363, 1993.

30. Warren J. B., Loi, K. R., and Wilson, A. J., PGD_2 is an intermediate in agonist-induced nitric oxide release in rabbit skin microcirculation, *Am. J. Physiol., 226, (Heart Circ. Physiol. 35),* H1846, 1994.

31. Ruzicka, T. and Printz, M. P., Arachidonic acid metabolism in skin: experimental contact dermatitis in guinea pigs, *Int. Archs. Allergy Appl. Immunol.*, 69, 347, 1982.

32. Urade, Y., Ujihara, M., Hariguchi, Y., Ikai, K., and Hayaishi, O., The major source of endogenous prostaglandin D_2 production is likely antigen-presenting cells: localization of glutathione-requiring PGD synthetase in histiocytes, dendritic and Kupffer cells in various rat tissues, *J. Immunol.*, 143, 2982, 1989.

33. Ruzicka, T. and Aubock, J., Arachidonic acid metabolism in guinea pig Langerhans cells: studies of cyclooxygenase and lipoxygenase pathways, *J. Immunol.*, 138, 539, 1987.

34. O'Byrne, S., and Roberts, L. J., II, unpublished data, 1994.

35. Aktories, K. K., Jakobs, K. H., and Schultz, G., Nicotinic acid inhibits adipocyte adenylate cyclase in a hormone-like manner, *FEBS Letters*, 115, 11, 1980.

36. Aktories, K. and Jakobs, K. H., *In vivo* and *in vitro* desensitization of nicotinic acid-induced adipocyte adenylate cyclase inhibition, *Naunyn-Schmiedeberg's Arch. Pharmacol.*, 318, 241, 1982.

9

Agricultural Chemicals

Christopher J. Dannaker

CONTENTS

9.1 INTRODUCTION

Working in the agricultural industry typically requires contact with pesticide chemicals, frequently resulting in prolonged and concentrated exposures.[1] Currently, more than 600 active pesticide ingredients are used, yet adequate toxicologic information is available for only approximately 100.[2] The agricultural industry remains the greatest consumer of pesticide chemicals, and as such, farmers and field workers represent a high risk population for suffering from toxic or allergic reactions. Agriculture has consistently had the highest rates and numbers of occupational skin diseases reported.[3]

The acute toxic events related to pesticide exposure and issues of long term carcinogenicity have been the focus of most toxicologic reports.[4-6] Delayed contact allergy commonly occurs from pesticides. Fungicides are implicated as the causative agent much more than insecticides or herbicides.[7,8] There remains, however, a scarcity of reports relating to pesticide-induced contact urticaria.

An operational definition of "pesticide" includes chemicals utilized for control of fungi, insects, rodents, or weeds. In California, nearly one third of reported illnesses and injuries due to pesticides are associated with skin complaints.[3] Most of these reactions appear to be due to irritation, but allergic contact dermatitis has also been reported.[9] Contact or systemic urticarial reactions to pesticides are not often cited. The paucity of reports may relate to the transitory nature of an urticarial reaction or the lack of association of the adverse reaction with the pesticide exposure. Routine patch testing detects delayed type hypersensitivity but is an incorrect methodology to evaluate contact urticaria.

Chlorothalonil (tetrachloroisothalonitrile), a fungicide, is one of few pesticides documented to cause contact urticaria and anaphylactoid symptoms.[10,11] Dannaker and Maibach reported an affected nursery worker who experienced facial erythema with edema, accompanied by nasal congestion and chest tightness. Testing with 0.01% Chlorothalonil on intact skin resulted in an anaphylactoid reaction within minutes.

Immediate skin testing of controls was negative and the patient's reaction was assumed to be immunologically based. Subsequent negative patch testing of additional controls further supports this deduction.[12] Review of previous reports of contact dermatitis of the delayed type to Chlorothalonil, in retrospect, might suggest concomitant contact urticarial symptomatology.[13–15]

Zinc diethyldithiocarbamate (ZDC) is utilized in the process of rubber manufacture and also as an agricultural fungicide and insecticide. Its presence in rubber has been reported to cause immunologic contact urticaria of the hands.[16] Chemically related thiocarbamates may also be potential causes of contact urticaria but have yet to be reported as such. ZDC and other thiocarbamates are used as insecticides (maneb, carbofuran, carbaryl) and were found in one study to be the most frequent cause of delayed type allergic contact dermatitis among farmers with contact dermatitis.[9] It is noteworthy that this class of fungicides, although reported to cause contact urticaria in rubber, has not yet been reported to cause contact urticaria when exposure occurs as an insecticide.

9.2 MISCELLANEOUS PESTICIDES

Ueda et al. published the results of a questionnaire-based study of 3717 inhabitants from a rural Japanese district where potential exposure to pesticides was present. Based on this patient-reported questionnaire, 16% reported urticaria-like dermatoses. Of patients, 21% reported a past history of allergic disorders. Poultry farmers had the highest prevalence of allergic symptoms (62%), closely followed by those engaged in raising flowers and tobacco (58%). Of those with allergic symptoms, 12–38% associated farm work and possible pesticide exposure as exacerbating factors. This study does not, however, definitively establish a link between pesticide exposures and allergic symptoms.[17]

A recent controlled study by Cellini and Offidani evaluated 426 agricultural workers for skin disorders and found a higher prevalence of acute systemic "intoxication" from pesticides (6.8%). Not evaluated was if some of these reactions might have represented cases of contact urticaria.[18]

Assini et al. may have uncovered additional cases of contact urticaria-like systemic reactions to pesticides.[19] The authors describe symptoms of urticaria/angioedema, asthma, and oculorhinitis. Causative pesticides cited included Cynoxamil, Mancozeb Thiophanate, Seccatutto, Dodine, and Paraquat.

Occupational asthma induced by trialkyltin-type fungicides used in carpet manufacture again suggests that an immunologically mediated immediate hypersensitivity reaction can develop due to pesticides.[20] Verified cases of pesticide-induced contact urticaria, though, remain rare.

Other chemical exposures among agricultural workers include building materials, such as cement and petroleum products; animal feed and additives; farm animal related medicaments; grooming supplies; rubber; and livestock waste products.[21] Numerous potential chemical allergens and irritants are necessarily contacted in the course of a farm laborer's work day. Pesticide applicators, veterinarians, nursery workers, exterminators, and some food handlers may also have potential exposure to agricultural chemicals.

O'Malley and Mathias identified horticultural specialties among all agricultural job titles, reporting the greatest number of claims for chemical exposures. Claims for adverse reactions attributed to plant and food products were also frequent among agriultural workers. This occupational group is recognized to be exposed to a complex range of chemicals. (See Table 9.1.)[22]

TABLE 9.1 Causes of Contact Urticaria Among Agricultural Workers[25,26,27,28a]

Animal products

Amniotic fluid	Hair
Blood	Saliva
Dander textbook reference	

Veterinary Medicaments and Feed Additives

Antibiotics:	Capsaicin[NI]
ampicillin	DMSO[NI]
bacitracin	Fragrances:
cephalosporins	Balsam of Peru[NI,I]
gentamicin	Menthol
neomycin	Cinnamic acid[NI]
nitrofuroximine	Cinnamic aldehyde[NI]
penicillin	Iodine[NI]
streptomycin	Tincture of Benzoin[NI]
Benzocaine[NI,I]	Tocopherol

Preservatives and Disinfectants

Chlorhexidine	Parabens
Chlorocresol[NI,I]	Sodium hypochlorite
Formaldehyde[NI,I]	Dannaker
Gentian Violet	

Miscellaneous

Acrylic monomers	Methyl ethyl ketone
Chlorothalonil	Plants

TABLE 9.1 (continued)   Causes of Contact Urticaria Among Agricultural Workers[25,26,27,28a]

Miscellaneous (continued)

Diethyltouluamide (DEET)	Rubber
Epoxy resin	Sulfur dioxide
Grains	Turpentine (non-immunologic)
Grain Mites	Wood
Insects	Zinc diethyldithiocarbamate

[a]Immunologically mediated (I) unless otherwise specified as nonimmunologically mediated (NI).

Erythema, stinging, pruritus without urticaria (suburticariogenic urticaria), eyelid edema, and respiratory complaints may all be presenting signs of the contact urticaria constellation.[23] Contact urticaria may be an explanation for some poorly categorized reactions to pesticides. In addition to cutaneous contact, urticarial symptoms due to respiratory pesticide exposure should be considered.

Our present knowledge of contact urticaria to agricultural chemicals, and pesticides in particular, remains deficient. As testing methodology of potential causes of contact urticaria become standardized, conjoined with improved accuracy of physician diagnosis, reports of pesticide-induced contact urticaria will undoubtedly increase.

REFERENCES

1. Hogan D.J., Pesticides and other agricultural chemicals. *Occupational Skin Disease*, 2nd ed., Adams, R.M., Eds., W.B. Saunders, Philadelphia, 1990, 546-577.
2. Weisenburger, D.D., Human health effects of agrichemical use. *Hum. Pathol.*, Jun 24(6):571-576, 1993.
3. Mathias, C.G. and Morrison, J.H., Occupational skin diseases, United States. Results from the Bureau of Labor Statistics Annual Survey of Occupational Injuries and Illnesses, 1973 through 1984. *Arch. Dermatol.*, Oct 124(10):1519-1524, 1988.
4. Mehler, L.N., O'Malley, M.A., and Krieger, R.I., Acute pesticide morbidity and mortality: California. *Rev. Environ. Contam. Toxicol.*, 129:51-66, 1992.
5. Edmiston, S. and Maddy, K.T., Summary of illnesses and injuries reported in California by physicians in 1986 as potentially related to pesticides. *Vet. Hum. Toxicol.*, 29:391-397, 1987.
6. Lessenger, J.E., Estock, M.D., and Younglove, T., An analysis of 190 cases of suspected pesticide illness. *J. Am. Bd. Fam. Prac.*, Jul-Aug 8(4):278-282, 1995.
7. Lisi, P., Caraffini, S., and Assalve, D., A test series for pesticide dermatitis. *Contact Dermatitis*, Nov 15(5):266-269, 1986.
8. Lisi, P., Caraffini, S., and Assalve, D., Irritation and sensitization potential of pesticides. *Contact Dermatitis*, Oct 17(4):212-218, 1987.
9. Sharma, V.K. and Kaur, S., Contact sensitization by pesticides in farmers. *Contact Dermatitis*, Aug 23(2):77-80, 1990.

10. Dannaker, C.J. and Maibach, H.I., Contact urticaria and anaphylaxis to Chlorothalonil. *Am. J. Contact Derm.,* 1:65, 1990 (abst).

11. Dannaker, C., Maibach, H.I., and O'Malley, M., Contact urticaria and anaphylaxis to the fungicide Chlorothalonil, *Cutis,* 52:312-5, 1993.

12. O'Malley, M., Rodriguez, P., and Maibach, H.I., Pesticide patch testing: California nursery workers and controls. *Contact Dermatitis,* Jan 32(1), 1995.

13. Bach, B. and Pedersen, N.B., Contact dermatitis from a wood preservative containing tetrachloroisophthalonitrile. *Contact Dermatitis,* 6:142, 1980.

14. Spindeldreier, A. and Deichmann, B., Kontaktdermatitis auf ein Holzschutzmittel mit neuer fungizider wirksubstanz. *Dermatosen,* 28:88-90, 1980.

15. Linden, C., Facial dermatitis caused by chlorothalonil in a paint. *Contact Dermatitis,* Apr 22(4):206-211, 1990.

16. Helander, I. and Makela, A., Contact urticaria to zinc diethyldithiocarbamate (ZDC). *Contact Dermatitis,* Jul 9(4):327-328, 1983.

17. Ueda, A., Ueda, T., Matsushita, T., Uano, T., and Nomura, S., Prevalence rates and risk factors for allergic symptoms among inhabitants in rural districts. *Jap. J. Indus. Health,* Jan 29(1):3-16, 1987.

18. Cellini, A. and Offidani, A., An epidemiological study on cutaneous diseases of agricultural workers authorized to use pesticides. *Dermatology,* 189(2):129-132, 1994.

19. Assini, R., Fracchiolla, F., Ravalli, C., and Nava, C., Allergic diseases caused by pesticides: 3 case reports. *Medicina del Lavoro,* Jul-Aug, 85(4):321-326, 1994.

20. Shelton, D., Urch, B., and Tarlo, S.M., Occupational asthma induced by a carpet fungicide--tributyl tin oxide. *J. Allergy Clin. Immunol.,* Aug 90(2):274-275, 1992.

21. Abrams, K., Hogan, D.J., and Maibach, H.I., Pesticide-related dermatoses in agricultural workers. *Occup. Med.,* Jul-Sep 6(3):463-492, 1991.

22. O'Malley, M.A. and Mathias C.G., Distribution of lost work time claims for skin disease in California agriculture: 1978-1983. *Am. J. Ind. Med.,* 14(6):715-720, 1988.

23. Kligman, A.M., The spectrum of contact urticaria. Wheals, erythema, and pruritus. *Dermatologic Clinics,* 8(1):57-60, 1990.

24. Maibach, H. and Lahti, A., Immediate contact reactions, *Exogenous Dermatoses: Environmental Dermatitis,* 1st Edition, Menne, T. and Maibach, H., Eds., CRC Press, Boca Raton, 1990, Chap. 2.

25. Harvell, J., Bason, M., and Maibach, H., Contact urticaria and its mechanisms. *Food Chem. Toxicol.,* Feb, 32(2):103-112, 1994.

26. Fumagalli, M. and Gibelli, F., Occupational contact urticaria. *Clinics in Dermatology,* 10(2):205-211, 1992.

27. Maibach, H.I., Dannaker, C.J., and Lahti, A., Contact skin allergy, in *Allergy Principals and Practice,* Vol II, 4th Edition, Middleton, E. et al., Eds., Mosby, St. Louis, 1993, Chap. 64.

10

Animals and Animal Products

Päivikki Susitaival and Matti Hannuksela

CONTENTS

10.1   GENERAL ASPECTS

Allergy to animals or animal products can appear as contact urticaria (CU) and protein contact dermatitis (PCD). In animal dander or hair allergy, CU is often accompanied by respiratory symptoms. In U.S. statistics, seafood and poultry plants are among the top industries yielding occupational skin diseases.[1] In Finland, about 100 work-related cases of PCD are reported to be caused by animal allergy yearly. They account for half of all reported work-related PCD cases (Finnish Register of Occupational Diseases). Skin prick tests (SPT) have been found to be positive to laboratory animals in 15 to 21% of persons who work with animals in laboratories,[2-4] and to cows in 5 to 14% of some farmer populations.[5-7]

10.2 LABORATORY ANIMAL WORKERS

Laboratory animals (rats, mice, guinea pigs, rabbits, hamsters, cats, dogs, and toads) have been reported to cause rashes and CU.[3,4,8-13] In the Finnish Register of Occupational Diseases from 1990 to 1994, the causes of PCD included rabbit (2 cases), mouse, rat, and guinea pig (each 1 case). Rats and mice have been reported to cause CU more often than other animals, probably because of the abundance of their use as compared with that of other laboratory animals. Laboratory animal allergy and CU seem to be more common in persons carrying out experiments with animals than in those tending them.[9,12] The former involves more direct handling of the animals, themselves, their secretions, and their internal organs. Symptoms are often reported only on scratched skin, and some types of contact, like the tail of rats and the urine of mice, have caused problems more often than others.[3,10] Protective measures are often effective in controlling CU symptoms.[10]

In a study by Weissenbach et al., one third of those handling cats or rats daily were sensitized, while the figures for other animals were somewhat lower.[4] Multiple sensitization to laboratory animals is common.[3,4,10] CU is the only symptom in only about one in ten cases of laboratory animal allergy, and almost half of those with respiratory symptoms from laboratory animals have also had skin symptoms.[3,4,12] Hand eczema has been uncommon in persons with laboratory animal allergy.[4,10] One probable reason is the exclusion or selection of those with hand eczema from laboratory animal work.

Allergen sources used in skin tests have included animal hair and dander, and also rat tail and mouse liver.[2,4,8,10,13,14] According to Hunskaar and Fosse, the main allergens of rats and mice are serum and urinary proteins, which are also present in hair, skin, feces, and other tissues.[15] There is no significant cross-reactivity between the species.[15] SPT and RAST results with animal proteins correlate well with skin symptoms.[10] In Agrup and Sjöstedt's study, 17% of the persons working with rats had symptoms of CU, and rats caused more severe CU reactions than mice.[10] Other laboratory animals, for example, guinea pigs, rabbits and cats, seem to cause more respiratory symptoms than skin reactions.[10,12]

10.3 VETERINARIANS

There are no recent reports of epidemiological studies on contact allergy in veterinary work. Case reports of veterinarians with CU or contact dermatitis and allergy deal mostly with cow hair, dander, amniotic fluid, blood, serum, and placenta.[16-21] CU and flaring hand dermatitis are the most important symptoms, and in many cases they have existed for a long time.[17,18,20,21] Symptoms of hand dermatitis have often been connected with obstetric work.[17,18,20] Positive SPTs and RASTs to cow dander and sometimes also positive SPTs to bovine amniotic fluid have been common findings for these patients.[17,18] In the study by Kalveram et al., veterinarians had positive scratch tests (ST) and RASTs to cow and swine sera and to cow amniotic fluid, but RASTs to animal danders were negative.[20] In many of these cases, the total IgE of serum was high (198 to 851 kU/l). There is also a report of a veterinarian with recurrent hand dermatitis and a positive patch test (PT) on day 4 (D4), together with a positive intradermal test to cow amniotic fluid.[21]

10.4 FARMERS

In 1948, Epstein described the typical clinical picture of "milker's eczema" for 42 patients (sharply outlined chronic dermatitis, radial aspect of index finger, thumb, and wrist, right hand first and more severely involved, flexor side of the right lower arm, face, neck, or legs, worse in winter).[22] In 1961, Spencer called the dermatitis "atopic dermatitis due to sensitivity to cattle."[23] The location of the dermatosis corresponds to the areas which touch the cow in the cleaning and milking process, also in modern dairying, or are exposed to airborne cattle dust. Patients connect the dermatosis almost invariably to cattle.[22,23] Such a connection was also found in most of the cases in a Finnish study.[24] Epstein's patients complained of itching and redness within 2 to 12 hours after milking. Among his 42 patients, 28 had positive skin test reactions to cow dander. Of Epstein's patients, 15 had positive immediate (STs or intradermal test) and 13 had delayed (intradermal or PTs) skin test reactions to cow dander. Some of the PTs of Epstein's patients were positive only on the hands or forearms.[22] The timing (appearing at 12 hours) and the morphology (often papulo-follicular) of the delayed reactions to cow dander in Epstein's study were similar to the findings in the study of Finnish farmers.[22,24] Epstein concluded his report by connecting most of the milkers' eczema to cattle dander allergy. He wondered why this common condition, with a typical clinical picture, has not been described in the literature or in textbooks.[22]

In Finland, where occupational diseases are compensated for farmers, cow dander allergy has accounted for more than a quarter of all occupational dermatoses and for more than half of all the allergic dermatoses occurring in farming during the past 5 years (Finnish Register of Occupational Diseases) (Table 10.1). Four cases of delayed contact dermatitis to cow dander are included in the figures in Table 10.1. In the Finnish Register of Occupational Diseases from 1990 to 1994, cases of PCD have been reported as caused by allergy to other animals, for example, pigs (8 cases), poultry (3 cases), fox (2 cases), horse (1 case), or other animals (4 cases).

The epidemiology of hand eczema among dairy farmers has been studied thoroughly in Finland.[25] The prevalence of hand dermatosis was three to four times higher for those with a history of skin atopy than for those with no history of atopy, while a history of hay fever or asthma doubled the prevalence. In a population of 2005 Finnish farmers, 8.6% reported hand or forearm dermatoses in a self administered questionnaire, and 138 (80%) of them attended a clinical examination. Cow epithelium elicited positive SPT reactions in one fifth of all farmers with hand eczema, and cow dander was the most common allergen in both the SPTs and PTs.[24] Positive reactions in SPTs to fodder flours (barley and oats) were common for women and positive reactions to molds, chicken feather, and lamb wool were fairly common for both genders. Everyone reacting to lamb wool in an SPT also had a positive SPT to cow epithelium. Prahl found cross-allergy to sheep and goat allergen preparations

TABLE 10.1   Causes of Occupational Dermatoses Reported for Farmers in 1990–1994 According to the Register of Occupational Diseases in Finland (N).

	Year						
	1990	1991	1992	1993	1994	All	%
Animal dander[a]	58	71	85	72	86	372	*28*
Detergents	53	53	47	43	61	257	*20*
Wet and dirty work	29	32	21	38	17	137	*10*
NRL[b] and rubber chemicals	24	33	22	32	25	136	*10*
Ringworm	19	25	17	10	9	80	*6*
Other	65	73	54	64	68	324	*25*
All occupational dermatoses reported for farming	248	287	246	259	266	1306	

[a] Predominantly cow dander.

[b] Natural rubber latex.

in persons with immediate allergy to cow dander. He also found similar allergens in allergen preparations from these animals.[26]

One third of the Finnish farmers with positive reactions to cow dander had a positive immediate skin test reaction in an SPT or in a 20 minute PT, but no delayed reaction in a 24 hour PT.[24] Another one third of these farmers had a positive delayed reaction, but no immediate reaction, and the remaining third had both immediate and delayed positive reactions. It is noteworthy that a third of the farmers with a positive immediate reaction to cow dander reacted only to patch testing (= contact urticaria). These contact urticarial reactions were obviously of an allergic nature because 20 minute PTs with cow dander were negative for all 50 of the nonfarming controls.[24]

In addition to Epstein's report and the Finnish study, there are other case reports of hand dermatitis with either immediate or delayed allergy to cattle.[22-24,27-33] Van Ketel and van Diggelen reported the case of a farmer who had hand eczema together with positive intracutaneous and STs with cow hair and dander extracts, as well as a positive RAST to cow hair.[30] Recently, Lings described a Danish dairy farmer with hand and forearm eczema, negative prick tests, and a positive PT on D4 to cow dander.[32] Similarly, Timmer and Coenraads reported the case of a farmer's son with eczema on his hands, arms, and face in relation to cow contact, and a positive PT from D2 to dander from the farmer's cow.[33] In Müller's report, a farm woman was found to be allergic to her brown cows but not to her black and white ones.[28] Veien reported some cases of hand dermatitis due to cow allergy in farmers.[31] According to him, a diagnostic work-up can be difficult since traditional tests may be negative. He recommended a challenge test by brushing the skin on the cow. There is also a report of one farmer's contact eczema from cow saliva.[34] All other PTs and RASTs (not specified) were negative, except the PT to cow saliva.

Farmers usually tend cattle for years before they start having skin symptoms. Only some of them have an earlier history of atopy, but many have noticed respiratory symptoms coinciding with the skin symptoms. If contact with cattle continues without protection, intense itch and only minor relief from topical corticosteroid is typical. Sometimes the symptoms are only urticaria, and in these cases the symptoms are often relieved by washing the skin. In cold climates, summer brings temporary relief, probably because the cattle are generally outdoors then. Moreover, ultraviolet light helps cure the dermatitis. The dermatitis subsides in about 1 month after protective measures begin. Motivation for strict protection with clothing, and as recommended with vinyl protective gloves, is of great importance, even though farmers often consider it impossible. We have had good experience in protecting the face and neck from airborne allergens with the use of powered respirators, equipped with a hood. It is important to advise farmers to change, store, and wash their work clothes outside their living quarters.

In Finland, cow allergy is also a major cause for occupational respiratory diseases, accounting for about 150 asthma cases every year, which is about one third of all reported cases of occupational asthma. According to our recent survey, about 40% of the farmers with cow allergic asthma also have hand dermatitis.[35]

Sensitization with CU has been reported for horse hair, dog saliva, and horse saliva.[27,36,37] Schneider et al. have described a case of allergy to horse and cow hair in a veterinarian who also farmed.[27] Both 10-minute and 24-hour PTs were positive for this patient, who started to suffer from rhinitis and urticaria after having had brucellosis. Roth has described a farm woman with eczema on her hands and face and positive immediate and delayed reactions to sheep, cow, goat, and pig (3 minute and 24 hour) and also horse (20 minute and 12 hour).[29] There is a report of contact eczema with a positive PT to scrapings of pig epithelia.[38] Delayed allergy to ewe's wool with hand eczema associated with milking or lambing ewes has been reported with and without wool alcohol allergy.[39,40]

10.5 SLAUGHTERHOUSE WORKERS AND OTHER WORKERS HANDLING MEAT OR SEAFOOD

In 1951, Seeberg paid attention to three patients with eczematous reactions from handling meat.[41] They all had relapsing vesicopapular rashes appearing 2 to 15 hours after contact with meat. All the patients had vesicopapular reactions in PTs, to both boiled and raw meats, but intracutaneous tests were negative. The PTs were later negative when the dermatitis had healed.[41] Any part of animals handled for food preparation will probably give rise to allergic PCD. Almost a quarter of slaughterhouse workers cutting and cleaning pigs reported a history of PCD, while 12% had positive scratch-patch tests to small intestine or mesenteric fat of pigs.[42] Raw meat (beef, pork, lamb, chicken) or other animal parts, like skin (chicken, turkey), liver (calf, chicken), gut (pig), and blood (cow, pig), have been found to cause either immunologic or nonimmunologic CU in cooks, kitchen workers, butchers, and slaughterhouse workers.[43-53] Many types of both salt and freshwater fish and other seafood (Table 10.2) have also been reported to cause CU and PCD.[49,50,54-58] Generalized urticaria has rarely been reported in connection with contact reactions from animal products.[53]

TABLE 10.2   Seafood Reported to Cause CU or PCD

Seafood	Symptom	Positive tests, if any	Reference
		One case	

Lobster
Shrimp
Herring
Plaice
Cod
	PCD	20 minute OT on
		  affected skin,
		ST protein
		  extract (cod, herring)
			*Hjort and Roed-
			Petersen 1976*

		One case	
Herring	PCD	20 minute OT on affected skin	*Hjort and Roed- Petersen 1976*
		One case	

Plaice
Cod
Herring
	PCD	20 minute OT on
		  affected skin,
		ST dialyzed
		  protein extract (cod)
			*Hjort and Roed-
			Petersen 1976*

		One case	

Plaice
Herring
	PCD	ST fresh fish,
		  ST dialyzed
		  protein extract
			*Hjort and Roed-
			Petersen 1976*

		One case	
Plaice Cod	PCD, swelling of mouth and throat after eating fish	SPT fish (commercial) RAST fish (commercial) OT fresh fish (in 5 minutes)	*Göransson 1981*
		Several cases	
Mackerel Cod Herring Plaice Other fish	CU	ST	*Veien et al. 1983*
		One case	

Anchovy
Cod
Mullet
Pilchard
	CU, edema on
	lips and tongue
	when eating fish
		20 minute PT, normal
		  and affected skin
		
		20 minute PT on
		  affected skin
			Melino et al. 1987

TABLE 10.2 (continued)   Seafood Reported to Cause CU or PCD

Seafood	Symptom	Positive tests, if any	Reference
		One case	
Anchovy	PCD	20 minute OT on previously affected skin	*Tosti and Guerra 1988*
		One case	
Shrimp Cuttlefish	PCD	20 minute OT on previously affected skin	*Tosti and Guerra 1988*
		One case	
Lobster Shrimp Scallops	CU	ST with extracts from lobster, shrimp and scallops	*Nethercott and Hollness 1989*
		One case	
Several salt and fresh water fish, shellfish	CU	20 minute OT with 12 fish species	*Abeck et al. 1990*
		One case	
Cuttlefish	PCD	OT on hands	*Tosti et al. 1990*

Note: ST = scratch test.

OT = open test.

PT = patch test.

SPT = skin prick test.

SPTs or open skin tests with pertinent animal products have often been negative on intact skin. In such cases, the suspected materials should be tested on the site of the dermatitis or on scratched skin.[42-45,47,48,50,51,55,58] Hjort and Roed-Petersen skin tested sandwich makers who associated their hand dermatitis with handling fish or chicken meat, and found positive reactions in STs, open patch tests on affected skin, and also in patch tests on D2 with fresh materials.[43] RASTs were often positive, and dialyzed protein extracts elicited positive ST reactions in several persons allergic to fish.[43] Most of the patients with food allergy have had chronic hand eczema rather than relapsing symptoms of CU, which probably reflects continuous contact with the allergens. Some patients with meat or fish allergy have also been reported to have urticarial symptoms on lips, tongue, or throat when eating the allergenic material.[47,54,55] Some cases of delayed allergy to animal products (swine and cow blood, chicken skin and meat, chicken liver and heart) have also been published.[46,59,60]

There are some reports of positive PT reactions to cooked meat and chicken products.[41,59]

10.6   OTHER OCCUPATIONS

In a case report by von den Driesch et al. a cosmetician contracted severe hand dermatitis from calf placenta extract. A scratch chamber test produced only a delayed reaction.[61]

10.7   CONCLUDING REMARKS

In the diagnosis of contact allergy to animals, SPTs and RASTs with animal danders often reveal immediate allergy to the allergens in question. For allergy to meat or seafood, the diagnostic-tests may have to be made with patient-supplied materials. In such cases, attention should be paid to contagious diseases possibly present in fresh materials. When "new" sterile materials are tested without prior knowledge from one's own experience or the literature, at least 20 control persons should be tested. Testing with fresh materials (animal danders, meat, fish, shrimp, etc.) should be avoided for controls. If SPTs, RASTs, and conventional skin test sites do not elicit responses even though the evidence is strong, tests should be done on scratched or diseased skin, and patch tests should be performed for immediate and delayed allergies.

REFERENCES

1. Wang, C. L., Occupational skin disease continues to plague industry, *Monthly Labor Rev.,* 102, 17, 1979.
2. Slovak, A. J. M. and Hill, R. N., Laboratory animal allergy: a clinical survey of an exposed population, *Br. J. Ind. Med.,* 38, 38, 1981.
3. Cockcroft, A., McCarthy, P., Edwards, J., and Andersson, N., Allergy in laboratory animal workers, *Lancet,* April 11, 827, 1981.
4. Weissenbach, T., Wüthrich, B., and Weihe, W. H., Labortier-Allergien, *Schweiz med. Wschr.,* 118, 930, 1988.
5. Rautalahti, M., Terho, E. O., Vohlonen, I., and Husman, K., Atopic sensitization of dairy farmers to work-related and common allergens, *Eur. J. Respir. Dis.,* (Suppl.) 152, 155, 1987.
6. Larmi, E., Reijula, K., Hannuksela, M., Pikkarainen, S., and Hassi J., Skin disorders and prick and patch test positivity in Finnish reindeer herders, *Dermatosen in Beruf und Umwelt;* 36 (3), 83, 1988.
7. Iversen, M. and Pedersen, B., The prevalence of allergy in Danish farmers, *Allergy,* 45, 347, 1990.
8. Rudzki, E., Contact urticaria due to hairs from a rat's tail, *Contact Dermatitis,* 1, 252, 1975.
9. Burrows, D., Urticaria from rats, *Contact Dermatitis,* 5, 122, 1979.
10. Agrup, G. and Sjöstedt, L., Contact urticaria in laboratory technicians working with animals, *Acta Derm. Venereol. (Stockh.),* 65, 111, 1985.

11. Thomsen, R. J. and Honsinger, R. W., Immediate hypersensitivity reaction to amphibian serum manifesting as eczema, *Arch. Dermatol.,* 123, 1436, 1987.

12. Aoyama, K., Ueda, A., Manda, F., Matsushita, T., and Ueda, T., Allergy to laboratory animals: an epidemiological study, *Br. J. Ind. Med.,* 49, 41, 1992.

13. Karches, F. and Fuchs, T., A strange manifestation of occupational contact urticaria due to mouse hair, *Contact Dermatitis,* 28, 200, 1993.

14. Kauppinen, K., Occupational contact urticaria provoked by mouse liver, *Contact Dermatitis,* 6, 444, 1980.

15. Huskaar, S. and Fosse, R. T., Allergy to laboratory mice and rats: a review of the pathophysiology, epidemiology and clinical aspects, *Laboratory Animals,* 24, 358, 1990.

16. Schmidt, H., Contact urticaria (Letters to the Editor), *Contact Dermatitis,* 4, 230, 1978.

17. Prahl, P. and Roed-Petersen, J., Type I allergy from cows in veterinary surgeons, *Contact Dermatitis,* 5, 33, 1979.

18. Hjorth, N. and Roed-Petersen, J., Allergic contact dermatitis in veterinary surgeons, *Contact Dermatitis,* 6, 27, 1980.

19. Degreff, H., Bourgeois, M., Naert, C., Van de Kerckhove, M., and Dooms-Goossens, A., Protein contact Dermatitis with positive RAST caused by bovine blood and amniotic fluid, *Contact Dermatitis,* 11, 129, 1984.

20. Kalveram, K-J., Kästner, H., and Forck, G., Nachweis von spezifischen IgE-Antikörpern bei Tierärzten mit Kontakturticaria, *Z. Hautkr.,* 61, 75, 1986.

21. Roger, A., Guspi, R., Garcia-Patos, V., Barriga, A., Rubira, N., Nogueiras, C., Castells, A., and Cadahia, A., Occupational protein contact Dermatitis in a veterinary surgeon, *Contact Dermatitis,* 32, 248, 1995.

22. Epstein, S., Milker's Eczema — An analysis of forty-two cases, *J. Allergy,* 19, 333, 1948.

23. Spencer, M. C., Occupational Dermatitis and eczema among farmers, *Illinois Med. J.,* 119, 136, 1961.

24. Susitaival, P., Husman, L., Hollmén, A., Horsmanheimo, M., Husman, K., and Hannuksela, M., Hand eczema in Finnish farmers — A questionnaire based clinical study, *Contact Dermatitis,* 32, 150, 1995.

25. Susitaival, P., Epidemiological study of hand dermatoses and other skin diseases in a cohort of Finnish farmers, Kuopio University Publications D. Medical Sciences 93, Kuopio 1996, 1-104 (Thesis).

26. Prahl, P., Allergens in cow hair and dander, *Allergy,* 36, 561, 1981.

27. Schneider, W., Coppenrathu, R., and Ruther, H., Über Tierhaar-Allergie, *Berufsdermatosen,* 8 (1), 1, 1960.

28. Müller, H., Über seltene Berufsdermatosen bei Landwirten und Schlachthofarbeitern, *Dermatol Wochenschr,* 151 (29), 820, 1965.

29. Roth, W. G., Ekzem und Asthma durch Rinder- und Pferdehaare, *Berufsdermatosen,* 16 (5), 278, 1968.

30. van Ketel, W. G. and van Diggelen, M. W., A farmer with allergy to cows, *Contact Dermatitis,* 8, 279, 1982.

31. Veien, N., Occupational dermatoses in farmers, in *Occupational and Industrial Dermatology,* Maibach, H., Ed., Yearbook Medical Publishers Inc., Chicago 1987 (Second edition), 436.

32. Lings, S., Malkehånd, Ugeskr Læger, 156 (47), 7028, 1994.

33. Timmer, C. and Coenraads, P-J., Allergic contact dermatitis from cow hair and dander, *Contact Dermatitis,* 34, 292, 1996.

34. Camarasa, J. G., Contact eczema from cow saliva, *Contact Dermatitis,* 15, 117, 1986.

35. Susitaival, P., Husman, K., Taattola, K., and Louhelainen, K., Prognosis of compensated occupational asthma in Finnish farmers using a powered respirator, presented at The Third Annual NIOSH Agricultural Health and Safety Conference, Iowa City, Iowa, March 24-26, 1996.

36. Valsecchi, R. and Cainelli, T., Contact urticaria from dog saliva, *Contact Dermatitis,* 20, 62, 1989.

37. van der Mark, S., Contact urticaria from horse saliva, *Contact Dermatitis,* 9, 145, 1983.

38. Malanin, G. and Kalimo, K., Occupational contact dermatitis due to delayed allergy to pig epithelia, *Contact Dermatitis,* 26, 134, 1992.

39. Sirieix-Sorhouet, M., Sirieix, P., and Ducombs, G., Ewe milkers and hand eczema, *Contact Dermatitis,* 25, 135, 1991.

40. Quirce, S., Olaguibel, J. M., Muro, M. D., and Tabar, A. I., Occupational dermatitis in a ewe milker, *Contact Dermatitis,* 27, 56, 1992.

41. Seeberg, G., Eczematous Dermatitis from contact with, or ingestion of beef, pork and mutton (4 case reports), *Acta Derm. Venereol.,* 32 (Suppl. 29), 320, 1952.

42. Hansen, K. S. and Petersen, H. O., Protein contact Dermatitis in slaughterhouse workers, *Contact Dermatitis,* 21, 221, 1989.

43. Hjorth, N. and Roed-Petersen, J., Occupational protein contact dermatitis in food handlers, *Contact Dermatitis,* 2, 28, 1976.

44. Maibach, H., Immediate Hypersensitivity in Hand Dermatitis, *Arch. Dermatol.,* 112, 1289, 1976.

45. Fisher, A. A. and Stengel, F., Allergic occupational hand dermaitis due to calf's liver; An urticarial "immediate" type hypersensitivity, *Cutis,* 19, 561, 1977.

46. Göransson, K., Occupational contact urticaria to fresh cow and pig blood in slaughtermen, *Contact Dermatitis,* 7, 281, 1981.

47. Fisher, A. A., Contact urticaria from handling meats and fowl, *Cutis,* 30, 726, 1982.

48. Moseng, D., Urticaria from Pig's gut, *Contact Dermatitis,* 8, 135, 1982.

49. Veien, N. K., Hattel, T., Justesen, O., and Nørholm, A., Causes of eczema in the food industry, *Dermatosen,* 31 (3), 84, 1983.

50. Tosti, A. and Guerra, L., Protein contact dermatitis in food handlers, *Contact Dermatitis,* 19, 149, 1988.

51. Zenarola, P. and Lomuto, M., Protein contact Dermatitis with positive RAST in a slaughterman, *Contact Dermatitis,* 24, 134, 1991.

52. Jovanovic, M., Oliwiecki, S., and Beck, M. H., Occupational contact urticaria from beef associated with hand eczema, *Contact Dermatitis,* 27, 188, 1992.

53. Judd, L., A descriptive study of occupational skin disease, *New Zealand Med. J.,* 107, 147, 1994.

54. Göransson, K., Contact urticaria to fish, Contact Dermatitis, 7, 282, 1981.

55. Melino, M., Toni, F., and Riguzzi, G., Immunologic contact urticaria to fish, *Contact Dermatitis,* 17, 182, 1987.

56. Nethercott, J. R. and Holness, D. L., Occupational dermatitis in food handlers and bakers, *J. Am. Acad. Dermatol.,* 21, 485, 1989.

57. Abeck, D., Korting, H. C., and Ring, J., Kontakturtikaria mit Übergang in eine Protein-Kontaktdermatitis bei einem Koch mit atopisher Diathese, *Dermatosen,* 38 (1), 24, 1990.

58. Tosti, A., Fanti, P. A., Guerra, L., Piancastelli, E., Poggi, S., and Pileri, S., Morphological and immunohistochemical study of immediate contact dermatitis of the hands due to foods, *Contact Dermatitis,* 22, 81, 1990.

59. Harrington, C. I., Chicken sensitivity, *Contact Dermatitis,* 7, 126, 1981.

60. Beck, H. I. and Nissen, B. K., Type I and type IV allergy to specific chicken organs, *Contact Dermatitis,* 8, 217, 1982.
61. von den Driesch, P., Fartasch, M., Diepgen, T. L., and Peters, K. P., Protein contact dermatitis from calf placenta extracts, *Contact Dermatitis,* 28, 46, 1993.

11

Antibiotics

Matti Hannuksela

CONTENTS

11.1   INTRODUCTION

Delayed-type contact allergy to antibiotics is usually manifested as eczematous contact dermatitis. Internal exposure to the same agent causes a rash resembling both exanthema and eczematous dermatitis also known as systemic contact dermatitis.

Contact urticaria (CU) to antibiotics is uncommon and is usually reported in case reports or letters to the editor. Local and generalized CU and occasionally anaphylactic shock are usual symptoms in antibiotic-induced CU,[1] and angioedema may also occur.[2]

11.2   ANTIBIOTICS CAUSING CONTACT URTICARIA

11.2.1   Penicillins

A nurse handling penicillins experienced localized rashes of CU in her daily work.[1] Penicillin taken perorally produced generalized urticaria. Penicilloyl RAST was negative. When an open epicutaneous test with 25 nmol of penicilloyl polylysine de

**TABLE 11.1 Antibiotics Causing Contact
Urticaria Syndrome**

Penicillins
  Penicillin G
  Ampicillin
  Amoxycillin
  Cloxacillin
  Mezlocillin
Cephalosporins
  Cephalotin
  Cefotiam hydrochloride
Aminoglycocides
  Streptomycin
  Neomycin
  Gentamycin
Rifamycin
Rifampicin
Bacitracin
Chloramphenicol

Weck was done, local urticaria developed and she also developed systemic symptoms. Other authors have also described CU from skin testing with pencillins.[3]

Minor determinants of ampicillin, amoxicillin, and cloxacillin were found to cause immediate allergic skin reactions more often than major and minor determinants of benzylpenicillin and its derivatives, when skin prick tests were made an average of 4.9 years after an allergic reaction to any of the penicillins taken internally.[4] This result stresses the importance of caution when performing skin tests with drugs that may cause anaphylactic reactions.

Mezlocillin was the cause of CU and dyspnea in a nurse handling the drug.[5] In an open patch test, a 1% solution of mezlocillin first produced local urticaria and within 2 days also produced eczematous dermatitis. This patient might have had both type I and type IV allergy to mezlocillin.

11.2.2 Cephalosporins

A chemist handling cephalotin powder frequently in his work began to suffer from itching, redness, and hives on the backs of the hands, the arms, and the face.[6] During several months, the reaction was aggravated and the urticaria was accompanied by lacrimation, sneezing, and watery nasal discharge. In an epicutaneous test with cephalotin, a huge weal and flare reaction appeared within minutes, and the patient began to sneeze. Ampicillin, penicillin G, and erythromycin were negative when tested similarly.

Cefotiam hydrochloride was the cause of localized CU and, subsequently, systemic urticaria in two nurses of the same hospital who had been preparing parenteral antibiotics for drip infusion.[7] One nurse also got paresthesia on her hands and the other had paresthesia in her mouth. In both cases, in an epicutaneous test with cefotiam, a wheal and flare reaction appeared in 20 minutes. Skin tests with other antibiotics used in the hospital were negative in both cases.

11.2.3 Other Antibiotics

Streptomycin, an aminoglycoside, was the cause of itching and swelling of the hands of a nurse giving streptomycin injections in a tuberculosis sanatorium.[8] When applied in an open manner on her arm, streptomycin drops produced a wheal and flare reaction. The open test was repeated 5 years later on the arm, and rhinitis and lacrimation appeared within minutes together with a local urticarial reaction.

Neomycin and gentamycin are also aminoglycocides. Both of them have been reported to cause CU, even anaphylaxis.[9,10] A 21-year-old male patient had experienced an anaphylactic-type reaction from neomycin gel applied to the face. Later on, he experienced a local CU from neomycin powder and from a steroid cream with neomycin. An open epicutaneous test with 0.35% neomycin sulphate solution produced a wheal and flare reaction which disappeared in 30 minutes.[10] Gentamycin but neither paromomycin nor kanamycin, produced a similar immediate reaction.[10]

Rifamycin SV, an antibiotic derived from *Streptomyces mediterranei*, has been reported to cause contact urticaria in sporadic cases only. Rifamycin compresses produced generalized urticaria in a leg ulcer patient.[11] An open test with 1% rifamycin solution was positive in 20 minutes, but an occluded patch test with 10% rifamycin was negative at 48–96 hours. The corresponding responses to 1% and 10% rifampicin were similar. The authors considered the immediate reaction to rifampicin to be due to cross-sensitivity to rifamycin, because these two antibiotics have the same nucleus. Another leg ulcer patient treated with rifamycin dressings also experienced a local CU reaction around the wound followed by generalized urticaria and anaphylactic shock.[12] Open tests with 0.05, 0.5, and 5% rifamycin were positive in 20 minutes. The authors also made a Prausnitz-Küstner (P-K) test with a positive result, demonstrating the allergic nature of the reaction.

Topical administration of bacitracin may lead to generalized urticaria and anaphylactic shock.[13-16] A positive P-K test has proven the reaction to be IgE-mediated.[14]

Urticaria and angioedema from 3% chloramphenicol ointment was thought to be caused by chloramphenicol itself in two patients.[2] Unfortunately, no tests were performed to verify the role of chloramphenicol in these reactions.

11.3 GENERAL ASPECTS

Immediate reactions to topical antibiotics, including anaphylaxis, may be severe. Most, if not all, of them seem to be mediated by IgE. As a diagnostic procedure, an open (patch) test with a very dilute chemical can be recommended as the first test. An increase of the test concentration and skin prick tests are the next steps. One should be prepared to treat anaphylactic test reactions.

The demonstration of a specific IgE in the patient's serum is possible in many cases, but a negative result in it does not exclude the possibility of an immediate allergic reaction. This has been demonstrated especially in penicillin allergy. A P-K test is another method for demonstrating humoral allergy. Tests for HIV, hepatitis, and other infectious diseases must be done before making the P-K test, and only first-degree relatives should be used as test subjects. Specific serum IgE does not inevitably mean that the administration of an antibiotic onto the the skin produces allergic CU. Lopez Serrano et al.[17] made the skin prick test and patch test in a case of urticaria from peroral erythromycin. In this particular patient, the former was positive and the latter negative.

REFERENCES

1. Böttger, E. M., Mücke, Chr., and Tronnier, H., Kontaktdermatitis auf neuere Anti-mykotika un Kontakturticaria, *Aktuelle Dermatologie,* 7, 70, 1981.
2. Schewach-Millet, M. and Shpiro, D., Urticaria and angioedema due to topically applied chloramphenicol ointment, *Arch. Dermatol.,* 121, 587, 1985.
3. Burdick, A. E. and Mathias, C. G. T., The contact urticaria syndrome, *Dermatologic Clinics,* 3, 71, 1985.
4. Silviu-Dan, F., McPhillips, S., and Warrington, R. J., The frequency of skin test reactions to side-chain penicillin determinants, *J. Allergy Clin. Immunol.,* 91, 694, 1993.
5. Keller, K. and Schwanitz, H. J., Combined immediate and delayed hypersensitivity to mezlocillin, *Contact Dermatitis,* 27, 348, 1992.
6. Tuft, L., Contact urticaria from cephalosporins, *Arch. Dermatol.,* 111, 1609, 1975.
7. Miyahara, H., Koga, T., Imayama, S., and Hori, Y., Occupational contact urticaria syndrome from cefotiam hydrochloride, *Contact Dermatitis,* 29, 210, 1993.
8. Rudzki, E., Rebandel, P., and Rogozinski, T., Contact urticaria from rat tail, guinea pig, streptomycin and vinyl pyridine, *Contact Dermatitis,* 7, 186, 1981.
9. Eriksen, H. C., Anaphylactic shock caused by neomycin treated with external cardiac massage, *Ugeskrift for Laeger,* 125, 1077, 1963.
10. Maucher, O. M., Anaphylaktische Reaktionen beim Epicutantest, *Hautarzt,* 23, 139, 1972.
11. Grob, J. J., Pommier, G., Robaglia, A., Collet-Villette, A. M., and Bonerandi, J. J., Contact urticaria from rifamycin, *Contact Dermatitis,* 16, 284, 1987.
12. Mancuso, G. and Masarà, N., Contact urticaria and severe anaphylaxis from rifamycin SV, *Contact Dermatitis,* 27, 124, 1992.
13. Comaish, J. S. and Cunliffe, W. J., Absorption of drugs from varicose ulcers: A cause of anaphylaxis, *Br. J. Clin. Prac.,* 21, 97, 1967.
14. Roupe G. and Strannegård, Ö., Anaphylactic shock elicited by topical administration of bacitracin, *Arch. Dermatol.,* 100, 450, 1969.
15. Vale, M. A., Connolly, A., Epstein, A. M., and Vale, M. R., Bacitracin-induced ana-phylaxis, *Arch. Dermatol.,* 114, 800, 1978.
16. Schechter, J. F., Wilkinson R. D., and Del Carpio, J., Anaphylaxis following the use of bacitracin ointment: Report of a case and review of the literature, *Arch. Dermatol.,* 120, 909, 1984.
17. Lopez Serrano, C., Quiralte Enriquez, J., and Martinez Altamora, F., Urticaria from erythromycin, *Allergia et Immunopathologia (Madrid),* 21, 225, 1993.

12

Cosmetics, Cosmetic Ingredients, Emulsifiers, and Moisturizers

Matti Hannuksela

CONTENTS

12.1 INTRODUCTION

Symptoms of contact urticaria (CU) from cosmetics and cosmetic ingredients vary from redness to widespread urticaria and, in rare cases, to anaphylactic shock. We do not know the frequency of such reactions, but we can assume that 20–30% of the population have some experience of immediate contact reactions (ICRs) to everyday cosmetics and personal hygiene products. The causes of cosmetic contact urticaria are numerous, sorbic and benzoic acids and fragrances being the most common among them.

Most cases of CUs are obviously nonimmunologic. There is some evidence to suggest that in rare instances the mechanism might be immunologic, even if specific IgE has not been demonstrated.

Many external substances influence the severity of ICRs. Some emulsifiers, e.g., sorbitan esters, may enhance the penetration of substances causing ICR, and salicylates may be able to alleviate the symptoms. Ultraviolet light inhibits nonimmunologic ICRs for up to 3 weeks. This is another reason why people are sometimes confused about the occurrence and severity of ICRs.

12.2 OCCURRENCE OF CONTACT URTICARIA REACTIONS

In his extensive work on nonimmunologic CU (NICU), Lahti[1] found that 39% of Caucasian people living in Finland reacted with edema and redness and 19% with redness only to 2.5% sorbic acid in petrolatum in an open application test. Of 26 persons, 16 reacted with CU to 2.5% sorbic acid in a w/o cream and 10 persons showed only redness in response to 0.25% sorbic acid in the same cream base. This finding means that as many as 50% of people may get harmful immediate skin symptoms from a cosmetic or dermatologic formulation containing 0.2% sorbic acid.

Fragrances are also able to produce ICRs. Usual patch test concentrations of cinnamic alcohol, cinnamic aldehyde, geraniol, eugenol, balsam of Peru, anisyl alcohol, benzyl alcohol, and coumarin produced wheal and flare reactions or redness only in 36–78% of 50 persons (31 patch test clinic patients and 19 controls) tested with an open application method.[2] The other cosmetic ingredients causing immediate reactions included formaldehyde, imidazodinyl urea, bronopol, Kathon CG, and paraben mixture. No correlation between the open application test result and the cosmetic sensitivity reported by the patients was found.

In another study on fragrance materials, 80 housewives without a history of cosmetic intolerance reacted with erythema to 2% cinnamic aldehyde, 2% sorbic acid, and 2% eugenol in petrolatum in a 20-minute occluded Finn Chamber test.[3] In the same population, 76 (95%) reacted to 2% benzoic acid. Sixteen also showed edema from cinnamic aldehyde and 15 from benzoic acid. This particular study did not answer the question of how many people would have reacted to these or other fragrance materials at the concentrations usually present in everyday cosmetics.

The occurrence of ICRs from sunscreens was studied in a random sample of subjects aged over 40 years using sunscreens to treat or prevent actinic keratoses.[4] One of the 603 people had generalized urticaria of unknown cause, one had possible contact urticaria with a weakly positive scratch test to the sunscreen used, and one obviously had a NICU reaction without any knowledge of the causative agent.

Halpern[5] conducted a study among the subjects attending his dermatological practice on Kauai, the most westerly of the major Hawaiian islands. The study population comprised 1020 sequential patients, who filled in a questionnaire on ICRs. Of these patients, 26% were aware of the substances that elicited immediate symptoms. None of them mentioned cosmetics as a possible cause of such reactions. The mode of questioning may have played a role in the lack of cosmetic intolerance in this particular study, but the abundance of ultraviolet radiation on the Hawaiian islands may also have prevented the wheal and flare reactions, redness, and itching from cosmetics.

12.3   MECHANISMS OF CONTACT URTICARIA REACTIONS TO COSMETICS AND THEIR INGREDIENTS

Most CU reactions to cosmetics and their ingredients are obviously nonimmunologic. Benzoic and sorbic acids are typical examples of substances producing NICU in most people exposed to them. In rare cases, however, the reaction to benzoic acid may be immunologic.[6] Immunologic CU is produced by proteins and protein derivatives used in cosmetics.[7,8] Some low molecular weight substances, such as formaldehyde, are also able to cause the production of specific IgE.[9] An immediate reaction to formaldehyde is not always mediated by IgE in spite of the fact that histamine is released in the reaction.[10]

Persulfates are rare causes of CU, rhinitis, and asthma. The reaction itself and the rarity of such reactions speak in favor of an immunologic reaction, but specific IgE has not been demonstrated. Therefore, persulfates are among the substances causing CU of unknown mechanism.

The mechanism of NICU is not yet fully understood. It is obviously mediated by prostaglandins, because systemic and topical inhibitors of prostaglandin synthesis also inhibit the NICU reaction to several NICU substances.[11-13] Peroral antihistamines have usually been found to be ineffective in the inhibition of NICU to common NICU substances,[1,11] but some effect has also been reported from clemastine.[14] Topical antihistamines partially abolished the skin reactivity to benzoic and sorbic acids in children.[15]

From the practical point of view, it is noteworthy that ultraviolet (UV) radiation diminishes skin reactivity to benzoic acid and other NICU substances. UVB is much more effective than UVA, and the skin only normalizes its reactivity more than 3 weeks after an erythemogenic UVB dose.[16] Suberythemogenic doses of UVB on 5 consecutive days produced an inhibitory effect comparable to that of one erythemogenic dose.[17] UVA was also effective from the second week onwards when 20 J was given 3 times a week for 1 month. The non-UVA-irradiated skin site also became less sensitive to benzoic acid, indicating a systemic effect of UVA.[17]

12.4   COSMETIC SUBSTANCES CAUSING IMMEDIATE CONTACT REACTIONS

The chemicals and other substances in cosmetics and personal hygiene products known to cause ICRs are listed in Table 12.1. Many of the substances listed in the table can only cause a nonimmunologic reaction. There is some evidence to suggest that many chemicals may produce immunologic reactions, but the final proof is still lacking. Sorbitan esters, for example, which are used as emulsifiers, are reported to cause widespread acute skin reactions. These reactions might be due to an impurity in the sorbitol anhydrides rather than to the esters themselves.[31] Alcohols (ethanol, butanol, and propanol) have been shown to produce immunologic reactions, and the patients react both to a topical application and to oral intake of these particular alcohols.[44]

TABLE 12.1   Chemicals and Other Substances in Cosmetics and Personal Hygiene Products Causing Immediate Contact Reactions with Special Reference to Their Mode of Action

Substance/chemical	Type of reaction[a]	Ref.
1. Preservatives		
Benzoic acid	N, I?	1, 14, 18–20
Sorbic acid	N	1, 11, 14, 18–21
Chlorocresol	N, I?	22, 23
Parabens	I?	2, 24
Bronopol®	N	2
Kathon CG®	N	2
Imidazodinyl urea	N	2
Formaldehyde	I, U	2, 9, 10
2. Fragrance materials		
Balsam of Peru	N, I?	1, 2, 14, 20, 25
Fragrance mix	N	19
Cinnamic aldehyde	N	2, 14, 19, 20, 26
Cinnamic alcohol	N	2, 19
Cinnamic acid	N	1, 14, 20
α-Amyl cinnamic aldehyde	N	2
Coumarin	N	2
Benzyl alcohol	N	2
Anisyl alcohol	N	2
Eugenol	N	2, 19
Geraniol	N	2, 19
Hydroxycitronellal	N	19
Cassia oil	N	21, 27
3. Emulsifiers		
Cetyl alcohol	U	28
Stearyl alcohol	U	28
Sorbitan monolaurate	I?	29
Sorbitan monostearate	I?	30
Sorbitan sesquioleate	I?	31
4. Other substances		
Wool alcohols	U	32
Chlorhexidin	I	33–36
Pyrrolidone carboxylate	N	37
Lecithin	I?	8
Allantoin	I?	8
Aloe gel	I?	8
Chamomile extract	I?	8
Melissa extract	I?	8
Protein hydrolysate	I?	7

TABLE 12.1 (continued)   Chemicals and Other Substances in Cosmetics and Personal Hygiene Products Causing Immediate Contact Reactions with Special Reference to Their Mode of Action

Substance/chemical	Type of reaction[a]	Ref.
Persulfates	U	38–40
Butylhydroxytoluene	I?	41, 42
Paraphenylene diamine	U	43
Ethanol	I, N	44–46
Propanol	I	44
Butanol	I	44
Propylene glycol	N	47

[a] N = nonimmunologic contact urticaria; I = immunologic contact urticaria; U = unknown mechanism.

In the 1970s and even in the 1980s, sorbic acid was one of the most important ingredients of cosmetics causing CU. Its importance has diminished during the recent years, because it has lost its popularity as a preservative. Benzoic acid and benzoates are also used very seldom as preservatives in cosmetic skin preparations.

Chlorhexidine is widely used as an antiseptic in cosmetic preparations, especially ones used to treat acne. Severe IgE-mediated reactions have been described from topical antiseptics used for preoperative skin cleansing.[34-36] Case reports of untoward reactions to chlorhexidine in cosmetics are lacking, but this possibility should be kept in mind.

The green wave in the cosmetic industry has brought an increasing variety of plant and animal products into everyday cosmetics. These substances contain natural or modified proteins capable of causing IgE-mediated allergy. The concentration of immunologic proteins in commercial products is usually so low that the risk of sensitization cannot be high. Another concern may be due to the natural fragrances present in flowers and their extracts. The concentrations of single separate chemicals are, however, so low that the risk of ICRs is usually minimal.

In addition to the substances presented in Table 12.1, many other chemicals are able to produce redness of the skin within tens of minutes after the application of the substance to the skin. Such reactions cannot be regarded as NICU, unless at least some of the test persons get contact urticarial lesions.

12.5   FACTORS INFLUENCING THE SEVERITY OF CONTACT URTICARIA REACTIONS

Lahti[1] found that the back skin is more sensitive to benzoic acid than the hands, the ventral aspects of the forearms, or the soles. Gollhausen and Kligman[20] applied 2.5–5.0% sorbic acid and 2.5–5.0% benzoic acid to various body areas and found the following rank order of diminishing reactivity: face > antecubital space > upper back > upper arm > inner forearm > lower back > leg. Buccal mucosa and scalp were nonreactive. Larmi and co-workers[37] showed the cheek to be more reactive to benzoic acid than the forehead, neck, or upper back. Sodium pyrrolidone carboxylate, the most important component of a substance called the natural moisturizing factor, caused redness in the back skin, but not in the face or the neck.[37] Shampoos and toothpastes, diluted with water at 1:100, caused contact urticaria in the face but not on the other areas of the body in a patient who also reacted to synthetic cassia oil and to sorbic acid (0.2% in ethanol and 5% in petrolatum) when these substances were chamber-tested on the forearm. The face thus seems to be more sensitive than the other parts of the body to the common NICU substances, but not to all, as was shown by sodium pyrrolidone carboxylate.

"Quenching" refers to the ability of a substance to reduce the potential of another substance to sensitize or to cause contact urticaria. Eugenol has been shown to reduce the severity of ICRs to benzoic acid, sorbic acid, and cinnamic aldehyde.[19,20,48,49] This quenching action can be demonstrated by a simultaneous application of eugenol and a NICU substance or by pretreating the skin with eugenol prior to a NICU test.

Repeated open application of 5% benzoic acid at 2-hour intervals diminished significantly the skin reaction during the first day of repeated applications. The effect was still seen early on the second day, and it was further increased by further repeated applications of the same test material.[1] This may explain some cases of a fluctuating response to NICU substances.

Pretreatment of the skin for 2 days with a 20:80 mixture of sorbitan sesquioleate and petrolatum increased the skin response to benzoic acid applied to the skin in yellow petrolatum.[50] When benzoic acid was applied in a mixture of sorbitan ses-quioleate and petrolatum, the skin response was significantly weaker than that to benzoic acid in petrolatum. These results also emphasize the importance of other substances used in skin care for the skin reactivity to NICU substances.

REFERENCES

1. Lahti, A., Non-immunologic contact urticaria, *Acta Dermatovenereologica (Stockh.)*, 60, Suppl. 91, 1, 1980.
2. Emmons, W. W. and Marks, J. G., Immediate and delayed reactions to cosmetic ingredients, *Contact Dermatitis*, 13, 258, 1985.
3. Safford, R. J., Basketter, D. A., Allenby, C. F., and Goodwin, B. F. J., Immediate contact reactions to chemicals in the fragrance mix and a study of the quenching action of eugenol, *Br. J. Dermatol.*, 123, 595, 1990.
4. Foley, P., Nixon, R., Marks, R., Frowen, K., and Thompson, S., The frequency of reactions to sunscreens: results of a longitudinal population-based study on the regular use of sunscreens in Australia, *Br. J. Dermatol.*, 128, 512, 1993.
5. Halpern, D. J., The syndrome of immediate reactivities (contact urticaria syndrome). An historical study from a dermatology practice. I. Age, sex, race, and putative substances, *Hawaii Med. J.*, 44, 426, 1985.
6. Pevny, I., Rauscher, E., Lechner, W., and Metz, J., Exzessive Allergie gegen Benzoesäure mit anaphylaktischem Schock nach Expositionstest, *Dermatosen*, 29, 123, 1981.
7. Niinimäki, A., Hannuksela, M., and Moilanen, M., Protein hydrolysates of hair cosmetic products as causes of contact urticaria in hair dressers. *Abstract book of Second Congress of the European Society of Contact Dermatitis*, Barcelona 6.-8.10. 1994, 57.

8. West, I. and Maibach, H. I., Contact urticaria syndrome from multiple cosmetic compounds, *Contact Dermatitis,* 32, 121, 1995.

9. Gehse, M., Gehring, W., and Gloor, M., Berufsbedingte Formaldehyd-Allergie vom Soforttyp, *Dermatosen,* 36, 101, 1988.

10. Lindskov, R., Contact urticaria to formaldehyde, *Contact Dermatitis,* 8, 333, 1982.

11. Soschin, D. and Leyden, J. J., Sorbic acid induced erythema and edema, *J. Am. Acad. Dermatol.,* 14, 234, 1986.

12. Lahti, A., Väänänen, A., Kokkonen, E.-L., and Hannuksela, M., Acetylsalicylic acid inhibits non-immunologic contact urticaria, *Contact Dermatitis,* 16, 133, 1987.

13. Johansson, J. and Lahti, A., Topical non-steroidal anti-inflammatory drugs inhibit non-immunologic immediate contact reactions, *Contact Dermatitis,* 19, 161, 1988.

14. Forsbeck, M. and Skog, E., Immediate reactions to patch tests with balsam of Peru, *Contact Dermatitis,* 3, 201, 1977.

15. Clemmensen, O. and Hjorth, N., Perioral contact urticaria from sorbic acid and benzoic acid in a salad dressing, *Contact Dermatitis,* 8, 1, 1982.

16. Larmi, E., Lahti, A., and Hannuksela, M., Ultraviolet light inhibits nonimmunologic immediate contact reactions to benzoic acid, *Arch. Dermatol. Res.,* 280, 420, 1988.

17. Larmi, E., Systemic effect of ultraviolet irradidiation on nonimmunologic immediate contact reactions to benzoic acid and methyl nicotinate, *Acta Dermatovenereologica (Stockh.),* 69, 296, 1989.

18. Hjorth, N. and Trolle-Lassen, C., Skin reactions to preservative in creams, *American Perfumer,* 77, 43, 1962.

19. Safford, R. J., Basketter, D. A., Allenby, C. F., and Goodwin, B. F. J., Immediate contact reactions to chemicals in the fragrance mix and a study of the quenching action of eugenol, *Br. J. Dermatol.,* 123, 595, 1990.

20. Gollhausen, R. and Kligman, A. M., Human assay for identifying substances which induce nonallergic contact urticaria: the NICU-test, *Contact Dermatitis,* 13, 98, 1985.

21. Rietschel, R. L., Contact urticaria from synthetic cassia oil and sorbic acid limited to the face, *Contact Dermatitis,* 4, 347, 1978.

22. Freitas, J. P. and Brandão, F. M., Contact urticaria to chlorocresol, *Contact Dermatitis,* 15, 252, 1986.

23. Goncalo, M., Goncalo, S., and Moreno, A., Immediate and delayed sensitivity to chlorocresol, *Contact Dermatitis,* 17, 46, 1987.

24. Henry, H. C., Tschen, E. H., and Becker, L. E., Contact urticaria to parabens, *Arch. Dermatol.,* 115, 1231, 1979.

25. Temesvári, E., Soos, G., Podányi, B., Kovács, I., and Nemeth, I., Contact urticaria provoked by balsam of Peru, *Contact Dermatitis,* 4, 65, 1978.

26. Mathias, C. G. T., Chappler, R. R., and Maibach, H. I., Contact urticaria from cinnamic aldehyde, *Arch. Dermatol.,* 116, 74, 1980.

27. Rudzki, E. and Grzywa, Z., Immediate reactions to balsam of Peru, cassia oil and ethyl vanillin, *Contact Dermatitis,* 2, 360, 1976.

28. Gaul, L. E., Dermatitis from cetyl and stearyl alcohols, *Arch. Dermatol.,* 99, 593, 1969.

29. Boyle, J. and Kennedy, C. T. C., Contact urticaria and dermatitis to Alphaderm®, *Contact Dermatitis,* 10, 178, 1984.

30. Maibach, H. I. and Conant, M., Contact urticaria to a corticosteroid cream: polysorbate 60, *Contact Dermatitis,* 3, 350, 1977.

31. Hardy, M. P. and Maibach, H. I., Contact urticaria syndrome from sorbitan sesquioleate in a corticosteroid ointment, *Contact Dermtitis,* 32, 114, 1995.

32. von Liebe, V., Karge, H.-J., and Burg, G., Kontakturtikaria, *Hautarzt,* 30, 544, 1979.
33. Nishioka, K., Doi, T., and Katayama, I., Histamine release in contact urticaria, *Contact Dermatitis,* 11, 191, 1984.
34. Okano, M., Nomura, M., Hata, S., Okada, N., Sato, K., Kitano, Y., Tashiro, M., Yoshimoto, Y., Hama, R., and Aoki, T., Anaphylactic symptoms due to chlorhexidine gluconate, *Arch. Dermatol.,* 125, 50, 1989.
35. Fisher, A. A., Contact urticaria from chlorhexidine, *Cutis,* 43, 17, 1989.
36. Susitaival, P. and Häkkinen, L., Anaphylactic allergy to chlorhexidine cream, in *Current Topics in Contact Dermatitis,* Frosch, P. J., Dooms-Goossens, A., Lachapelle, J.-M., Rycroft, R. J. G., and Scheper, R. J., Eds., Springer-Verlag, Berlin, 1989, 99.
37. Larmi, E., Lahti, A., and Hannuksela, M., Immediate contact reactions to benzoic acid and the sodium salt of pyrrolidone carboxylic acid. Comparison of various skin sites, *Contact Dermatitis,* 20, 38, 1989.
38. Brubaker, M. M., Urticarial reaction to ammonium persulfate, *Arch. Dermatol.,* 106, 413, 1972.
39. Calnan, C. D. and Shuster, S., Reactions to ammonium persulfate, *Arch. Dermatol.,* 88, 812, 1963.
40. Fisher, A. A. and Dooms-Goossens, A., Persulfate hair bleach reactions, *Arch. Dermatol.,* 112, 1407, 1976.
41. Roed-Petersen, J. and Hjorth, N., Contact dermatitis from antioxidants, *Br. J. Dermatol.,* 94, 233, 1976.
42. Osmundsen, P. E., Contact urticaria from nickel and plastic additives (*Butylhydroxytoluene, oleylamide*), *Contact Dermatitis,* 6, 452, 1980.
43. Edwards, E. K. Jr. and Edwards, E. K., Contact urticaria and allergic contact dermatitis caused by paraphenylenediamine, *Cutis,* 34, 87, 1984.
44. Rilliet, A., Hunziker, N., and Brun, R., Alcohol contact urticaria syndrome (Immediate-type hypersensitivity), *Dermatologica,* 161, 361, 1980.
45. Kanzaki, T. and Hori, H., Late phase allergic reaction of the skin to ethyl alcohol, *Contact Dermatitis,* 25, 252, 1991.
46. Wilkin, J. K. and Fortner, G., Ethnic contact urticaria to alcohol, *Contact Dermatitis,* 12, 118, 1985.
47. Funk, J. O. and Maibach, H. I., Propylene glycol dermatitis: re-evaluation of an old problem, *Contact Dermatitis,* 31, 236, 1994.
48. Guin, J. D., Meyer, B. N., Drake, R. D., and Haffley, P., The effect of quenching agents on contact urticaria caused by cinnamic aldehyde, *J. Am. Acad. Dermatol.,* 10, 45, 1984.
49. Allenby, C. F., Goodwin, B. F. J., and Safford, R. J., Diminution of immediate reaction to cinnamic aldehyde by eugenol, *Contact Dermatitis,* 11, 322, 1984.
50. Larmi, E., Lahti, A., and Hannuksela, M., Effects of sorbitan sesqioleate on nonimmunologic immediate contact reactions to benzoic acid, *Contact Dermatitis,* 19, 368, 1988.

13

Contact Urticaria from Dental Products

Lasse Kanerva

CONTENTS

13.1   INTRODUCTION

Dental personnel have a high risk to develop occupational allergic diseases. Patients treated for dental problems are exposed to the same substances and have the risk to develop allergy to the same compounds as the dental personnel. The present report gives a check-list on agents (Table 13.1) that putatively could elicit contact urticaria in dental personnel and patients and is based on previous summaries.[1,2] On the other hand, contact urticaria to the many agents in Table 13.1 has been reported from dental work and products in only a few cases.

TABLE 13.1   Agents Which Could Produce Immediate Contact Reactions in Dental Personnel and Their Patients

	Ref.		Ref.
1. Biologic products			
Blood		Saliva	
Dander	7	Serum	
Hair	7	Sweat	6
2. Fragrances and flavorings			
Balsam of Peru	15	Cinnamic aldehyde	14
Benzaldehyde	14	Menthol	42
Benzoic acid	16	Eugenol	12, 13
3. Medicaments			
Acetylsalicylic acid		Benzocaine	17
Aminophenazone & Pyrazolones	25, 26	Benzoyl peroxide	20
Antibiotics		Clobetasol-17-propionate	
Ampicillin		Etofenamate	27, 28
Bacitracin		Dinitrochlorobenzene	
Cephalosporins		Fumarates	28
Chloramphenicol		Phenothiazines	
Gentamicin		Propylene glycol	23
Iodochlorhydroxyquin		Sorbitan monolaurate	21
Neomycin		Sorbitan sesquioleate	22
Nifuroxime			
Rifamycin	24		
Streptomycin			
4. Metals and their salts			
Cobalt	31	Nickel	22, 32
Copper		Palladium	38, 39
Iridium	37	Platinum	34–36
Mercury	40	Rhodium	38, 39
5. Plant products			
Abietic acid	45	Lilies	49
Algae		Natural rubber latex	
Chrysanthemum	50	Perfumes	
Colophony	44	Spathe flower	48
Corn starch	43	Tobacco	51
Ficus benjamina	47	Tulips	49
6. Preservatives and disinfectants			
Alcohols (amyl, butyl, ethyl, isopropyl)	58	Methamizole	
Benzoic acid		Propylphenazone	

TABLE 13.1 (continued)   Agents Which Could Produce Immediate Contact Reactions in Dental Personnel and Their Patients

	Ref.		Ref.
Benzyl alcohol		Tocopherol	
Chlorhexidine	52, 53	p-Hydroxybenzoic acid	
Chloramine T	54–57	Parabens	
Chlorocresol		Phenylmercuric propionate	
1,3-diiodo-2-hydroxypropane		o-Phenylphenate	
Formaldehyde		Polysorbates	
Gentian violet		Sodium benzoate	59
Hexanetriol		Sodium hypochlorite	
Pyrazolones		Sorbitan monolaurate	
Aminophenazone		Tropicamide	

7. Rubber chemicals

	Ref.		Ref.
Mercaptobenzothiazol	60	Thiurams	62
Para-phenylenediamine	60	Zinc diethyldithiocarbamate	61

8. Acrylics					**63–67**

9. Miscellaneous

	Ref.		Ref.
Acetyl acetone		Naphthylacetic acid	
Ammonia		Nylon	
Ammonium persulphate		Oleylamide	
Aminothiazole		Patent blue dye	
Benzophenone		Perlon	
Butylated hydroxytoluene		Phosphorus sesquisulphide	
Carbonless copy paper		Polypropylene	
Cu(II)-acetyl acetonate		Polyethylene glycol	
Denatonium benzoate		Potassium ferricyanide	
Diethyltoluamide		Sodium sulphide	
Epoxy resin		Sulphur dioxide	
Formaldehyde resin		Terpinyl acetate	
Lanolin alcohols		Textile finish	69
Methyl ethyl ketone		Vinyl pyridine	
Monoamylamine		Xylene	68

13.2   STATISTICS

In Finland, dental assistants were the sixth most common occupational group with occupational contact urticaria during 1990-1994 (28 cases), and dentists the 21st (5 cases).[3] In regard to the frequency of occupations with occupational contact urticaria per 100,000 employed workers, in a "ranking list" dental assistants were the third most affected (102), and dentists the 14th most commonly affected group (23).[4] Most of the cases were due to natural rubber latex.

Compared to the numbers in Finland, Rudzki et al.[5] reported a very low incidence of contact urticaria in Poland. Among 574 patients with urticaria in an occupational dermatology clinic, only five (=1.1%) had contact urticaria; these were caused by rat tail, guinea pig, streptomycin, vinyl pyridine, and penicillin.

No data on the frequency of contact urticaria in dental patients are available.

13.3 CAUSATIVE PRODUCTS (TABLE 13.1)

13.3.1 Biologic Products

The exposure of hairdressers to biologic products such as hair, dander, and sweat[6] has been dealt with in this book.[7] Dental personnel used to be very much exposed to saliva, but this has diminshed due to the use of disposable gloves. Contact allergy from dog,[8] horse,[9] and cockroach saliva[10] has been reported.

13.3.2 Fragrances and Flavorings

Eugenol is a common allergen and is the essential chemical constituent of clove oil. It is also present in cinnamon oil, perfumes, soaps, bay rum, oil of carnation (hyacinth), pimento oil (allspice), flower oils, food spices, and flavors. In dentistry, eugenol is used in the zinc oxide-eugenol cement, toothache drops, and in antiseptics. It may also be combined with colophony.[11] When eugenol is used in dental preparations, such as impression pastes, surgical packing, and cements, it may produce stomatitis, eczema, or contact urticaria.[11] Contact urticaria from eugenol is probably nonimmunological.[12,13]

Contact urticaria may possibly be induced by many other fragrances, too,[13] although reports are scarce. Recently, contact urticaria was reported from cinnamic aldehyde and benzaldehyde.[14] Benzaldehyde may cross-react with Balsam of Peru,[15] as may benzoic acid.[16]

13.3.3 Medicaments

Dentists were earlier frequently sensitized to local anesthetics,[11] e.g., benzocaine, tetracaine, and procaine. These are used in a great number of products including preparations for toothache and teething.[11]

Benzocaine is a para-aminobenzoic acid (PABA) derivative. It cross-reacts with local anesthetic agents such as procaine, tetracaine, piperocaine, and cocaine. Benzocaine also cross-reacts with hair dyes, aniline dyes, and drugs such as para-aminobenzoic acid, parasalicylic acid, antidiabetic medications, and sulfonamides.[11]

LIDOCAINE (XYLOCAINE) is used as a local anesthetic and as an antiarrhythmic agent. It does not cross-react with benzocaine or tetracaine. Lidocaine is usually safe to use because allergic reactions are rare, but have been reported.[11]

Benzocaine has induced contact urticaria,[17] whereas the other "caines" have caused allergic contact dermatitis, but evidently very seldom contact urticaria.

BENZOYL PEROXIDE. In addition to its use in the treatment of acne and stasis ulcers, benzoyl peroxide is a catalyst for acrylic and polyester resins. Benzoyl peroxide in acne preparations and baking additives is a rare sensitizer, but when used on leg ulcers it is more common.[11] Benzoyl peroxide has caused stomatitis,[11] and two cases of allergic contact dermatitis (ACD) from manufacturing dental prostheses were reported by Calnan and Stevenson.[18] Recently, Quirce et al. reported airborne ACD from benzoyl peroxide.[19] Topical benzoyl peroxide for acne has caused contact urticaria.[20]

Corticosteroids may elicit both delayed and immediate allergies. Other components in corticosteroid ointment, e.g., sorbitan monolaureate[21] and sorbitan sesquioleate, have caused contact urticaria.[22] Propylene glycol is widely used in medical lotions and creams and may induce immediate skin reactions.[23] Various antibiotics, used or not used by dentists, e.g., rifamycin,[24] may cause contact urticaria. Pain-relieving chemicals, e.g., aminophenazone, have caused contact urticaria.[25,26] Dental personnel may develop contact urticaria from their patients' topical medicaments, or vice versa, e.g., from anti-inflammatory ointments, such as etofenamate,[27,28] or from monoethyl fumarate.[29]

13.3.4 Metals

Vilaplana et al.[30] charted the metals used in dental prostheses. They are: gold, platinum, palladium, silver, copper, zinc, tin, indium, gallium, cobalt, chrome, nickel, titanium, molybdenum, iron, beryllium, manganese, wolfram, aluminum, and yttrium. Table 13.1 lists metals that have caused contact urticaria, e.g., cobalt[31] and nickel.[32,33] Nickel is a rare cause of contact urticaria.[32,33] Platinum is a strong type I allergen,[34-36] and recently iridium, one of the platinum group metals, was reported to induce respiratory allergy and contact urticaria.[37] Other metals in the platinum group that have caused immediate allergy are ruthenium, rhodium, and palladium.[38,39]

Mercury salts[40] and sodium fluoride,[41] which was present in 31% of the toothpastes sold in Finland,[42] have caused contact urticaria.

13.3.5 Plant Products

Natural rubber latex (NRL) is the most common cause of contact urticaria in health care personnel, including dental personnel. NRL-allergic dental patients may develop serious reactions, because the strongest reactions have usually occurred from mucosal exposure. Contact urticaria due to corn-starch glove powder seems to be rare,[43] but has caused anaphylactic reactions.

Colophony is widely used in dentistry. In addition to colophony,[44] contact urticaria has been reported from one of the allergens in colophony, namely abietic acid.[45]

Decorative plants at work places have caused serious, unexpected allergic eruptions,[46,47] and should be remembered as a source of occupational[48] or nonoccupational allergy.[49,50] Even tobacco has caused contact urticaria.[51]

13.3.6   Preservatives and Disinfectants

Chlorhexidine recently caused anaphylactic reactions in two dental patients in Denmark.[52,53] Both patients were healthy and unaware of their sensitivity. One patient developed anaphylaxis when chlorhexidine liquid was sprayed into the cavity after extraction of a wisdom tooth. The other patient suffered from pericoronitis, and developed anaphylaxis when Hibitane Dental Gel 1% (i.e., chlorhexidine) was applied to the gingival pocket.

In Finland, the use of chloramine-T has greatly increased among health care personnel, including dental personnel. Four patients with asthma and allergic rhinitis were recently reported from our institute.[54] Immediate allergic reactions[55] caused by chloramine-T are IgE-mediated.[56,57]

Various types of alcohols, including ethanol, may elicit contact urticaria.[58] Sodium benzoate caused airborne contact urticaria to a worker at a pharmaceutical plant.[59]

13.3.7   Rubber Chemicals

On rare occasions, chemicals, and not the natural rubber latex proteins, have been reported to cause contact urticaria from rubber products.[60-62]

13.3.8   Acrylics

Immediate hypersensitivity, such as contact urticaria (see below), pharyngitis, and/or bronchial asthma from cyanoacrylates, methyl methacrylate, acrylic acid, and non-specified acrylics has been reported,[63-67] but the mechanism of action is not known. We reported 18 cases of respiratory hypersensitivity from acrylics, mainly asthma,[64] but prick tests have not been positive, indicating that other than IgE-mediated mechanisms may be involved.

13.3.9   Miscellaneous

A large number of products that dental personnel and their patients could come into contact with have caused contact urticaria (Table 13.1). For example, xylene, used in medical laboratories, has caused contact urticaria.[68] Even clothes and textile finish have caused strong contact urticaria reactions.[69]

13.4   CONCLUDING REMARKS

It is not very unusual that patients develop immediate skin and mucosal reactions during dental treatment, but the reason often remains unknown. The present chapter may help to clarify possible causes.

REFERENCES

1. Lahti, A., Immediate contact reactions, In: Rycroft, R.J.G., Menné, T. and Frosch, P.J., Eds., *Textbook of Contact Dermatitis,* 2nd ed., Springer Verlag, 62, 1995.
2. Kanerva, L., Estlander, T. and Jolanki, R., Occupational skin allergy in the dental profession, *Derm., Clin.,* 12, 517, 1994.
3. Kanerva, L., Toikkanen, J., Jolanki, R. and Estlander, T., Statistical data on occupational contact urticaria, *Contact Dermatitis,* 35, 229, 1996.
4. Kanerva, L., Jolanki, R., Toikkanen, J. and Estlander, T., Statistics on occupational contact urticaria, In: Amin, S., Lahti, A. and Maibach H. I., Eds., *Contact Urticaria Syndrome,* CRC Press Inc, Boca Raton, FL, 1997.
5. Rudzki, E., Rebandel, P. and Grzywa, Z., Incidence of contact urticaria, *Contact Dermatitis,* 13, 279, 1985.
6. Freeman, S., Woman allergic to husband's sweat and semen. *Contact Dermatitis,* 14, 110, 1985.
7. Leino, T. and Kanerva, L., Contact urticaria from hairdressing products, In: Amin, S., Lahti, A. and Maibach H. I., Eds., *Contact Urticaria Syndrome,* CRC Press Inc, Boca Raton, FL, 1997.
8. Calnan, C.D., Allergy to dog saliva, *Contact Dermatitis Newsletter,* 3, 40, 1968.
9. van der Mark, S., Contact urticaria from horse saliva, *Contact Dermatitis,* 9, 145, 1983.
10. Kanerva, L., Tarvainen, K., Tupasela, O., Kaarsalo, K. and Estlander, T., Occupational allergic contact dermatitis caused by cockroach *(Blaberus giganteus), Contact Dermatitis,* 33, 445, 1995.
11. Fisher, A.A., *Contact Dermatitis,* 3rd ed., Philadelphia, Lea & Febiger, 1986.
12. Warin, R.P. and Smith, R.J., Chronic urticaria. Investigations with patch and challenge tests, *Contact Dermatitis,* 8, 117, 1982.
13. Safford, R.J., Basketter, D.A., Allenby, C.F. and Goodwin, B.F.J., Immediate contact reactions to chemicals in the fragrance mix and a study of the quenching effect of eugenol, *Br. J. Dermatol.,* 123, 596, 1990.
14. Seite-Bellezza, D., el-Sayed, F. and Bazex, J., Contact urticaria from cinnamic aldehyde and benzaldehyde in a confectioner, *Contact Dermatitis,* 31, 272, 1994.
15. Hjorth, N., Eczematous allergy to balsams, allied perfumes and flavouring agents, *Acta Derm. Venereol. (Stockh),* 41, suppl 46, 1961.
16. Lahti, A., Oikarinen, A., Viinikka, L., Ylikorkala, O. and Hannuksela, M., Prostaglandins in contact urticaria induced by benzoic acid, *Acta Derm.-Venereol. (Stockh),* 63, 425, 1983.
17. Ryan, M.E., Brian, M.D. and Marks, J.G., Contact urticaria and allergic contact dermatitis to benzocaine gel, *J. Am. Acad. Dermatol.,* 2, 221, 1980.
18. Calnan, C.D. and Stevenson, C.J., Studies in contact dermatitis XV: Dental materials, *Trans. St John's Hosp. Dermatol. Soc.,* 49, 9, 1963.
19. Quirce, S., Olaguibel, J.M. and Garcia, B.E., et al., Occupational airborne contact dermatitis due to benzoyl peroxide, *Contact Dermatitis,* 29, 165, 1993.
20. Tkach, J.R., Allergic contact urticaria to benzoyl peroxide, *Cutis,* 29, 187, 1982.
21. Boyle, J. and Kennedy, C.T.C., Contact urticaria and dermatitis to Alphaderm®/R, *Contact Dermatitis,* 10, 178, 1984.
22. Hardy, M. and Maibach, H.I., Contact urticaria syndrome from sorbitan sesquioleate in a corticosteroid ointment, *Contact Dermatitis,* 32, 360, 1995.
23. Funk, J.O. and Maibach, H.I., Propylene glycol dermatitis: re-evaluation of an old problem, *Contact Dermatitis,* 31, 236, 1994.

24. Mancuso, G. and Masara, N., Contact urticaria and severe anaphylaxis from rifamycin SV, *Contact Dermatitis,* 27, 124, 1992.

25. Lombardi, P., Giorgini, S. and Achille, A., Contact urticaria from aminophenazone, *Contact Dermatitis,* 9, 428, 1983.

26. Maucher, O.M. and Fuchs, A., Kontakturtikaria im Epikutantest bei Pyrazolonallergie, *Hautarzt,* 34, 383, 1983.

27. Pinol, J. and Carapeto, F., Contact urticaria to etofenamate, *Contact Dermatitis,* 11, 132, 1984.

28. Götze, A., Teikemeier, G. and Goerz, G., Contact dermatitis from etofenamate, *Contact Dermatitis,* 26, 209, 1992.

29. Ducker, P. and Pfeiff, B., Zwei Fälle von Nebenwirkungen einer Fumarsäureester Lokaltherapie, *Z. Hautkr.,* 65, 734, 1990.

30. Vilaplana, J., Romaguera, C. and Cornellana, F., Contact dermatitis and adverse oral mucous membrane reactions related to the use of dental prostheses, *Contact Dermatitis,* 30, 80, 1994.

31. Smith, J.D., Odom, R.B. and Maibach, H.I., Contact urticaria from cobalt chloride, *Arch. Dermatol.,* 111, 1610, 1975.

32. Jones, T.K., Hansen, C.A., Singer, M.T. and Kessler, H.P., Dental implications of nickel hypersensitivity, *J. Prosthet. Dent.,* 56, 507, 1986.

33. Estlander, T., Kanerva, L., Tupasela, O., Keskinen, H. and Jolanki, R., Immediate and delayed allergy to nickel with contact urticaria, rhinitis, asthma and contact dermatitis, *Clin. Exp. Allergy,* 23, 306, 1993.

34. Hunter, D., Milton, R. and Perry, K., Asthma caused by the complex salts of platinum, *Br. J. Ind. Med.,* 2, 92, 1945.

35. Baker, D.B., Gann, P.H., Brooks, S.M., Gallagher, J. and Bernstein, I.L., Cross-sectional study of platinum salts sensitization among precious metals refinery workers, *Am. J. Ind. Med.,* 18, 653, 1990.

36. Schena, D., Barba, A. and Costa, G., Occupational contact urticaria to cisplatin, *Contact Dermatitis,* 34, 220, 1996.

37. Bergman, A, Svedberg, U. and Nilsson, E., Contact urticaria and anaphylactic reactions caused by occupational exposure to iridium salt, *Contact Dermatitis,* 32, 14, 1995.

38. Murdoch, R.D., Pepys, J. and Hughes, E.G., IgE-antibody responses to platinum group metals: a Large scale refinery survey, *Br. J. Ind. Med.,* 43, 37, 1986.

39. Murdoch, R.D. and Pepys, J., Platinum group metal sensitivity: Reactivity to platinum group metal salts in platinum halide salt-sensitive workers, *Ann. Allergy,* 59, 464, 1987.

40. Torresani, C,. Caprari, E., Manara, G.C., Contact urticaria syndrome due to phenyl-mercuric acetate, *Contact Dermatitis,* 29, 282, 1993.

41. Camarasa, J.G., Serra-Baldrich, E., Lluch, M. and Malet A., Contact urticaria from sodium fluoride, *Contact Dermatitis,* 28, 294, 1993.

42. Sainio, E-L. and Kanerva, L., Contact allergens in toothpastes and a review of their hypersensitivity, *Contact Dermatitis,* 33, 100, 1995.

43. Fisher, A.A., Contact urticaria due to cornstarch surgical powder, *Cutis,* 38, 307, 1986.

44. Rivers, J.K. and Rycroft, R.J.C., Occupational allergic contact urticaria from colophony, *Contact Dermatitis,* 17, 181, 1987.

45. El-Sayed, F., Manzur, F., Bayle, P., Marquery, M.S. and Bazek, J., Contact urticaria from abietic acid, *Contact Dermatitis,* 32, 361, 1995.

46. Lidén, C., Contact allergy: a cause of facial dermatitis among visual display operators, *Am. J. Contact Dermatitis,* 1, 171, 1990.

47. Schmid, P., Stoger, P. and Wütrich, B., Severe isolated allergy to Ficus benjamina after bedroom exposure, *Allergy,* 48, 466, 1993.

48. Kanerva, L., Mäkinen-Kiljunen, S., Kiistala, R. and Granlund, H., Occupational allergy caused by spathe flower (Spathiphyllum wallisii), *Allergy,* 50, 174, 1995.

49. Lahti, A., Contact urticaria and respiratory symptoms from tulips and lilies, *Contact Dermatitis,* 14, 317, 1986.

50. Tanaka, T., Moriwaki, S.I. and Horio, T., Occupational dermatitis with simultaneous immediate and delayed allergy to chrysanthemum, *Contact Dermatitis,* 16, 152, 1987.

51. Tosti, A., Melino, M. and Veronesi, S., Contact urticaria to tobacco, *Contact Dermatitis,* 16, 225, 1987.

52. Petersen, J.K., Et tilfaelde af akut anafylaktisk shock efter mundskyldning med klorhexidinoplosning, *Tandlaegebladet,* 98, 335, 1994 (in Danish).

53. Petersen, J.K. and Heiden, M., Nyt tilfaelde af anafylaktisk shock over for klorheksidin, *Tandlaegebladet,* 99, 733, 1995 (in Danish).

54. Nordqvist, E., Keskinen, H., Tuppurainen, M. and Pekkarinen, E., Kloramiini-T ja sen aiheuttamat hengitystieallergiat Suomessa, In: Kanerva, L., Jolanki, R., Toikkanen, J. and Keskinen, H., Työperäiset allergiat v. 1993, *Työterveyslaitos,* 147, 1994, (in Finnish).

55. Dooms-Goossens, A., Gevers, D., Mertens, A. and Vanderheyden, D., Allergic contact urticaria duo to chloramine, *Contact Dermatitis,* 9, 319, 1983.

56. Beck, H., Type 1 reaction to chloramine, *Contact Dermatitis,* 9, 155, 1983.

57. Wass, U., Belin, L. and Eriksson, N.E., Immunological specificity of chloramine-T-induced IgE antibodies in serum from sensitized worker, *Clin. Exp. Allergy,* 19, 463, 1989.

58. Ophaswongse, S. and Maibach, H.I., Alcohol dermatitis: allergic contact dermatitis and contact urticaria syndrome, A review, *Contact Dermatitis,* 30, 1, 1994.

59. Nethercott, J.R., Lawrance, M.J., Roy, A.M. and Gibson, B.L., Airborne contact urticaria due to sodium benzoate in a pharmaceutical manufacturing plant, *J. Occup. Med.,* 26, 734, 1984.

60. Belsito, D.V., Contact urticaria caused by rubber. Analysis of seven cases, *Dermatol. Clin.,* 8, 61, 1990.

61. Helander, I. and Mäkelä, A., Contact urticaria to zinc diethyldithiocarbamate (ZDC), *Contact Dermatitis,* 9, 327, 1983.

62. van Ketel, W. G., Contact urticaria from rubber gloves after dermatitis from thiurams, *Contact Dermatitis,* 11, 323, 1984.

63. Kanerva, L., Estlander, T., Jolanki, R., et al., Occupational pharyngitis associated with allergic patch test reactions from acrylics, *Allergy,* 47, 571, 1992.

64. Savonius, B., Keskinen, H. Tuppurainen, M. and Kanerva, L., Occupational respiratory disease caused by acrylics, *Clin. Exp. Allergy,* 23, 416, 1993.

65. Taylor, J.S., Acrylic reactions — ten years' experience, In: Frosch, P.J., Dooms-Goossens, A., Lachapelle, J-M., Rycroft, R.J.G. and Scheper, R.J., Eds., *Current Topics in Contact Dermatitis,* Springer, Berlin, 346, 1989.

66. Fowler, J.F., Immediate contact hypersensitivity to acrylic acid, *Dermatol. Clin.,* 8, 193, 1990.

67. Daecke, C., Schaller, S., Schaller, J. and Gos, M., Contact urticaria from acrylic acid in Fixomull tape, *Contact Dermatitis,* 29, 216, 1993.

68. Palmer, K.T. and Rycroft, R.J.C., Occupational airborne contact urticaria due to xylene, *Contact Dermatitis,* 28, 44, 1993.
69. de Groot, A.C. and Gerkens, F., Contact urticaria from a chemical textile finish, *Contact Dermatitis,* 20, 63, 1989.

14

Contact Urticaria, Dermatitis, and Respiratory Allergy Caused by Enzymes

Lasse Kanerva and Jonas Brisman

CONTENTS

14.1 INTRODUCTION

Chemical reactions in biological systems often occur in the presence of catalysts, called enzymes. Enzymes are proteins or glycoproteins, and accelerate biological reactions by factors of at least a million.

This report is based on a recent document by Brisman,[1] and is focused on immunologically mediated adverse effects of enzymes on the skin. As most data on enzyme allergy come from studies on the respiratory tract, these are also reviewed. General aspects of enzymes, such as occurrence, production, and use, are included.

The available documentation reflects the way of describing the toxic effects of environmental factors: first come case reports, then cross-sectional studies. Unfortunately, studies on enzymes with a longitudinal epidemiologic design are rare.[1]

14.2 OCCURRENCE, PRODUCTION, AND USE

Enzymes have been used since prehistoric times, when it was discovered that juice extracted from grapes could be turned into wine.[2] Similar observations, such as how to leaven bread and brew beer, were made during the later centuries. In the 19th century, scientists studying the process of fermentation discovered the existence of enzymes. In 1833, Anselm Payen and Jean Francois Persoz isolated a substance from malt which converted starch into sugar. This substance was an amylase enzyme. In 1876 William Kühne proposed the word "enzyme," which comes from Greek words "en" meaning "in," and "zyme," meaning "yeast," i.e., *in the yeast*.[1,2]

Enzymes have had an important role in the detergent industry during this century, although enzyme-containing animal bile is said to have been used in washing since ancient times. The first commercial enzyme-containing washing powder, *Burnus,* was marketed in 1913. This trypsin-containing powder was not a success, because it was unstable.

In 1959, the Swiss Ferment Company in Basel marketed the washing powder Bio 40. The enzyme was a protease from one of the species of *Bacillus subtilis.* This was a major advance in enzyme technology, since the bacteria could be fermented in large tanks, thus permitting mass production without dependence upon animal organs.[1]

Meanwhile, the Danish firm Novo Industry A/S developed a subtilisin preparation stable under the conditions of heat and alkalinity existing in normal laundering. Alcalase was introduced in 1962. The breakthrough for enzyme-containing washing powders came when Novo, in collaboration with Swiss and Dutch firms, put their products on the European market in 1965 and in America in the following years.[1] By the end of the 1960s, half of the European and North American textile detergents contained enzymes.[1-5]

The market for enzymes has an estimated turnover of USD 1 billion yearly[3] with an annual increase of 8–12%.[1] By the year 2000, the market may be USD 1.5 billion.[3-5] In Scandinavia, there is enzyme production in Denmark and Finland.[1] The production is mainly based on fermentation in tanks with *Bacillus, Aspergillus, Streptomyces,* or *Trichoderma microorganisms.*[1,3,4] Extraction from plants (papain,

TABLE 14.1   Industrial Enzymes and Their Major Applications[1,3]

Acylase	pharmaceuticals
Amylase	alcohol production, animal feed, baking, brewing, detergents, pulp and paper, starch- and sugar production, textile industry, wine and fruit juice
Amyloglucosidase	baking, brewing
Cellulase (cellobiohydrolases, endoglucanes, beta-glukosidases)	alcohol production, animal feed, brewing, protein industry, pulp and paper, textile industry, baking
Chymotrypsin	pharmaceuticals
Glucanase	animal feed, brewing, wine and fruit juice
Glucosidase	alcohol production
Glucoseisomerase	starch- and sugar production
Glucoseoxidase	baking
Lactase	dairy
Lipase	dairy, leather production, oils and fat, starch and sugar production, wine and fruit juice
Pectinase	wine and fruit juice
Protease	alcohol production, animal feed, baking, brewing, detergents, leather production, meat portioning, protein industry
Pullulase	starch- and sugar production
Streptokinase	pharmaceuticals
Trypsine	pharmaceuticals
Urokinase	pharmaceuticals
Xylanase (Hemicellulase)	pulp and paper

bromelain) and animal pancreases also occurs. With the use of modern molecular biology and genetic technology, more purified and effective enzymes can be produced in large quantities using microbes, bacteria, and molds. More than 2000 enzymes are known,[3] and the currently used enzymes and their applications are given in Table 14.1.

14.3   OCCUPATIONAL EXPOSURE

Enzymes can be found today in a wide range of occupational settings. Bakers are probably the largest exposed occupational group since enzyme, mainly alfa-amylase, is routinely added to flour in many countries.[6] The major enzyme applications are listed in Table 14.2.

14.4   TOXICOKINETICS AND MECHANISMS OF TOXICITY

Enzyme exposure occurs from dust or liquid aerosols.[1] The particles are deposited on the skin or on the mucous membranes of the airways. When an enzyme comes into contact with the skin or the respiratory tract, antibodies to this enzyme may be

TABLE 14.2 Major Enzyme Applications and Used Enzymes or Enzyme Groups.[1,3,26]

Alcohol production	amylase	Leather production	lipase
	cellulase		protease
	glukoamylase	Meat portioning	protease
	glucosidase	Oils and fat	lipase
	protease	Pharmaceuticals	acylase
Animal feed	amylase		alkaline phosphatase
	cellulase		bromelin
	glucanase		chymotrypsin
	hemicellulase		glucose oxidase
	phytase		papain
	protease		penicillinase
Baking	amylase		peroxidase
	amyloglucosidase		protease
	cellulase		streptokinase
	glucoseoxidase		trypsine
	hemicellulase		urokinase
	protease	Protein industry	cellulase
Brewing	amylase		protease
	amyloglucosidase	Pulp and paper	amylase
	carbohydrase	industry	hemicellulase
	cellulase		cellulase
	glucanase		lipase
	glucoamylase		pectinase
	papain		xylanase
	peptidase	Starch and sugar	amylase
	protease	production	cellulase
Cheese	pepsin		glucanase
manufacturing	rennin (chymosin)		glucoamylase
Composting	cellulase		glucoseisomerase
Contact lens	catalase		lipase
detergent	lipase		pullulase
	mucinase	Textile industry	amylase
	papain		cellulase
	protease	Wine and fruit juice	amylase
Cosmetology	papain		glucanase
Dairy	lactase		lipase
	lipase		pectinase
Detergents	amylase		
	cellulase		
	lipase		
	protease		

formed, resulting in IgE-mediated sensitization. Other isotypes may be formed, mainly IgG, but they seem to be markers of exposure rather than mediating symptoms. An allergic contact dermatitis may arise if there is a cell-mediated allergic reaction in the skin. Direct enzymatic action may cause irritant effects in enzyme-exposed tissue.[1]

14.5   SKIN

14.5.1   Irritant Dermatitis

Irritant dermatitis from pineapples, apparently from bromelain, was reported more than four decades ago.[7] After the introduction of enzyme-containing washing powders, there was much concern about possible dermatological effects among users. These effects were regarded as irritative, caused by nonenzymatic ingredients,[8-10] or a combination of enzymatic and detergent action.[11]

Ducksbury and Dave in 1970 reported a cross-sectional questionnaire study among home-helps.[12] The prevalence of detergent-associated dermatitis was 5%. Patch tests with enzyme-containing detergents were negative. Bolam concluded in 1970 after a study among housewives that enzymatically active washing powders were not more of an irritant than conventional powders.[13] In 1972, Göthe et al. reported on 50 workers exposed to enzymes during detergent production;[14] 47% reported work-related skin symptoms, and the reactions were regarded as irritative. Generalized urticaria upon enzyme contact, probably reflecting the contact urticaria syndrome, was reported in one case.[14] Irritant dermatitis was also reported from Switzerland, Finland, Japan, and Denmark.[11,15-18] Zachariae et al. in 1973 reported 79 workers with skin symptoms and exposure in enzyme production, and 12 unexposed controls.[17] Patch tests with subtilisin were negative. A high enzyme concentration was considered to cause irritant dermatitis.

14.5.2   Allergic Reactions

Then, for a long time, there were very few reports on skin symptoms from enzymes, but in 1987 Schirmer et al. described one baker with dermatitis.[19] He had positive skin prick tests to alfa-amylase and various bread improvers. The immediate test reaction to alfa-amylase persisted for 48 hours. A patch test with alfa-amylase was also positive, as well as RAST to alfa-amylase, malt, and bread improvers.

Four cases of contact urticaria developing after 0.5–4 years of exposure to the enzymes cellulase and xylanase were reported in 1990 by Kanerva and Tarvainen.[20] All cases later developed rhinitis and asthma, and two of them an allergic contact dermatitis.[21] Skin prick tests were positive to cellulase and xylanase in all cases (Table 14.3). A patch test was positive to cellulase in one case and to xylanase in the other. By the end of 1993, 25 cases of occupational allergy had been detected at the Institute of Occupational Health, Helsinki, Finland: 19 had asthma and allergic rhinitis, and 6 had allergic rhinitis.[3] During chamber provocation tests, 5 developed symptoms of contact urticaria. Probably contact urticaria was much more frequent, as many patients complained of such symptoms at work. Several patients also had pharyngitis or laryngitis related to enzyme exposure.[22] Most of the 25 cases with occupational allergy[3] had been exposed to enzymes in the enzyme production

**TABLE 14.3	Characteristics and Test Results of Four Patients Allergic to Enzymes**

	1	2	3	4
Age(Y)/Sex	49/F	38/F	25/M	29/F
Occupation	Lab. Assistant	Lab. Assistant	Process Worker	Lab. Assistant
Enzymes Exposed to	Xylanase Cellulase Amylase	Cellulase	Cellulase	Xylanase Cellulase
Duration of Exposure (Y)	4	2	2	0.5
Causative Enzyme	Xylanase	Cellulase	Cellulase	Xylanase
Symptoms	Asthma Rhinitis Urticaria	Rhinitis Urticaria Dermatitis	Asthma Urticaria	Asthma Urticaria Dermatitis
Prick Tests				
Cellulase	0.01%; Neg	0.001%; 3+	0.01%; 3+	0.001%; 2+
Xylanase	0.01%; 3+	0.001%; 3+	ND	0.001%; 3+
Own/Family Atopy	–/+	+/+	+/+	–/+
Total IgE (kU/L)	72	4500	1000	110
Patch Tests				
Cellulase	ND	3.3%; 3+ 1%; 3+ 0.33%; 3+	ND	Neg
Xylanase	ND	Neg	ND	3.3%; 3+ 1%; 3+ 0.33%; 3+
Standard Series	Neg	Neg	Neg	Neg
Specific IgE (Normal Below 0.35 PRU/ml)				
Cellulase (PRU/ml)	6.2	1200	175	3.6
Xylanase (PRU/ml)	6.5	490	68	1.4

Abbreviations:	ND, Not Done; Neg, Negative; PRU, Phadebas RAST Units; Y, years.

From Tarvainen, K., *Clin. Exp. Allergy,* 21, 609, 1991. With permission.

industry, where the total number of exposed workers was only 300–400, indicating the great potential of enzymes to sensitize.[3]

Contact urticaria from papain has been reported by Baur et al.[23] in papain workers, and by Bernstein et al.,[24] Santucci et al.,[25] and Podmore and Storrs,[26] from contact lens cleansing solutions. Papain persists in the soft lens matrix despite careful rinsing.[27] In a factory manufacturing papain, Baur[23] reported 17 out of 33 workers who developed type-1 reactions such as periorbital edema, conjunctival irritation, or allergic asthma.

In a cross-sectional study, Brisman and Belin reported in 1991 on 20 amylase-exposed workers who had significantly more skin symptoms than the controls.[28] In 1993, Morren et al.[29] reported on 32 consecutive bakers patch tested with alfa-amylase. Seven had an immediate reaction, and two had a positive delayed skin test. Four of the seven were skin prick tested to alfa-amylase and they were all positive.

14.5.2.1 Clinical Symptoms

Contact urticaria may present as whealing on the contact sites[30] but may also present as generalized symptoms. Apparently the mild form, i.e., "non-visible" contact urticaria[30] is only seldom diagnosed, but may be much more common.

14.5.3 Systemic Contact Allergic Reactions and Food Allergy

Mansfield and Bowers[31] reported a man who developed periorbital edema on ingestion of papain-treated meat. Recently, Del Pozo and co-workers[32] described a patient who developed generalized dermatitis after taking digestive tablets containing amylase, protease, and cellulase enzymes. Type IV hypersensitivity was believed to be involved. On the other hand, only some people who have allergic contact dermatitis develop systemic reactions after ingesting the allergen.[33] Therefore, patients with type IV hypersensitivity may be able to eat products containing the allergen. Since 1989, it has been permissible in Finland to add, e.g., cellulase to white bread dough to break up roughage. Four patients, allergic to cellulase, could eat white bread without any symptoms.[21] On the other hand, recently it has been suspected that enzymes in bread may cause food allergy.[34,35]

Detergent enzymes are currently unusual causes of occupational allergies.[36,37]

14.6 RESPIRATORY TRACT

14.6.1 Detergent Enzymes in Occupational Settings

The first adverse effects from handling detergent enzymes were reported in 1969 by Flindt.[38,39] He observed an epidemic among the workers in a detergent powder factory in 1967: 28 patients had symptoms of the respiratory tract. Positive skin prick tests and precipitating antibodies with detergent enzyme extract indicated an immediate allergy.[38] Pepys and co-workers reported immunological findings in three selected patients referred from Flindt.[40] Apart from reproducing the skin prick tests, they found immediate and late asthmatic reactions to inhalation tests with enzyme powder.[40] Occupational asthma was also reported the same year in the German literature.[41]

Since then, numerous studies dealing with respiratory allergy have been published. The interested reader is referred to the original reports (for references, see Brisman[1]).

14.6.2 Nonoccupational Exposure to Detergent Enzymes

In 1970, Belin et al. reported three cases of enzyme allergy in housewives.[42] They had symptoms while handling detergent enzymes, were positive to skin prick tests, and presented with IgE antibodies, but no IgG antibodies. Falleroni and Schwartz reported a similar case.[43] Shapiro and Eisenberg tested 35 consecutive allergic housewives without occupational exposure to enzymes.[44] Four had strongly positive intradermal tests, including one with asthma from detergent powders.

TABLE 14.4   Allergy from Proteolytic Enzymes

Enzyme	Ref.
Papain	50–57
Chymotrypsin	58–62
Pepsin	63–64
Bromelain	65–66
Pancreatic proteases	67
Proteolytic enzyme from *Aspergillus Niger*	68

Bernstein found positive skin tests to enzymes in 25% of 353 consecutive allergic patients in the U.S.,[45] but the enzyme extracts used for skin testing may have been too concentrated, causing nonspecific reactions.[46,47]

Zetterström and Wide tested 1132 patients of whom 21 (1.9%) had a positive RAST to subtilisin.[48] Pepys et al. studied 2500 consective patients, and only 2 had weak prick test reactions to enzyme preparations.[49] RAST tests were performed on sera from enzyme-exposed workers (with negative prick tests) and the 2500 consecutive patients. The latter were interviewed about the use of detergents and divided into unexposed, light, or heavy exposure groups. There were significant differences in RAST counts between the unexposed and light exposed, between light-and heavy exposed, as well as between heavy exposed patients and exposed workers. Table 14.4 lists references of reports on allergy from other proteolytic enzymes.[50-68]

14.6.3   Nonproteolytic Enzymes

The first report on adverse effects from the nonproteolytic enzyme alfa-amylase was reported by Flindt.[54] Eight workers in an enzyme-handling factory had respiratory symptoms. Five of them were skin prick test positive to α-amylase. Adverse effects from α-amylase as a baking additive were reported by Baur et al.[69] 118 sera from bakers were studied: 91 were screened at random and 27 because of work-related respiratory complaints. 34% of the symptomatic bakers had positive RAST to α-amylase, but none of the symptom-free ones. Skin prick tests and bronchial provocation tests in selected individuals were also positive.

The same author tested 140 sera from symptomatic bakers with RAST to a number of enzymes.[9] Of these, 24% were positive to α-amylase, 8% to hemicellulase or cellulase, 5% to amyloglycosidase, and 1% to papain or subtilisin. Quirce reported five cases of α-amylase sensitized bakers.[71] Different immunologic tests and bronchial provocations were positive. Four were also sensitized to cellulase.

Brisman and Belin reported four cases (all with rhinitis and three with asthma) from an enzyme handling factory.[28] A subsequent cross-sectional study in the same factory showed significantly more work-related nasal and skin problems in 20 exposed workers compared with controls.[28] Six exposed workers had positive skin prick tests. Nasal challenge tests validated three cases of α-amylase rhinitis. Specific IgG antibodies to α-amylase were detected in two nonsymptomatic workers.

TABLE 14.5   Prevalence of Positive Skin Tests to Enzymes According to Atopic Status

Number of tested workers	Percent with positive test		Author
	Atopics	Non-atopics	
121	64	33	Greenberg et al. (77)
640	43	13	Flood et al. (78)
459	26	18	Flood et al. (78)
1614	24	13	Flood et al. (78)
56	28	11	Göthe et al. (79)
1642	37	15	Juniper et al. (80)
155	77	45	Mitchell and Gandevia (81)
103	82	37	Newhouse and Foster (82)
65	83	23	Pepys et al.(49)

Losada reported a cross-sectional study of 83 pharmaceutical workers exposed to powdered α-amylase.[72] Of them, 59% reported rhinitis and 30% reported asthma. Their mean working time was 9.5 years, and 26 (31%) were skin prick test positive to α-amylase, but 6 of these were nonsymptomatic.

Tarvainen et al. reported four persons who were RAST-positive to both cellulase and xylanase.[21,73] There was cross-reactivity between the two enzymes. Losada described two cases from the packing department of a pharmaceutical firm, both with asthma.[74] They had immediate hypersensitivity to cellulase.

In a recent Finnish cross-sectional study in four bakeries,[3,75] one flour mill and one crisp bread factory, 12 workers in the bakeries (8%), 3 (5%) in the flour mill, and 4 (3%) in the crisp bread factory were skin prick positive to α-amylase and cellulase. The corresponding percentages of positive reactions to flours were 12, 5, and 8%, indicating that industrial enzymes in, e.g., bakeries, pose a considerable risk of sensitization.[75] In another recent study it was shown that enzymes with the same name (i.e., α-amylase) may have different antigenic characteristics.[76] A patient had occupational allergic contact urticaria from fungal but not bacterial α-amylase.[76]

14.7   ATOPICS AND ENZYME ALLERGY

Atopy, defined as having a history of atopy (childhood eczema, asthma, hay fever) and/or a positive prick test to one or more of common allergens, usually is a risk for developing IgE-mediated allergy to proteins. Studies in which the sensitization rate to enzymes is given in relation to atopic status are listed in Table 14.5,[49,77-82] indicating that both atopics and nonatopics can be sensitized to enzymes, but atopy increases the risk for sensitization. However, many researchers consider it unjustified to exclude atopics from work with proteins, e.g., enzymes.

The present knowledge of skin or respiratory allergy does not permit the setting of a NOAEL (No Observable Adverse Effect Level) for any industrial enzyme. Respiratory sensitization has been observed at levels of about 0.012 µg subtilisin/m^3 and 0.2–7.3 µg α-amylase/m^3, with commercial enzyme preparations as standards.[1]

14.8 CONCLUDING REMARKS

Skin irritation has been demonstrated for proteolytic enzymes, but patch tests in the 1960s and 1970s were negative. Recent case reports show positive patch tests to non-proteolytic enzymes (i.e., cellulase, amylase, xylanase). It is worth noting that these persons also have positive prick tests to the same enzymes. This may indicate that the observed patch test reactions in fact are IgE-mediated allergic reactions and not necessarily the classical type IV reactions, at least in some cases. This may also indicate that these enzymes are causative agents in developing contact urticaria, and that this urticaria may proceed to an allergic contact dermatitis.

When evaluating allergy caused by enzymes, it should be remembered that commercial enzymes are crude products, which may contain remnants of the growth material and the microorganism used for fermentation. They may also contain preservatives, e.g., benzoates, sorbates, and parabens, in addition to the main enzyme,[83,84] and other enzymes produced by the microbes.[3] These additional compounds may be the cause of enzyme allergy in some cases.[85]

Enzymes may be more prone to cause sensitization than other proteins because of their enzymatic capacity. Several common allergens, e.g., house dust mites, storage mites, ragweed, pollens, *Alternaria,* cats, and bee venoms are, in fact, enzymes.[86]

When performing skin tests, it is important to use test extracts with an appropriate concentration in order not to induce false positive reactions. Unfortunately, commercial test substances are not available, and tests must also be performed in nonexposed controls. Open tests on intact skin may give false negative results, and may not reflect the situation *in situ,* where coexisting exogenous factors may impair the function of the skin barrier.

REFERENCES

1. Brisman, J., Industrial enzymes, *Arbete och Hälsa,* 28, 1, 1994.
2. Brodeur, P., The Enigmatic Enzyme, *The New Yorker Magazine,* Jan 16, 1971.
3. Vanhanen, M., Nordman, H., Tuomi, T., Tupasela, O., et al., Teollisuusentsyymien käyttö ja entsyymiallergia Suomessa, (The use of industrial enzymes and allergy to enzymes in Finland, in Finnish), *Työsuojelurahaston loppuraportti,* Helsinki, 1, 1994.
4. Gerhartz, W., (Ed.), Enzymes in industry, Weinheim, *VCH Verlagsgesellschaft,* 1990.
5. Jokinen, O., Entsyymisovellutusten tulevaisuudennäkymät sellu- ja paperiteollisuudessa, (Prospects of enzyme applications in cellulose and paper industry, in Finnish), *Kemia-Kemi,* 3, 180, 1993.
6. Linko, Y.Y. and Linko, P., Enzymes in baking, In: Blanshard, J.M.V., Frazier, P.J. and Galliard, T., Eds., *Chemistry and Physics of Baking,* London, Royal Societ Cop, 1986.
7. Polunin, I., Pineapple dermatosis, *Br. J. Dermatol.,* 63, 441, 1951.
8. McMurrain, K.D., Dermatologic and pulmonary responses in the manufacturing of detergent enzyme products, *J. Occup. Med.,* 12, 416, 1970.
9. Jensen, N.E., Severe dermatitis and "biological" detergents, *Br. Med. J.,* 1, 299, 1970.
10. Smith, D.J., Mathias, C.G.T. and Greenwald, D.I., Contact dermatitis from *B. subtilis*-derived protease enzymes, *Contact Dermatitis,* 20, 58, 1989.

11. Wütrich, B., Schwarz, K. and Eichenbergern-De Beer, H., Zur Pathogenese von Hautschäden durch biologisch aktive, proteasenhaltige Waschmittel, *Dermatologica,* 142, 265, 1971.

12. Ducksbury, C.F.J. and Dave, V.K., Contact dermatitis in home helps following the use of enzyme detergents, *Br. Med. J.,* 1, 537, 1970.

13. Bolam, R.M., Severe dermatitis and "biological" detergents (letter), *Br. Med. J.,* 1, 817, 1970.

14. Göthe, C-J., Nilzén, Å., Holmgren, A., Szamosi, A., Werner, M. and Wide, L., Medical problems in the detergent industry caused by proteolytic enzymes from bacillus subtilis, *Acta Allergologica,* 27, 63, 1972.

15. Stubb, S., Entsyymipesuaineet hengitystie- ja iho-oireiden aiheuttajana, (Enzymes in detergents as cause of respiratory and skin symptoms, in Finnish), *Duodecim,* 88, 721, 1972.

16. Okamoto, K., Futami, T. and Kanda, Y., Skin irritation and allergy inductivity due to alkaline proteinases, *Eisei Kagaku,* 8, 304, 1972.

17. Zachariae, H., Thomsen, K. and Gowertz Rasmussen, O., Occupational enzyme dermatitis, *Acta Dermatovener* (Stockholm), 53, 145, 1973.

18. Niinimäki, A. and Saari, S., Dermatologic and allergic hazards of cheesemakers, *Scand. J. Work Environ. Hlth,* 4, 262, 1978.

19. Schirmer, R.H., Kalveram, K-J., Kalveram, C-M., Siebert, J. and Kunze, J., Chronisch lichenoide Dermatitis bei Sensibilisierung gegen Alpha-Amylase bei einem Bäcker, *Z. Hautkr.,* 62, 791, 1987.

20. Kanerva, L. and Tarvainen, K., Allergic contact dermatitis and contact urticaria from cellulolytic enzymes, *Am. J. Contact Dermatitis,* 1, 244, 1990.

21. Tarvainen, K., Kanerva, L., Tupasela, O., Grenquist-Nordén, B., Jolanki, R., Estlander, T. and Keskinen, H., Allergy from cellulase and xylanase enzymes, *Clin. Exp. Allergy,* 21, 609, 1991.

22. Hytönen, M., Vanhanen, M., Nordman, H., Keskinen, H., Tuomi, T. and Tupasela, O., Pharyngeal edema caused by occupational exposure to cellulase enzyme. *Allergy,* 49, 782, 1994.

23. Baur, X., König, G. Bencze, K. and Fruhmann, G., Clinical symptoms and results of skin test, RAST and bronchial provocation test in thirty three papain workers: evidence for strong immunogenic potency and clinically relevant "proteolytic effects of airborne papain", *Clin. Allergy,* 12, 9, 1982.

24. Bernstein, D.I., Gallagher, J.S., Grad, M. and Bernstein, I.L., Local ocular anaphylaxis to papain enzyme contained in a contact lens solution, *J. Allergy Clin. Immunol.,* 74, 258, 1984.

25. Santucci, B., Cristando, A. and Picarto, M., Contact urticaria from papain lens solution, *Contact Dermatitis,* 12, 233, 1985.

26. Podmore, P. and Storrs, F.J., Contact lens intolerance; allergic conjunctivitis, *Contact Dermatitis,* 20, 98, 1989.

27. Fichman, S., Baker, V.V. and Horton, H.R., Iatrogenic red eyes in soft contact lens wearers, *Int. Contact Lens. Clinic.,* 5, 202, 1978.

28. Brisman, J. and Belin, L., Clinical and immunological responses to occupational exposure to alfa-amylase in the baking industry, *Br. J. Ind. Med.,* 48, 604, 1991.

29. Morren, M-A., Janssens, V., Dooms-Goossens, A., Van Hoeyveld, E., Cornelis, A., De Wolf-Peeters, C. and Heremans, A., Alfa-amylase, a flour additive: An important cause of protein contact dermatitis in bakers, *J. Am. Acad. Dermatol.,* 29, 723, 1993.

30. Kligman, A., The spectrum of contact urticaria: wheals, erythema, and pruritus, *Derm. Clin.*, 8, 57, 1990.

31. Mansfield, L. E. and Bowers, C. H., Systemic reaction to papain in a nonoccupational setting, *J. Allergy Clin. Immunol.*, 71, 371, 1983.

32. Del Pozo, M.D., Navarro, J.A., Gastaminza, G., Munoz, D., Fernandez, E. and de Corres, L.F., Delayed systemic dermatitis from amylase, cellulase and protease, *Am. J. Contact Dermatitis*, 6, 9, 1995.

33. Menné, T. and Hjorth, N., Reactions from systemic exposure to contact allergens, *Sem. Dermatol.*, 1, 15, 1982.

34. Kanny, G. and Moneret-Vautrin, D.A., Alfa-amylase contained in bread can induce food allergy, *J. Allergy Clin. Immunol.*, 95, 132, 1995.

35. Baur, X., Sander, I., Jansen, A. and Czuppon, A.B., Sind Amylasen von Backmitteln und Backmehl relevante Nahrungsmittelallergene?, *Schweiz. Med. Wschr.*, 124, 846, 1994.

36. Kanerva, L., Jolanki, R., Toikkanen, J., Tarvainen, K. and Estlander, K., Statistics on occupational dermatoses in Finland. In: *Curr. Probl. Dermatol.*, vol 23, Karger Verlag, 28, 1995.

37. Kanerva, L., Jolanki, R., Toikkanen, J. and Keskinen, H., Työperäisten sairauksien rekisteriin ilmoitetut uudet tapaukset v. 1990-1994 (New cases reported to Register 1990-1994, in Finnish), In: Kanerva, L., Jolanki, R., Toikkanen, J. and Keskinen, H., Eds., *Työterveyslaitos*, 13, 1996.

38. Flindt, M.L.H., Pulmonary disease due to inhalation of derivatives of bacillus subtilis containing proteolytic enzyme, *Lancet*, i, 1177, 1969.

39. Flindt, M.L.H., Biological miracles and misadventures: identification of sensitization and asthma in enzyme detergent workers, *Am. J. Industr. Med.*, 29, 99, 1996.

40. Pepys, J., Longbottom, J.L., Hargreave, F.E. and Faux, J., Allergic reactions of the lungs to enzymes of Bacillus subtilis, *Lancet*, i, 1181, 1969.

41. Wütrich, B., Ott, F., Berufsasthma durch proteases in der Waschmittelindustrie, *Schweiz. Med. Wochenschr.*, 99, 1584, 1969.

42. Belin, L., Hoborn, J., Falsen, E. and André, J., Enzyme sensitisation in consumers of enzyme-containing washing powder, *Lancet*, i, 1153, 1970.

43. Falleroni, A.E. and Schwartz, D.P., Immediate hypersensitivity to enzyme detergents, *Lancet*, i, 548, 1971.

44. Shapiro, R.S. and Eisenberg, B.C., Sensitivity to proteolytic enzymes in laundry detergents, *J. Allergy*, 47, 76, 1971.

45. Bernstein, I.L., Enzyme allergy in populations exposed to long-term, low-level concentrations of household laundry products, *J. Allergy Clin. Immunol.*, 49, 219, 1972.

46. Belin, L. and Norman, P., Diagnostic tests in the skin and serum of workers sensitized to Bacillus subtilis enzymes, *Clin. Allergy*, 7, 55, 1977.

47. Pepys, J., Allergic asthma to Bacillus subtilis enzyme: A Model for the effects of inhalable proteins, *Am. J. Ind. Med.*, 21, 587, 1992.

48. Zetterström, O. and Wide, L., IgE-antibodies and skin test reactions to a detergent-enzyme in Swedish consumers, *Clin. Allergy*, 4, 273, 1974.

49. Pepys, J., Wells, I.D., D'Souza, M.F. and Greenberg, M., Clinical and immunological responses to enzymes of Bacillus subtilis in factory workers and consumers, *Clin. Allergy*, 3, 143, 1973.

50. Baur, X. and Fruhmann, G., Papain-induced asthma: diagnosis by skin test, RAST and bronchial provocation test, *Clin. Allergy*, 9, 75, 1979.

51. Beecher, W., Hyperaesthetic rhinitis and asthma due to digestive ferments, *Illinois Medical J.,* 59, 343, 1931.

52. Eyermann, C.H., Food allergy as the cause of nasal symptoms, *J. Am. Med. Assoc.,* 91, 312, 1928.

53. Flindt, M.L.H., Respiratory hazards from papain, *Lancet,* i, 430, 1978.

54. Flindt, M.L.H., Allergy to alfa-amylase and papain, *Lancet,* i, 1407, 1979.

55. Milne, J. and Brand, S., Occupational asthma after inhalation of dust of the proteolytic enzyme papain, *Br. J. Ind. Med.,* 32, 302, 1975.

56. Novey, H.S., Keenan, W.J., Fairshter, R.D., Wells, I.D., Wilson, A.F. and Culver, B.D., Pulmonary disease in workers exposed to papain: clinico-physiological and immunological studies, *Clin. Allergy,* 10, 721, 1980.

57. Tarlo, S.M., Shaikh, W., Bell, B., Cuff, M., Davies, G.M., Dolovich, J. and Hargreave, F.E., Papain-induced allergic reactions, *Clin. Allergy,* 8, 207, 1978.

58. Colten, H.R., Polakoff, P.L., Weinstein, S.F. and Strieder, D.J., Immediate hypersensitivity to hog trypsin resulting from industrial exposure, *N. Engl. J. Med.,* 292, 1050, 1975.

59. Hartmann, A.L., Wüthrich, B. and Baur, X., Allergisches Asthma auf Enzyme in Arzneimitteln, *Schweiz. Med. Wschr.,* 114, 916, 1984.

60. Howe, C., Erlanger, B.F., Beiser, S.M., Ellison, S.A. and Cohen, W., Hypersensitivity to purified trypsin and chymotrypsin, *New Eng. J. Med.,* 265, 332, 1961.

61. McLaren, W.R. and Aladjem, F., Allergy to chymotrypsin, *J. Allergy,* 28, 89, 1957.

62. Zweiman, B., Green, G., Mayock, R.L. and Hildreth, E.A., Inhalation sensitization to trypsin, *Allergy,* 39, 11, 1967.

63. Cartier, A., Malo, J.L., Pineau, L. and Dolovich, J., Occupational asthma due to pepsin, *J. Allergy Clin. Immunol.,* 73, 574, 1984.

64. Maisel, F.E., Pepsin allergy, Case report, *J. Allergy,* 11, 607, 1940.

65. Baur, X. and Fruhmann, G., Allergic reactions, including asthma, to the pineapple protease bromelain following occupational exposure, *Clin. Allergy,* 9, 443, 1979.

66. Galleguillos, F. and Rodrigues, J.C., Asthma caused by bromelain inhalation, *Clin. Allergy,* 8, 21, 1978.

67. Wiessmann, K.J. and Baur, X., Occupational lung disease following long-term inhalation of pancreatic extracts, *Eur. J. Respir. Dis.,* 66, 13, 1985.

68. Pauwels,R., Devos, M., Callens, L. and Van der Straeten, M., Respiratory hazards from proteolytic enzymes (letter), *Lancet,* i, 669, 1978.

69. Baur, X., Fruhmann, G., Haug, B., Rasche, B., Reiher, W. and Weiss, W., Role of Aspergillus amylase in baker's asthma (letter), *Lancet,* i, 43, 1986.

70. Baur, X., Weiss, W., Sauer, W., et al., Backmittel als Mitursache des Bäckerasthmas, *Dtsch. Med. Wochenschr.,* 11, 1275, 1988.

71. Quirce, S., Cuevas, M., Díes-Gómez, M.L., Fernández-Rivas, M., Hinojosa, M., Gonzáles, R. and Losada, E., Respiratory allergy to Aspergillus-derived enzymes in baker's asthma, *J. Allergy Clin. Immunol.,* 90, 970, 1992.

72. Losada, E., Hinojosa, M., Quirce, S., Sánchez-Cano, M. and Moneo, I., Occupational asthma caused by alfa-amylase inhalation: Clinical and immunologic findings and bronchial response patterns, *J. Allergy Clin. Immunol.,* 89, 118, 1992.

73. Tarvainen, K., Kanerva, L., Grenquist-Nordén, B. and Estlander, T., Berufsallergien durch Cellulase, Xylanase und Alpha-Amylase, *Z. Hautkr.,* 66, 964, 1991.

74. Losada, E., Hinojosa, M., Moneo, I., Dominguez, J., Gomez, M.L.D. and Ibanez, M.D., Occupational asthma caused by cellulase, *J. Allergy Clin. Immunol.,* 77, 635, 1986.

75. Vanhanen, M., Tuomi, T., Hokkanen, H., Tupasela, O., Tuomainen, A., Holmberg, P.C., Leisola, M. and Nordman, H., Enzyme exposure and enzyme sensitization in the baking industry, *Occup. Environ. Med.,* 53, 670, 1996.

76. Kanerva, L., Vanhanen, M. and Tupasela, O., Occupational allergic contact urticaria from fungal but not bacterial α-amylase, *Contact Dermatitis,* (in press).

77. Greenberg, M., Milne, J.F. and Watt, A., Survey of workers exposed to dusts containing derivatives of Bacillus Subtilis, *Br. Med. J.,* 2, 629, 1970.

78. Flood, D.F.S., Blofeld, R.E., Bruce, C.F., Hewitt, J.I., Juniper, C.P. and Roberts, D.M., Lung function, atopy, specific hypersensitivity, and smoking of workers in the enzyme detergent industry over 11 years, *Br. J. Ind. Med.,* 42, 43, 1985.

79. Göthe, C-J., Westlin, A. and Sundquist, S., Air-borne B. Subtilis enzymes in the detergent industry, *Int. Arch. Arbeitsmed.,* 29, 201, 1972.

80. Juniper, C.P., How, M.J., Goodwin, B.F.J. and Kinshott, A.K., Bacillus subtilis enzymes: a 7-year clinical, epidemiological and immunological study of an industrial allergen, *J. Soc. Occup. Med.,* 27, 3, 1977.

81. Mitchell, C. and Gandevia, B., Respiratory symptoms and skin reactivity in workers exposed to proteolytic enzymes in the detergent industry, *Am. Review. Respir. Dis.,* 104, 1, 1971.

82. Newhouse, M.L., Tagg,. B. and Pocock, S.J., An epidemiological study of workers producing enzyme washing powders, *Lancet,* i, 689, 1970.

83. Pariza, M.W. and Foster, E.M., Determining the safety of enzymes used in food processing, *J. Food Protect.,* 46, 453, 1983.

84. Tiikkainen, U., Louhelainen, K. and Nordman, H., Flour dust, *Arbete och Hälsa,* 27, 1, 1996.

85. Moneo, I., Alday, E., Sanchez-Agudo, L., Curiel, G., Lucena, R. and Calatrava, J.M., Skin-prick tests for hypersensitivity to alfa-amylase preparations, *Occup. Med.,* 45, 151, 1995.

86. Chabane, M.H., Abuaf, A. and Leynadier, F., Pourquoi certains allergenes sont-ils des enzymes, *Ann. Biol. Clin.,* 52, 425, 1994.

15

Contact Urticaria from Epoxy Resins

Riitta Jolanki, Lasse Kanerva, and Tuula Estlander

CONTENTS

15.1   INTRODUCTION

The first epoxy resin product was an adhesive introduced in 1946. Large-scale production of epoxy resins began in 1952. Dermatitis caused by exposure to epoxy resin compounds was observed in the 1950s, shortly after the introduction of epoxy resins.[1-2]

15.2   CHEMISTRY AND USE

Epoxy resins contain at least two epoxy groups in their molecules. The term "epoxy resin" may refer to the resin in both the uncured thermoplastic and cured thermoset states. The uncured resins can be cross-linked through the use of a variety of curing agents (hardeners) to form cured plastics. The reaction products of epichlorohydrin and bisphenol A resulted in the first commercial epoxy resins, which are generally mixtures of glycidyl ether of bisphenol A (DGEBA), with a molecular weight (MW) of 340, and oligomers with higher MW. The average number of repetitive parts in the oligomers range from 0 to approximately 25 (Figure 15.1).[3] Resins with a low

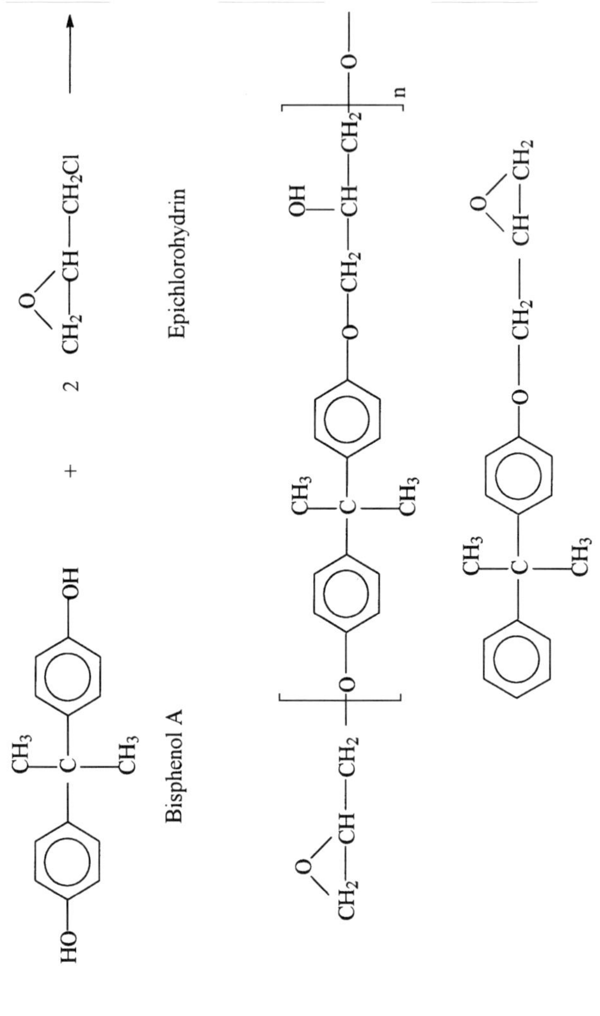

FIGURE 15.1 DGEBA epoxy resin.

average MW of 350–400 are liquid with a relatively high viscosity, and they contain monomeric DGEBA up to more than 90%. Resins with an average MW of more than 900 are solid but may contain even more than 15% DGEBA.[2-4]

DGEBA epoxy resins possess a unique combination of properties, such as easy cure, low shrinkage, high adhesive strength, high electrical insulation, good chemical and mechanical resistance, and versatility. The special properties of non-DGEBA epoxy resins have made the non-DGEBA epoxy resins competitive with the less expensive DGEBA resins for certain applications. However, the epoxy resin based on DGEBA still constitutes about three-quarters of the currently used epoxy resins.[5]

Epoxy resins are used in combination with other epoxy resin system compounds such as reactive diluents, hardeners, and other additives. Reactive diluents are used principally to reduce their viscosity. The reactive diluents are generally glycidyl ethers, sometimes glycidyl esters, which participate in the cross-linking reactions by their epoxy groups and become chemically linked to cured epoxy resins. Aliphatic diluents include such compounds as *n*-butyl glycidyl ether and 1,4-butanediol diglycidyl ether, whereas phenyl glycidyl ether and cresyl glycidyl ether are good examples of aromatic diluents. More than half of the epoxy resin products studied contained varying amounts of reactive diluents (0.1–20%).[4,6]

When epoxy resins are used in two-component products, the hardeners are added to the resins immediately preceding the application, and the subsequent cross-linking occurs at either an ambient or an elevated temperature. One-component products contain latent curing agents, which are inactive at storage temperatures but which initiate the cross-linking when heated. Examples of one-component products are epoxy or epoxy-polyester powder paints,[7] one-pack glues,[8] and prepregs.[9]

Currently a wide variety of curing agents is available. Aliphatic amines include, for example, ethylene diamine, diethylene triamine, and thiethylene tetramine; isophorone diamine is a cycloaliphatic amine, and 4,4'-diaminodiphenyl methane belongs to the group of aromatic amines.[5] Aliphatic and cycloalipahtic amines are low-viscosity liquids that react readily with epoxy resins at ambient temperatures; less reactive aromatic amines require an elevated curing temperature.[5] Polyamide and amine-epoxy adduct hardeners are less volatile, less reactive, and less irritating and sensitizing to the skin and respiratory tract. The polyamides and amine-epoxy adducts are synthetized using polyamines as raw materials resulting in products containing up to several percent of free polyamines.[10]

Tertiary polyamines, for example, 2,4,6-tris-(dimethylaminomethyl)phenol, are catalyst-type curing agents used for epoxy resin homopolymerization.[5] With the organic acid anhydrides, the cross-linking reaction is catalyzed by tertiary amines, and an elevated curing temperature (50–200°C) is used. The anhydrides include, for example, phthalic anhydride and phthalic anhydride derivatives[2,5] (See Chapter 21). The typical latent curing agents in epoxy powder paints are composed of about 4% hardener, such as dicyandiamide or pyromellitic anhydride, and of triglycidyl isocyanurate (TGIC) in polyester powder paints. The polymerization of the powder paints is achieved in a curing oven at about 200°C.[7]

Epoxy resin compounds are used in coatings, electronics, structural composites, and adhesives. Epoxy coatings are used where good resistance to chemicals, corrosion, or abrasion is needed. Epoxy resins are used in electronic applications to insulate or encapsulate. Structural composites include applicatons in pipes, vessels, electrical, aerospace, and sporting goods. Adhesives range from two-package consumer applications to high-performance sheet adhesives for aircraft assembly.[11]

15.3 CONTACT URTICARIA

Epoxy resins and their hardeners and reactive diluents are well-known causes of allergic contact dermatitis (delayed type contact allergy),[2,12] but only a few cases of immediate type contact urticaria due to the compounds have been reported. In 1974, a patch test with an epoxy resin was reported to induce generalized urticaria and an asthmatic reaction.[13] In 1983, Suhonen[14] reported on two patients who in a patch test showed immediate urticarial reactions, probably due to an impure DGEBA epoxy resin used in a ski pole factory. The DGEBA epoxy resin in the patch test standard series did not give an immediate reaction. The causative epoxy resin was not further identified. Kanerva et al.[15] described two patients with both immediate and delayed allergy to DGEBA epoxy resin. Prick tests with DGEBA epoxy resin conjugated to human serum albumin and specific immunoglobulin E determinations with purified DGEBA with a MW of 340 indicated that the DGEBA was the specific immediate type allergen in the two patients. The immediate type allergy of the patients appeared as respiratory symptoms and pruritus. Both patients complained of immediate pruritus from exposure to epoxy resin. According to the authors, it was evident that this occurrence was a sign of contact urticaria although hives were not present. Observations of the patient groups from an insulator factory[15] and a ski factory[16] indicate that immediate type allergy to epoxy resin is possibly rare, although the patients are heavily exposed to epoxy resins.

No cross-reactivity has been observed between the specific IgE determinations for DGEBA-based epoxy resins and non-DGEBA epoxy resins such as cycloaliphatic epoxy resins.[15]

A few cases of contact urticaria due to organic phthalic anhydride epoxy hardeners have been reported[6,17] (See Chapter 21). In addition, contact urticaria can be caused by aliphatic polyamine hardeners[18] and possibly by other amines.[19]

15.4 CONCLUSION

Epoxy resins are well-known delayed type contact allergens. The DGEBA epoxy resins have the ability to induce specific IgE-mediated sensitization. Only a few cases of immediate type contact urticaria from epoxy resins have been reported. Nevertheless, epoxy resins should be regarded as potential causes of the contact urticaria syndrome.

REFERENCES

1. Calnan, C. D., Studies in contact dermatitis, *Trans. St. John's Hosp. Dermatol. Soc.,* 40, 12, 1958.
2. Jolanki, R., Occupational skin diseases from epoxy compounds. Epoxy resin compounds, epoxy acrylates and 2,3-epoxypropyl trimethyl ammonium chloride, [Doctoral dissertation], *Acta Derm. Venereol.,* suppl. 159, 1991.
3. Bauer, R. S., Epoxy resins, in *Applied Polymer Science,* 2nd ed., Tess, R. W. and Poehlein, G. W., Eds., American Chemical Society, Washington, D.C., 1985, 931.
4. Henriks-Eckerman, M.-L. and Laijoki, T., Epoksituotteiden sisältämät glysidyylieetterit [Gysidyl ethers in epoxy resin products], *Työterveyslaitoksen tutkimuksia,* 4, 41 [English summary 70], 1986.
5. Muskopf, J. W. and McCollister, S. B., Epoxy resins, in *Ullmann's Encyclopedia of Industrial Chemistry,* 5th ed., Gerhartz, W., Yamamoto, Y. S., Kaudy, L., Rounsaville, J. F., and Schulx, G., Eds., VCH Verlagsgesellschaft, Weinheim, 1987, Vol. A9, 547.
6. Jolanki, R., Estlander, T., and Kanerva, L., Occupational contact dermatitis and contact urticaria caused by epoxy resins, *Acta Dermatol. Venereol.,* Suppl. 134, 90, 1987.
7. Peltonen, K., Thermal degradation of epoxy powder paints, [Doctoral dissertation], University of Kuopio, Finland, 1986.
8. Dahlquist, I., Fregert, S., Persson, K., and Trulsson, L., Epoxy resin in a one-pack glue, *Contact Dermatitis,* 5, 189, 1979.
9. Mathias, C. G. T., Allergic contact dermatitis from a nonbisphenol A epoxy in a graphite fiber reinforced epoxy laminate, *J. Occup. Med.,* 29, 754, 1987.
10. Henriks-Eckerman, M.-L. and Laijoki, T., Alifaattisten polyamiinien ja epoksioligomeerien sitoutuminen kylmäkovettumisessa [Aliphatic polyamines and epoxy oligomers in cold cured epoxy products], *Työterveyslaitoksen tutkimuksia,* 4, 37 [English summary 69], 1986.
11. Gardiner, T. H., Waechter, Jr., J. M., Wiedow, M. H., and Solomon, W. A., Glycidyloxy compounds used in epoxy resin systems: a toxicology review, *Regulatory Toxicology and Pharmacology,* 15, S1, 1992.
12. Jolanki, R., Kanerva, L., Estlander, T., and Tarvainen, K., Epoxy dermatitis, in *Occupational Skin Disease,* Nethercott, J. R., Ed., Occupational Medicine: State of the Art Reviews. Hanley & Belfus, Inc., Medical Publishers, Philadelphia, PA, 9 (1), 97, 1994.
13. Woytón, A., Wasik, F., and Blizanowska, A., Niezwykla reakcja anafilaktycna I wypryskowa po kontakcie z zywicami epoksydowymi [An uncommon anaphylactic and eczematous reaction after contact with epoxide resins], *Przegl. Dermatol.,* 61, 303, 1974.
14. Suhonen, R., Epoxy-dermatitis in a ski-stick factory, *Contact Dermatitis,* 9, 131, 1983.
15. Kanerva, L., Jolanki, R., Tupasela, O., Halmepuro, L., Keskinen, H., Estlander, T., and Sysilampi, M.-L., Immediate and delayed allergy from epoxy resins based on diglycidyl ether of bisphenol A, *Scand. J. Work Environ. Health.* 17, 208, 1991.
16. Jolanki, R., Tarvainen, K., Tatar, T., Estlander, T., Henriks-Eckerman, M.-L., Mustakallio, K. K., and Kanerva, L., Occupational dermatoses from exposure to epoxy resin compounds in a ski factory, *Contact Dermatitis,* 34, 390, 1996.
17. Tarvainen, K., Jolanki, R., Estlander, T., Tupasela, O., Pfäffli, P., and Kanerva, L., Immunologic contact urticaria due to airborne methylhexahydrophthalic and methyltetrahydrophthalic anhydride, *Contact Dermatitis,* 32, 204, 1995.
18. Fisher, A. A., *Contact Dermatitis,* 3rd ed., Lea & Febiger, Philadelphia, 1986.
19. Savonius, B., Keskinen, H., Tuppurainen, M., and Kanerva, L., Occupational asthma caused by ethanolamines, *Allergy,* 49, 877, 1994.

16

Fruits and Vegetables

Arto Lahti

CONTENTS

16.1 INTRODUCTION

Allergy to fruits, edible roots, and vegetables has been known for decades.[1,2] The symptoms are usually immediate, appearing within minutes after ingestion. Not only ingestion of fruits and vegetables, but also handling them may cause skin symptoms. Maibach (1976) reported a patient with immediate skin reactions to several foods,[3] and Hjorth and Roed-Petersen (1976) found immediate contact dermatitis to be fairly common among kitchen personnel.[4] Fruits and vegetables as causes of immediate contact reactions have attracted research interest not only from the clinical point of view but also for theoretical reasons because of the interesting cross-reactivities between taxonomically unrelated plants.

16.2 SYMPTOMS OF ALLERGY TO FRUITS AND VEGETABLES

The most common manifestation of fruit and vegetable allergy is the "oral allergy syndrome."[5] The symptoms include pharyngeal, palatal, gingival, and labial itching and tingling, hoarseness of the throat, rhinitis, conjunctivitis, swelling of the soft periorbital tissue, angioedema, wheezing, and gastrointestinal symptoms.[6-10] Perioral erythema, contact urticaria, generalized urticaria, and aggravation of atopic dermatitis are often seen. Immediate eczema-like reactions have been reported on the hands, especially on the fingers.[3,4,11] The most severe symptom is anaphylactic shock, which has often been reported after celery intake.[12]

16.3 FRUIT AND VEGETABLE ALLERGY CONNECTED TO POLLEN ALLERGY

Tuft and Blumstein (1942) reported four pollen-allergic patients who developed swelling and itching of the mouth and throat after eating fresh peaches, apples, bananas, and melons, but did not react to canned or cooked fruits.[13] Juhlin-Dannfelt (1948) was the first who reported the association between hypersensitivity to fruits and vegetables and allergy to birch pollen.[14] Since then, this observation has been amply confirmed.[6,7,15,16]

In Finland, Hannuksela and Lahti (1977) reported that 152 (66%) of 230 atopic patients allergic to birch pollen complained of itching, tingling, or edema of the lips and tongue and hoarseness or irritation of the throat when eating such raw fruits and vegetables as apple, potato, carrot, tomato, celery, and parsnip.[6] Positive results on scratch chamber tests with the suspected fresh fruits and vegetables were seen in 36% of the 230 patients. Apple, carrot, parsnip, and potato elicited skin reactions more often than swede (rutabaga), tomato, onion, celery, and parsley. It was also noticed that a patient usually reacted not only to one, but to many fruits and vegetables both in skin tests and in everyday life. The clinical relevance of the skin test results with apple, potato, and carrot was 80–90%. Only 7 out of 158 (4%) atopic patients who were not allergic to birch pollen had positive skin test reactions to any of the 9 fruits and vegetables tested. Other fruits and vegetables causing immediate contact reactions include apricot, mango, orange, plum, cherry, kiwi, beans, cabbage, chives, cucumber, endive, lettuce, soybean, garlic, lime, and strawberry.[10]

In the U.S., Anderson et al. (1970) studied 1447 patients with pollinosis.[17] They found that all the 90 patients complaining of oral pruritus after eating melons (cantaloupe, watermelon, honeydew melon) and banana were also sensitive to ragweed pollen. All of their melon-banana-sensitive patients showed varying degrees of skin test sensitivity to grass pollen in addition to ragweed. They state that grass pollen may also have a role in the syndrome. Melon-banana oral pruritus was not found in any of 620 nonpollinosis-allergic patients. As an explanation for this "melon, banana-sensitivity-ragweed pollinosis" syndrome, they suggested the presence of common antigenic determinants. Enberg et al. (1987) extended the association with ragweed allergy to the whole gourd family (watermelon, cantaloupe, honeydew melon, zucchini, and cucumber).[18]

In Italy, Ortolani et al. (1988) used skin prick tests and RASTs to study 262 patients suffering from hay fever and the oral allergy syndrome after fruit and vegetable ingestion.[19] They noticed a strong association between allergy to birch pollen and allergy to apple, pear, carrot, and cherry on the one hand and between allergy to grass pollen and melons and tomato on the other.

The observation that celery intake can induce hypersensitivity reactions was made 70 years ago.[20] Since then, many studies have shown the importance of celery allergy, which often causes severe urticarial and even life-threatening anaphylactic reactions.[6,12,21] Celery allergy is strongly associated with allergy to mugwort pollen and also to birch pollen.[12,21-23]

Ortolani et al. (1993) pointed out that in analyzing these associations one must bear in mind the topographic prevalence of the local flora inducing pollen allergy and the dietary habits influencing the intake of different fruits and vegetables in different countries.[24]

Not only allergy to fruits and vegetables, but also allergy to some spices seems to be associated with pollen allergy. Niinimäki and Hannuksela (1981) studied 1120 atopics and 380 nonatopic patients and showed that positive skin test reactions to spices were seen most often in atopic patients with allergy to birch pollen and fruits and vegetables.[25] The spices which most often gave positive reactions were paprika, coriander, caraway, cayenne, and mustard. These reactions were mostly reproducible in retesting.[26]

The first report on the association of banana allergy to natural rubber latex allergy was published by M´Raihi et al. (1991).[27] This observation has been confirmed by Mäkinen-Kiljunen (1994).[28] In addition to banana, latex allergy has also been associated to chestnut and avocado.[29-31]

16.4 MECHANISMS OF IMMEDIATE CONTACT REACTIONS TO FRUITS AND VEGETABLES

It was already noted in the early reports that a pollen-allergic patient usually reacted not only to one but to many fruits from different botanical groups.[13,14] Using the passive serum transfer technique described by Prausnitz-Küstner, Tuft and Blumstein (1942) were able to show that reagins in the serum of the patient were responsible for their allergic reactions to peach and melon (type I allergy).[13] More than 15 years ago, it was shown that IgE antibodies that cross-react with pollen and food proteins are responsible for the clustering of fruit and vegetable allergy to certain pollen allergies.[12,32-36] The early reports on fruit allergy already stressed that allergens (peach) are labile and easily destroyed by heat in cooking and canning processes or even by storing fresh juice in the refrigerator for 1 to 3 days.[13] In studies of apple allergens, it was shown that allergens are probably proteins and that they can be extracted in an active form only if their reactions with the phenolic compounds present in apple are inhibited by chelators.[33]

The research for the characterization of allergens in fruits, vegetables, and birch pollen, which can be responsible for the cross-reactions, took a big step forward when profilins were found in plants and connected to allergy to pollens and other plant products. Valenta et al. (1991) identified a birch pollen allergen, Bet v 2, as profilin.[37] Profilins constitute an ubiquitous group of proteins of the cytoskeleton and control actin polymerization in eukaryotic cells. It was shown that profilins may be prominent allergens that can be isolated from birch, timothy, and mugwort pollens.[38] The presence of an allergen homologous to the major birch pollen allergen Bet v 1 (17 kd) in apples has been demonstrated by the Northern blotting method.[39] By using recombinant Bet v 1 and Bet v 2 for IgE inhibition experiments as well as specific antibodies, the presence of Bet v 1 and Bet v 2 homologous allergens has been demonstrated in many fruits, vegetables, and spices.[40-42]

16.5 DIAGNOSIS OF IMMEDIATE CONTACT REACTIONS TO FRUITS AND VEGETABLES

Skin tests are usually reliable in detecting immediate type allergies and should belong to the diagnostic regime if the patient's history reveals symptoms of immediate contact reactions to fruits and vegetables.[43]

The skin prick test is the most convenient test method for confirming immunoglobulin E mediated allergy. Commercial test series are available, but self-prepared test solutions can also be used. Drops of allergen solutions are applied to the skin, usually on the forearm or the back, 3–5 cm apart and pierced with a special test lancet (e.g., Dome-Hollister-Stier prick test lancet). Histamine hydrochloride 10 mg/ml is used as a positive control and the vehicle solution as a negative control. After 15 min. the diameters of the weals are measured. Reactions larger than 3 mm and at least half the size produced by histamine are regarded as positive.[44,45]

Scratch and *scratch-chamber tests* are still used if nonstandardized food allergens, such as fruits and vegetables, are to be tested. A scratch approximately 5 mm long is made with a blood lancet or a venepuncture needle, avoiding bleeding. A small amount of allergen is applied to the scratch and the result is read and the possible weals measured 15 min. later. Powdered allergens are mixed with a drop of physiological saline or 0.1 N NaOH. Fruits and vegetables may dry out too quickly, but covering the allergen material on the scratch with a Finn Chamber (Epitest, Helsinki, Finland) prevents drying and enhances the sensitivity of the test.[6] Histamine hydrochloride (10 mg/ml) is used as the positive and the vehicle as the negative control. Weal reactions at least equal in size to the histamine weal are usually clinically significant.

The open application test, rub test, and use test are less standardized methods, where the allergen is applied to healthy or previously affected skin. As a positive reaction, an urticarial reaction, erythema, and itching appears usually within 20 min.[46]

The Radio-Allergo-Sorbent Test may aid in detecting specific IgE antibodies and *RAST-inhibition tests* have been useful in investigating cross-allergenity.[36]

16.6 CONCLUSION

In clinical practice, patients often report symptoms of immediate contact reactions after handling or eating edible roots, fruits, and vegetables. The symptomatology varies from weak local symptoms to severe life-threatening conditions. Detailed studies on the cross-allergies between fruits and vegetables have forced dermatologists and allergists to open their minds to new views in understanding the complexity of food allergies, while simultaneously facing a completely new area of problems in research and clinical work now that transgenic foods have appeared on the market.[47]

REFERENCES

1. Hansen, K., Exposition, in *Allergie*, Hansen, K., Ed., Georg Thieme Verlag, Stuttgart, 1957, 199.
2. Tuft, L. and Müller, H. L., in *Allergy in Children*, W. B. Saunders Company, Philadelphia, 1970, 128.
3. Maibach, H., Immediate hypersensitivity in hand dermatitis, *Arch. Dermatol.,* 112, 1289, 1976.
4. Hjorth, N. and Roed-Petersen, J., Occupational protein contact dermatitis in food handlers, *Contact Dermatitis,* 2, 28, 1976.
5. Amlot, P. L., Kemeny D. M., Zachary, C., Parkes, P. and Lessof, M. H., Oral allergy syndrome (OAS): symptoms of IgE-mediated hypersensitivity to foods, *Clin. Allergy,* 17, 33, 1987.
6. Hannuksela, M. and Lahti, A., Immediate reactions to fruits and vegetables, *Contact Dermatitis,* 3, 79, 1977.
7. Eriksson, N. E., Formgren, H. and Svenonius, E., Food hypersensitivity in patients with pollen allergy, *Allergy,* 37, 437, 1982.
8. Dreborg, S., Food allergy in pollen-sensitive patients, *Ann. Allergy,* 61, 41, 1988.
9. Kivity, S., Dunner, K. and Marian, Y., The pattern of food hypersensitivity in patients with onset after 10 years of age, *Clin. Exp. Allergy,* 24, 19, 1994.
10. Lahti, A., Immediate contact reactions, in *Textbook of Contact Dermatitis*, Rycroft, R. J. G., Menné, T. and Frosch, P. J., Eds., Springer-Verlag, Berlin, 1995, Chap. 2.3.
11. Hannuksela, M., Atopic contact dermatitis, *Contact Dermatitis,* 6, 30, 1980.
12. Pauli, G., Bessot, J. C., Dietemann-Molard, A., Braun, P. A. and Thierry, R., Celery sensitivity: clinical and immunological correlations with pollen allergy, *Clin. Allergy,* 15, 273, 1985.
13. Tuft, L. and Blumstein, G. I., Studies in food allergy. II. Sensitization to fresh fruits: clinical and experimental observations, *J. Allergy,* 13, 574, 1942.
14. Juhlin-Dannfeldt, C., About the occurrence of various forms of pollen allergy in Sweden, *Acta Med. Scand.,* 130, Suppl. 206, 563, 1948.
15. Eriksson, N. E., Food sensitivity reported by patients with asthma and hay fever, *Allergy,* 33, 189, 1978.
16. Eriksson, N. E., Clustering of foodstuffs in food hypersensitivity. An inquiry study in pollen allergic patients, *Allergol. Immunopathol.,* 12, 28, 1984.
17. Anderson, L. B., Dreyfuss, E. M., Logan, J., Johnstone, D. E. and Glaser, J., Melon and banana sensitivity coincident with ragweed pollinosis, *J. Allergy,* 45, 310, 1970.
18. Enberg, R. N., Leickly, F. E., McCullough, J., Nailey, J. and Ownby, D. R., Watermelon and ragweed share allergens, *J. Allergy Clin. Immunol.,* 79, 867, 1987.
19. Ortolani, C., Ispano, M., Pastorello, E., Bigi, A. and Ansaloni, R., The oral allergy syndrome, *Ann. Allergy,* 61, 47, 1988.

20. Jadassohn, W. and Zaruski M., Idiosyncrasie gegen Sellerie, *Arch. Dermatol. Syph.*, 151, 93, 1926.
21. Kauppinen, K., Kousa, M. and Reunala, T., Aromatic plants — a cause of severe attacks of angio-edema and urticaria, *Contact Dermatitis,* 6, 251, 1980.
22. Vallier, P., Dechamp, C., Vial, O. and Deviller, P., A study of allergens in celery with cross-sensitivity to mugwort and birch pollens, *Clin. Allergy,* 18, 491, 1988.
23. Wüthrich, B., Stäger, J. and Johansson, S. G. O., Celery allergy associated with birch and mugwort pollinosis, *Allergy,* 45, 566, 1990.
24. Ortolani, C., Pastorello, E. A., Farioli, L., Ispano, M., Pravettoni V., Berti C., Incorvaia, C. and Zanussi C., IgE-mediated allergy from vegetable allergens, *Ann. Allergy,* 71, 470, 1993.
25. Niinimäki, A. and Hannuksela, M., Immediate skin test reactions to spices, *Allergy,* 36, 487, 1981.
26. Niinimäki, A., Hannuksela, M. and Mäkinen-Kiljunen S., Skin prick tests and *in vitro* immunoassays with native spices and spice extracts, *Ann. Allergy,* 74, 280, 1995.
27. M'Raihi, L., Charpin, D., Pons, A., Bongrand, P. and Vervloet, D., Cross-reactivity between latex and banana, *J. Allergy Clin. Immunol.,* 87, 129, 1991.
28. Mäkinen-Kiljunen, S., Banana allergy in patients with immediate-type hypersensitivity to natural rubber latex: characterization of cross-reacting antibodies and allergens, *J. Allergy Clin. Immunol.,* 93, 990, 1994.
29. Añibarro, B., Garcia-Ara, M. C. and Pascual, C., Associated sensitization to latex and chestnut, *Allergy,* 48, 130, 1993.
30. de Corres, L. F., Moneo, I., Muñoz, D., Bernaola, G., Fernández, E., Audicana, M. and Urrutia, I., Sensitization from chestnuts and bananas in patients with urticaria and anaphylaxis from contact with latex, *Ann. Allergy,* 70, 35, 1993.
31. Ahlroth, M., Alenius, H., Turjanmaa, K., Mäkinen-Kiljunen, S., Reunala, T. and Palosuo, T., Cross-reacting allergens in natural rubber latex and avocado, *J. Allergy Clin. Immunol.,* 96, 167, 1995.
32. Lahti, A., Björksten, F. and Hannuksela, M., Allergy to birch pollen and apple, and cross-reactivity of the allergens studied with RAST, *Allergy,* 35, 297, 1980.
33. Björksten, F., Halmepuro, L., Hannuksela, M. and Lahti, A., Extraction and properties of apple allergens, *Allergy,* 35, 671, 1980.
34. Aalberse, R. C., Koshte, V. and Clemens, J. G., Immunoglobulin E antibodies that crossreact with vegetable foods, pollen, and Hymenoptera venom, *J. Allergy Clin. Immunol.,* 68, 356, 1981.
35. Halmepuro, L., Vuontela, K., Kalimo, K. and Björksten, F., Cross-reactivity of IgE antibodies with allergens in birch pollen, fruits and vegetables, *Int. Arch. Allergy Appl. Immunol.,* 74, 235, 1984.
36. Halmepuro, L. and Løwenstein, H., Immunological investigation of possible structural similarities between pollen antigens and apple, carrot and celery tuber, *Allergy,* 40, 264, 1985.
37. Valenta, R., Duchêne, M., Pettenburger, K., Sillaber, C., Valent, P., Bettelheim, P., Breitenbach, M., Rumpold, H., Kraft, D. and Scheiner, O., Identification of profilin as novel pollen allergen: IgE autoreactivity in sensitized individuals, *Science,* 253, 557, 1991.
38. Valenta, R., Duchene, M., Ebner, C., Valent, P., Sillaber, C., Deviller, P., Ferreira, F., Tejkl, M., Edelmann, H., Kraft, D. and Scheiner, O., Profilins constitute a novel family of functional plant pan-allergens, *J. Exp. Med.,* 175, 377, 1992.

39. Ebner, C., Birkner, T., Valenta, R., Rumpold, H., Breitenbach, M., Scheiner, O. and Kraft, D., Common epitopes of birch pollen and apples — studies by Western and Northern blot, *J. Allergy Clin. Immunol.,* 88, 588, 1991.

40. Vallier, P., Dechamp, C., Valenta, R., Vial, O. and Deviller, P., Purification and characterization of an allergen from celery immunochemically related to an allergen present in several other plant species. Identification as a profilin, *Clin. Exp. Allergy,* 22, 774, 1992.

41. van Ree, R., Voitenko, V., van Leeuwen, W.A. and Aalberse, R.C., Profilin is a cross-reactive allergen in pollen and vegetable food, *Int. Arch. Allergy Immunol.,* 98, 97, 1992.

42. Ebner, C., Hirschwehr, R., Bauer, L., Breiteneder, H., Valenta, R., Ebner, H., Kraft, D. and Scheiner, O., Identification of allergens in fruits and vegetables: IgE cross-reactivities with the important birch pollen allergens Bet v 1 and Bet v 2 (birch profilin), *J. Allergy Clin. Immunol.,* 95, 962, 1995.

43. Hannuksela, M., Skin tests for immediate contact reactions, in *Textbook of Contact Dermatitis,* Rycroft, R. J. G., Menné, T. and Frosch, P. J., Eds., Springer-Verlag, Berlin, 1995, Chap. 10.4.

44. Basompa, A., Sastre, A., Pelaez, A., Romar, A., Campos, A. and Garcia-Villalmanzo, A., Standardization of the prick test. A comparative study of three methods, *Allergy,* 40, 395, 1985.

45. Malling, H-J., Reproducibility of skin sensitivity using a quantitative skin prick test, *Allergy,* 40, 400, 1985.

46. Niinimäki, A., Scratch-chamber tests in food handler dermatitis, *Contact Dermatitis,* 16, 11, 1987.

47. Nestle, M., Allergies to transgenic foods — questions of policy, *N. Engl. J. Med.,* 334, 726, 1996.

17

Contact Urticaria from Hairdressing Products

Timo Leino and Lasse Kanerva

CONTENTS

17.1   INTRODUCTION

Hairdressers are exposed to a wide variety of hair care products containing substances that can cause both immediate and delayed allergic reactions. Hundreds of chemicals are used as basic ingredients for making hair cosmetics. Many of them are synthetic organic chemicals. Natural substances derived from plant, animal, and mineral sources are used as well. An inventory of cosmetic ingredients has been prepared by the European Community (Cosmetics Directive 76/768/EEC) using the nomenclature of the International Nomenclature of Cosmetic Ingredients (INCI).[1] The U.S., the EC member states, and increasing numbers of other countries are adopting INCI names for ingredient labeling.

Itching, wheals, flare, and sometimes microvesicles appear as symptoms of contact urticaria immediately or soon, usually within an hour, after skin contact with a substance. To a large extent, these symptoms resemble those of skin irritation and can be misinterpreted by a physician or even missed if the patient presenting hand eczema is not questioned properly. Skin and *in vitro* tests are needed to confirm the diagnosis. In this chapter, we review the agents that may cause contact urticaria among hairdressers and their clients (Table 17.1).

17.2   PREVALENCE

The true prevalence of contact urticaria among hairdressers is unknown. Recently, Kanerva et al. reported that according to cases reported by physicians to the Finnish Register of Work-Related Diseases, 11.8 cases of occupational contact urticaria per 100,000 hairdressers occurred in Finland 1990–1994.[2] Considering the high occurrence of hand dermatitis (mainly irritant type) among hairdressers, two separate cohort studies indicating a 1-year cumulative incidence of 25.7–27.9% among apprentice hairdressers,[3,4] it is likely that some of the irritant symptoms are, in fact, nonimmunological or immunological contact urticaria. Typical sites for contact urticaria among hairdressers are the fingers, dorsum of the hand, and forearms, whereas the scalp, forehead, face, and eyelids are more often the locations of their clients' contact urticaria. Generalized urticaria can spread over the whole body and may be accompanied by symptoms of anaphylactic shock.

17.3   TEST METHODS

Only a few prick tests and radioallergosorbent tests (RAST) are commercially available for products used by hairdressers. Usually the ingredients have to be tested with specially constructed tests and this procedure is time consuming and sometimes frustrating since reactions seldom appear. When a reaction appears, tests on control subjects are also mandatory in most instances. The RAST is problematic for low-molecular substances, because the haptens have to first be coupled with carrier molecules, usually proteins, and the test may not reflect the actual exposure situation or allergen on the skin.[5] An open test is an alternative and should be used more often, although the possibility of an incorrect reaction is considerable. Intracutaneous tests can provoke anaphylactic reactions. Scratch tests with ammonium persulphate can also elicit anaphylactic reactions and should be avoided.

TABLE 17.1 Agents that have Caused Contact Urticaria in Hairdressing

Agent	Causative ingredient	Ref.
Hair and dandruff	Human proteins	Mikkelsen 1978 (57), Leino 1995 (64)
Rubber gloves	Natural rubber latex proteins	Guerra 1992 (11), Van der Walle 1995 (12)
Shampoos and conditioners	Protein hydrolyzates	
	stearyl trimethylammonium	Pasche-Koo 1992 (25)
	hydroxypropyltrimonium-hydrolyzed collagen	Niinimäki 1994 (26)
	quaternized hydrolyzed milk protein	Niinimäki 1994 (26)
	quaternized collagen hydrolyzate	Kousa 1990 (24)
	hydrolyzed bovine collagen	Pfeiff 1989 (23), Pasche-Koo 1992 (25)
	Tilia (lime)	Picardo 1985 (18)
	eugenol	Picardo 1985 (18)
	sorbic acid	Rietschel 1978 (19)
	egg proteins	Braun-Falco 1984 (22)
Hair colorants	para-phenylenediamine	Calnan 1967 (44), Edwards 1984 (45), Temesvári 1984 (46)
	N'N'-bis-(4-aminophenyl)-2,5-diamino-1,4-quinonediimine	Goldberg 1987 (47a)
	Diaminotoluene	Pasche-Koo 1996 (47b)
	Para-aminodiphenylamine	Von Liebe 1979 (48a)
	Basic Blue 99	Wigger-Alberti 1996 (48b), Jagtman 1996 (48c)
	Ammonium persulphate	Calnan 1963 (28), Gaultier 1966 (29), Meindl 1969 (30), Fisher 1976 (32), Widström 1977 (33), Von Krogh 1981 (40) Fisher 1985 (34, 35), Pepys 1987 (36), Kleinhans 1989 (37), Scwaiblmair 1990 (38), Guerra 1992 (39)
	Henna	Frosch 1986 (49a), Majoie 1996 (49b)
Permanent wave fluid	Causative ingredient not specified	Von Liebe 1979 (48a)
Fixation fluid for permanent wave	Causative ingredient not specified	Von Liebe 1979 (48a)
Hair sprays	Causative ingredient not specified	Fisher 1973 (54)

17.4 CAUSATIVE FACTORS

17.4.1 Natural Rubber Latex Gloves

Natural rubber latex proteins, rubber chemicals, and also the corn starch used to dust gloves can cause contact urticaria.[6-10] In an Italian questionnaire study, 12.5% (30/240) of the hairdressers reported cutaneous lesions on their hands.[11] Gloves worsened the dermatitis of eight of these subjects, but the type of skin reaction was not reported. Of the 302 patch-tested hairdressers with dermatitis, 10 complained of swelling and itching after wearing latex gloves, and four of them were positive in a latex glove use test. In a Dutch study, 5 of 41 hairdressers who regularly used rubber gloves reacted positively to liquid or solid latex or to latex gloves.[12] The clinical symptoms were not reported. Due to a likely selection bias, it is not possible to draw any conclusions from the data about the true prevalence of contact urticaria among hairdressers. Among hospital workers, the prevalence of contact urticaria from exposure to natural rubber latex has been reported to be 2.5–10.7%.[13]

In some countries, the use of protective gloves in hairdressing is still rare.[11] It is also obvious that many hairdressers are not aware of the high allergy risk of latex gloves. An information campaign can lower the occurrence of contact urticaria among hairdressers. In our own questionnaire study, 81.5% (255/313) of Finnish hairdressers did not use rubber gloves at all.[14] The glove industry has also taken measures to reduce natural rubber latex allergens in gloves. Vinyl and polyethene gloves have been advocated as a substitute. However, one latex allergic patient experienced urticaria even when using latex gloves coated with a hypoallergenic polyurethane membrane.[15]

17.4.2 Shampoos and Conditioners

Shampoos are basically made of surfactant and water, but many other ingredients are used to make the product desirable (e.g., foam builders, refatting agents, thickeners, opacifiers, coloring agents, fragrances, buffers, and preservatives).[16] Conditioners are meant for restoring manageability, softness, and shine to the hair. Conditioning agents fall into three cathegories: cationic detergents, film formers, and proteins.[17]

Considering their wide use, shampoos and conditioners do not often seem to be a cause of contact urticaria among hairdressers. The low concentration of potential agents causing contact urticaria, like dyes, fragrances, and preservatives and their low potency to cause reactions make them less likely candidates, but the risk still exists. A shampoo containing *Tilia* (lime) caused facial edema and generalized urticaria in a young woman. Urticarial reactions were confirmed in patch tests with the shampoo, *Tilia* extract, perfume mix, and 1% eugenol, all of which were positive after 30 minutes.[18] The same symptoms occurred in a young student. The patch test with the individual ingredients of the shampoo revealed contact urticaria to sorbic acid.[19] Natural ingredients in shampoos and conditioning products, such as flowers, leaves, roots, seeds, and fruits of many herbs and shrubs, can also cause contact urticaria.

Allergies not originating from hair cosmetics can predispose a person to contact urticaria when the same allergen occur in hair preparations. Chronic urticaria in a 9-year-old girl was associated with a shampoo containing papaya; the allergen papain occurred in cleaning solutions used for contact lenses.[20] A hairdresser who experienced local and generalized urticaria when eating egg dishes showed contact urticaria reactions also when in contact with raw egg in the course of her work, and an egg shampoo caused contact urticaria in an atopic dermatitis patient.[20,21] In a similar manner, a person allergic to ragweed and flowers of the daisy family (*Compositae*) can react to camomile, and persons allergic to latex can react to hair cosmetics containing avocado.

Protein hydrolysates derived from animal and plant proteins are used increasingly in many hair care products, including hair conditioners and shampoos. They increase the volume of hair and make the hair easier to comb. Hydrolyzed bovine collagen, quaternized collagen hydrolyzate, stearyl trimethylammonium, hydroxypropyltrimonium-hydrolyzed collagen, and quaternized-hydrolyzed milk protein have caused contact urticaria in hairdressers.[23-26] According to limited experience, some protein hydrolyzates (e.g., keratine and collagen hydrolyzates) often give false irritative reactions in prick and scratch tests and therefore make it necessary to supplement them with a RAST and also include a control group.[26]

17.4.3 Hair Colorants

17.4.3.1 Hair Bleaches

Hair bleaches are used to lighten the natural color of hair. Ammonium persulphate and other persulphate salts are used extensively in hair bleaches to accelerate the oxidizing action of hydrogen peroxides. The concentration of persulphates in bleaches varies between 50 and 70%. They are the most common cause of contact urticaria reactions in hairdressers. Already in 1939 Bonnevie described ammonium persulphate as a causative factor for contact urticaria and since then several reports have been published on hairdressers' immediate-type skin and respiratory reactions.[25-38] Both localized and generalized urticarial reactions have occurred in hairdressers and their clients.[34,39] The mechanism behind these reactions has remained unsolved. Although the clinical picture of patients resembles an IgE-mediated reaction, IgE-class antibodies against ammonium persulphate have not been demonstrated.[40,41] Dipersulphate ion has been shown to liberate histamine from the mast cells, and therefore partly explains the urticariogenic action of persulphates.[42] Other agents causing potential contact urticaria in hair bleaches are sodium silicate (a filler material in bleaches), ammonia, and the colorants.

17.4.3.2 Hair Dyes

Hair colorants can be classified as temporary, semi-permanent, and permanent dyes. The permanent dyes are generally *p*-phenylenediamines and *p*-aminophenols.Their nitro derivates are used in semi-permanent dyes together with a selected number of azo dyes and aminoanthraquinone dyes. The temporary dyes are water-soluble acid or basic dyes.[43]

Contact urticaria caused by paraphenylenediamine (PPDA) is rare considering its wide use in hair cosmetics. Calnan reported a patient showing an immediate reaction with a 0.6% concentration of PPDA in a scratch test, but no delayed reaction.[44] The second case was a beautician, who was tested by applying 1.0% PPDA in petrolatum to her forearm. She had both an immediate contact urticaria reaction and a delayed reaction in the test equable to her symptoms at work.[45] PPDA has also elicited contact urticaria in other occupations.[46] The oxidation product of N′N′-bis-(4-aminophenyl)-2,5-diamino-1,4-quinonediimine and diaminotoluene have caused contact urticaria with anaphylaxis in one patient.[47a,b] Von Liebe et al. reported one hairdresser, who had urticarial eruptions on the dorsum of her hands, neck, face, and occasionally also in her upper chest when in contact with hair colorants and permanent wave fluids. In an open patch test, immediate contact urticarial reaction was shown to para-aminodiphenylamine.[48] Also Basic Blue 99 (CI 56059), a semi-permanent dye, has caused generalized urticaria in hairdressers and their clients.[48b,c]

Natural hair coloring agents have become popular. The plant extracts and grinded parts of plants can cause contact urticaria. Potential urticariogenic agents are, for example, henna, senna, camomile, rhubarb root, and tea. Henna has been used for coloring hair for centuries. It is derived from the leaves and stems of *Lawsonia alba*. The coloring molecule in henna is 2-hydroxy-1,4-naphtoquinone, but it may not be the allergen in the immediate allergic skin and respiratory reactions.[36;49a,b;50] Senna has also caused asthma and rhinoconjunctivitis in a factory worker mixing hair colorants, but the patient did not have urticaria.[51] Other potential agents in hair coloring preparations that can cause contact urticaria are some of the semi-permanent dyes, ammonia, preservatives, and fragrances.

17.4.4   Permanent Wave Preparations

Salts of thioglycolic acid in permanent wave preparations are a common cause of delayed allergic reactions in hairdressers, but they do not seem to cause contact urticaria.[52] Only one report exists of a 42-year-old hairdresser who experienced contact urticaria when using permanent wave fluid and its fixation solution, but the causative ingredient was not investigated.[48] Ammonium, which is used to control the pH of some wave preparations, has caused contact urticaria in other circumstances than in hairdressing. Other potential urticariogenic ingredients in permanent wave preparations are preservatives, fragrances, and hydrolyzed proteins.

17.4.5   Hair Sprays and Other Hair Styling Preparations

Hair styling preparations occur in many forms as hair sprays, foams, lotions, gels, and waxes. They are used to make the hair easier to style. They all consist of various types and amounts of film-forming polymers (e.g., polyvinylpyrrolidone and acrylate-acrylamide copolymers) dissolved in water or water-alcohol solution or mixed in oils. The flexibility of the polymer film is controlled with emollients, such as diethyl phthalate, silicones, lanolin derivates, or polyglycols. The most important solvents used in setting lotions and hair sprays are ethanol, 2-propanol, and acetone. Various hydrocarbons are used as propellants in sprays. Many preparations also contain emulgators, perfumes, dyes, vitamins, preservatives, and ultraviolet filters.[53]

No reports exist on contact urticaria caused by any specific ingredients in hair styling preparations, although hair sprays are mentioned to cause contact urticaria in Fisher's Contact Dermatitis book.[54] Nevertheless, hair styling products contain many potential urticariogenic substances, such as alcohols, acetone, lanolin, colophony, trace amounts of acrylic monomers, preservatives, perfumes, and in some, also emulgators, protein derivatives, vitamins, and coloring agents.[55]

17.4.6 Perfumes

Perfumes are used in almost all hair cosmetic products to give a distinctive and appealing scent, and sometimes also to mask the natural bad odor of ingredients. The actual concentration of perfume is low, usually less than 1% of the total volume of a product, even in perfumed Eau de Colognes and after shave lotions which are mostly alcohol solutions. Perfumes are a common cause of skin and respiratory complaints among hairdressers and their clients. Still, reports of immediate IgE-mediated hypersensitivity to perfumes are rare. This lack may partly be due to the difficulty of verifying a specific allergen among the thousands of different odor-emitting chemical substances in perfumes. There are several reports of contact urticaria in perfume-sensitive patients, but in most cases the mechanism involved was nonimmunological or uncertain.[56] Perfumes should be also considered possible causes of contact urticaria among hairdressers.

17.4.7 Hair and Dandruff

Hairdressers are constantly exposed to human hair, dandruff, sweat, and saprophytes of the clients' scalp. Small particles of cut hair can cause itching and redness of the skin and, when stuck to workclothes, continuous irritation and urticaria-like symptoms. In most cases, the reaction is an irritative one, but not always. One hairdresser experienced pruritic vesicles on her hands on contact with clients' hair and dandruff. A scratch test with acetone extract of human dandruff was positive and also gave a delayed reaction.[57] In a prick test, human hair has also elicited a positive reaction in a woman allergic to her husband's sweat.[58] In this case, the proteins in sweat or dandruff may have contaminated the hair samples. Immediate reactions to human dandruff have been reported to be common in patients suffering from atopic dermatitis. In a scratch test used in a Japanese study, 62% of atopic dermatitis patients reacted positively in a scratch test to crude extract of human dandruff and a fraction of 10-13 kD proteins obtained with the high-speed gel filtration chromatography.[59] Human sweat has also caused IgE-mediated allergy in atopics and has been claimed to be involved in cholinergic urticaria.[60,61] Reactions to human dandruff may also be induced by other organisms, for example, *Pityrosporum ovale* yeast — a common saprophyte of the scalp. *P. ovale* is associated with atopic dermatitis, particularly when it is located on the face, scalp, or neck.[62] It is also found in excess in seborrhoeic dermatitis patients.[63] Our recent observations indicate that hairdressers' frequency of immediate allergy to human dandruff and *P. ovale* is increased compared with that of nonoccupationally exposed controls. In prick tests with human dandruff, 8.6% (7/81) of hairdressers were positive to human dandruff and 11.2% to *P. ovale* (11/98), whereas among the controls only one showed a positive reaction to human dandruff (1/311) and 3.5% to *P. ovale* (26/711).[64]

17.4.8 Instruments

Nickel and cobalt are used in utensils, such as scissors and clips, from which small amounts can be released by the action of sweat on hands or alkaline waving solutions.[65] Nickel sulfate and cobalt chloride have caused contact urticaria in rare cases, but there are no data for hairdressers.[66-68]

17.4.9 Antimicrobials

Chlorhexidine is used in some hair care products and in disinfectants for cleaning instruments. It has caused contact urticaria, but not among hairdressers.[69,70] Although preservatives and disinfectants (mainly parabens, formaldehyde releasers, and Kathon CG™) are used widely in hair cosmetics, no reports exist on contact urticaria caused by them among hairdressers. This situation may reflect their low potency to cause contact urticaria in the concentrations these substances are used in hair cosmetics.

17.5 CONCLUDING REMARKS

We have reviewed the current literature on agents causing contact urticaria in hairdressing products (Table 17.1). Potentially, many other agents that have been reported to cause contact urticaria may also be present in hairdressing products, and accordingly elicit contact urticaria.[56,71,72] Table 17.2 has been formulated by cross checking the list of agents causing contact urticaria and the list of ingredients in hair cosmetics as presented in the International Cosmetic Ingredient Handbooks of the Cosmetic, Toiletry, and Fragrance Association (CTFA) and other sources.

TABLE 17.2 Potential Contact Urticaria Causing Agents in Hair Cosmetics According to Product Categories

Agent	Shampoos	Conditioners	Rinses	Bleaches	Dyes and Colors	Permanent Waves	Wave Sets	Straighteners	Shaving Creams	Aerosol Fixatives	Other Hair Styling Agents
Alcohols											
benzyl alcohol	X		X		X	X			X	X	X
butyl alcohol						X					
cetyl alcohol	X	X	X	X	X	X		X	X	X	X
ethyl alcohol	X	X					X		X	X	X
isopropyl alcohol	X	X		X	X	X	X	X	X	X	X
lanolin alcohol	X	X		X	X	X	X	X	X	X	X
propylene glycol	X	X	X	X	X	X	X	X	X	X	X
stearyl alcohol	X	X	X	X	X	X		X	X		X
Anti-dandruff agents											
salicylic acid	X							X			X
sulfur	X	X			X					X	X
tar extracts	X										X
Colorants											
henna	X	X	X		X		X			X	
p-phenylenediamine					X						
N-phenyl-p-phenylenediamine					X						
resorcinol	X				X						X
senna	X	X	X		X		X			X	
Persulfates											
ammonium persulfate				X	X						
potassium persulfate				X	X						
sodium persulfate				X	X						

TABLE 17.2 (continued)   Potential Contact Urticaria Causing Agents in Hair Cosmetics According to Product Categories

Agent	Shampoos	Conditioners	Rinses	Bleaches	Dyes and Colors	Permanent Waves	Wave Sets	Straighteners	Shaving Creams	Aerosol Fixatives	Other Hair Styling Agents
Proteins and hydrolyzates, and other ingredients from plant, fruit, vegetable and animal origin											
apricot (oil)		X									
avocado (oil)	X										
birch (extract, sap)	X	X		X		X	X				
beer	X										
carrot (oil)	X	X	X				X			X	
castor oil	X	X		X	X	X	X	X			X
chamomile (extract, oil)	X	X			X					X	X
collagen (hydrolyzed)	X	X	X			X	X	X		X	X
corn (oil, starch)	X	X	X				X		X		X
egg	X	X	X			X					X
gelatin	X	X				X	X	X			
honey	X	X	X			X	X			X	X
keratin (hydrolyzed)	X	X				X				X	X
malt (extract)	X	X									X
milk/casein (hydrolyzed)	X	X		X		X	X				X
orange (oil)	X	X							X		X
papaya (extract)	X										
parsley (extract)	X										

peach (oil)		X								X	
rhubarb root					X						
sesame (oil)	X	X							X		X
silk (hydrolyzed)	X	X	X							X	X
soy (hydrolyzed, oil)	X	X			X	X					X
sunflower (oil)	X								X		X
tea (oil)	X	X			X						
wheat (extract, oil, hydrolyzed)							X		X		X
Perfumes											
balsam Peru		X									
camphor	X								X		X
cinnamal											X
eugenol											X
lime	X										
menthol	X	X	X						X	X	X
vanillin									X		
Preservatives and Disinfectants											
benzoic acid	X		X			X		X			X
chlorhexidine		X			X						
formaldehyde	X	X				X	X				X
hexamine isethionate	X										
ethylparaben						X	X		X		X
methylparaben	X	X	X	X	X	X	X		X	X	X
sodium benzoate	X	X				X			X	X	X
sodium sulfite	X	X			X	X					
sorbic acid	X	X		X			X		X		X
Resins and Polymers											
acrylics					X		X			X	X
colophony (rosin)										X	X

TABLE 17.2 (continued)   Potential Contact Urticaria Causing Agents in Hair Cosmetics According to Product Categories

Agent	Shampoos	Conditioners	Rinses	Bleaches	Dyes and Colors	Permanent Waves	Wave Sets	Straighteners	Shaving Creams	Aerosol Fixatives	Other Hair Styling Agents
Surfactants											
cocamide DEA	X	X	X	X	X	X			X		X
oleamide DEA	X	X		X	X	X					X
polysorbate 60		X	X						X		X
sorbitan laurate	X					X					
Miscellaneous											
ammonia		X		X	X	X		X	X		
sodium silicate				X		X			X		
α-tocopherol	X	X			X	X			X	X	X

REFERENCES

1. Wenninger, J. A. and McEwen, G. N. Jr., Eds., *International Cosmetic Ingredient Dictionary*, The Cosmetic, Toiletry, and Fragrances Association, Washington D.C., 1993, Sec. 4.
2. Kanerva, L., Jolanki, R., Toikkanen, J. and Estlander, T., Statistics on occupational contact urticaria, in *The Contact Urticaria Syndrome*, Amin, S., Lahti, A. and Maibach, H. I., Eds., CRC Press, Boca Raton, 1997.
3. Smit, H. A., van Rijssen, A., Vandenbroucke, J. P. and Coenraads, P. J., Susceptibility to and incidence of hand dermatitis in a cohort of apprentice hairdressers and nurses, *Scand. J. Work Environ. Health.* 20, 113, 1994.
4. Uter, W., Gefeller, O. and Schwanitz, H. J., The influence of skin sensitivity (atopy) and skin protection on the development of hand eczema in hairdressers — first results of a prospective cohort study, *Allergologie*, 18, 312, 1995.
5. Tupasela, O. and Kanerva, L., Skin tests and spesific IgE determinators in the diagnosis of contact urticaria caused by low-molecular weight chemicals, in *The Contact Urticaria Syndrome*, Amin, S., Lahti, A. and Maibach, H. I., Eds., CRC Press, Boca Raton, 1997.
6. Nutter, A. F., Contact urticaria to rubber, *Br. J. Dermatol.*, 101, 597, 1979.
7. Kleinhans, D., Contact urticaria to rubber gloves, *Contact Dermatitis*, 10, 179, 1984.
8. Assalve, D., Cicioni, C., Perno, P. and Lisi, P., Contact urticaria and anaphylactic reaction from cornstarch surgical glove powder, *Contact Dermatitis*, 19, 61, 1988.
9. Maso, M. J. and Goldberg, D. J., Contact dermatitis from disposable glove use: a review, *J. Am. Acad. Dermatol.*, 23, 733, 1990.
10. Belsito, D. V., Contact urticaria caused by rubber, *Derm. Clin.*, 8, 61, 1990.
11. Guerra, L., Tosti, A., Bardazzi, F., Pigatto, P., Lisi, P., Santucci, B., Valsecchi, R., Schena, D., Angelini, G., Sertoli, A., Alaya, F. and Kokelj, F., Contact dermatitis in hairdressers: the Italian experience, *Contact Dermatitis*, 26, 101, 1992.
12. Van der Walle, H. B. and Brunsveld V. M., Latex allergy among hairdressers, *Contact Dermatitis*, 32, 177, 1995.
13. Turjanmaa K., Mäkinen-Kiljunen S., Reunala T., Alenius H., and Palosuo T., Natural rubber latex allergy, *Immunology and Allergy Clinics of North America*, 15, 71, 1995.
14. Leino, T., unpublished data, 1994.
15. Kwangsukstith, C. and Maibach, H. I., Contact urticaria from polyurethane-membrane hypoallergenic gloves, *Contact Dermatitis*, 33, 200, 1995.
16. Lang, G., Hair cleansing and care preparations, in *Ullmann's Encyclopedia of Industrial Chemistry*, 5th ed., Elvers, B., Hawkins, S., Ravenscroft, M., Rounsville, J. F. and Schulz, G., Eds., VCH Publishers, New York, 1989, 576.
17. Draelos, Z. K., Hair cosmetics, *Dermatol. Clinics*, 9, 19, 1991.
18. Picardo, M., Rovina, A., Cristaudo, A., Cannistraci, C. and Santucci, B., Contact urticaria from *Tilia* (lime), *Contact Dermatitis*, 13, 72, 1985.
19. Rietschel, R. L., Contact urticaria from synthetic cassia oil and sorbic acid limited to the face, *Contact Dermatitis*, 4, 347, 1978.
20. Fisher, A. A., Urticaria from papaya shampoo, *Am. J. Contact Dermatitis*, 4, 65, 1993.
21. Temesvári, E. and Varkonyi, V., Contact urticaria provoked by egg, *Contact Dermatitis*, 6, 143, 1980.
22. Braun-Falco, O. and Ring, J., Zur Therapie des atopischen Ekzems, *Hautarzt*, 35, 447, 1984.

23. Pfeiff, B. and Kalveram, C. M., Airborne contact urticaria by hydrolyzed collagen, *Aktuel Dermatol.,* 15 (1-2), 21, 1989.

24. Kousa, M., Strand, R., Mäkinen-Kiljunen, S. and Hannuksela, M., Contact urticaria from hair conditioner, *Contact Dermatitis,* 23, 279, 1990.

25. Pasche-Koo, F., Cleys, M. and Hauser, C., Contact urticaria with systemic symptoms caused by bovine collagen in a hair conditioner, *Am. J. Contact Dermatitis,* 7, 56, 1996.

26. Niinimäki, A., Hannuksela, M. and Moilanen M., Protein hydrolysates of hair cosmetic products as causes of contact urticaria in hairdressers, in *Abstracts of the Second Congress of the European Society of Contact Dermatitis,* European Society of Contact Dermatitis, Barcelona, 1994, 57.

27. Bonnevie, P., *Aetiologie und Pathogenese der Ekzemkrankheiten,* Nyt Nordisk Forlag, Kopenhagen, 1939.

28. Calnan, C. and Shuster, S., Reactions to ammonium persulphate, *Arch. Dermatol.,* 88, 812, 1963.

29. Gaultier, R., Gervaise, P. and Mellario, F., Two causes of occupational asthma and urticaria in hairdressers: persulphate salts and silk, *Arch. Mal. Prof.,* 27, 809, 1966.

30. Meindl, K. and Meyer R., Asthma and urticaria in hairdressers caused by bleaching agents containing persulphates, *Zentralbl. Arbeitsmed. Arbeitsschul.,* 3, 75, 1969.

31. Brubacker, M. M., Urticarial reactions to ammonium persulphate, *Arch. Dermatol.,* 106, 413, 1972.

32. Fisher, A. A. and Dooms-Goossens, A., Persulphate hair bleach reactions, *Arch. Dermatol.,* 112, 1407, 1976.

33. Widström, L., Allergic reactions to ammonium persulphate in hair bleach, *Contact Dermatitis,* 3, 343, 1977.

34. Fisher, A. A., The persulphates — a triple threat, *Cutis,* 35, 520, 1985.

35. Fisher, A. A., The persulphates — a triple threat, part II: occupational exposures, *Cutis,* 36, 25, 1985.

36. Pepys, J., Hutchcroft, B. J. and Breslin, A. B. X., Asthma due to immediate chemical agents — persulfate salts and henna in hairdressers, *Clin. Allergy,* 6, 399, 1987.

37. Kleinhans, D. and Ranneberg, K. M., Immediate-type reactions caused by ammonium persulphate hair bleaches, *Allergologie,* 12, 353, 1989.

38. Schwaiblmair, M., Baur, X. and Fruhmann, G., Bronchial asthma caused by hair bleach in a hairdresser, *Dtsch. Med. Wschr.,* 115, 695, 1990.

39. Guerra, L., Bardazzi, F. and Tosti, A., Contact dermatitis in hairdressers' clients, *Contact Dermatitis,* 26, 108, 1992.

40. Von Krogh, G. and Maibach, H. I., The contact urticaria syndrome — an update review, *J. Am. Acad. Dermatol.,* 5, 328, 1981.

41. Parra, F. M., Igea, J. M., Quirce, S., Ferrando, M. C., Martin J. A. and Losada E., Occupational asthma in a hairdresser caused by persulphate salts, *Allergy,* 47, 656, 1992.

42. Parsons, J. F., Goodwin B. F. J. and Safford R. J., Studies on the action of histamine release by persulphates, *Fd. Cosmet. Toxicol.,* 17, 129, 1979.

43. Zviak, C., Ed., *The Science of Hair Care,* Marcel Dekker, New York, 1986.

44. Calnan, C. D., Hair dye reactions, *Contact Derm. Newsl.,* 1, 16, 1967.

45. Edwards, E. K. Jr. and Edwards, E. K., Contact urticaria and allergic contact dermatitis caused by paraphenylenediamine, *Cutis,* 34, 87, 1984.

46. Temesvári, E., Contact urticaria from paraphenylenediamine, *Contact Dermatitis,* 11, 125, 1984.

47a. Goldberg, B. J., Herman, F. F. and Hirata, I., Systematic anaphylaxis due to an oxidation product of p-phenylenediamine in a hair dye, *Ann. Allergy,* 58, 205, 1987.

47b. Pasche-Koo, F., French, L., Piletta, P.-A., Saurat, J.-H. and Hauser, C., Contact urticaria and anaphylactic shock due to an oxidation product of diaminotoluene found in a hair dye, Abstracts of the Clinical Dermatology 2000 Congress, Vancouver, CCT Healthcare Communications Ltd., London, 1996, 151.

48a. Von Liebe, V., Karge H.-J. and Burg, G., Kontakturtikaria, *Hautarzt,* 30, 544, 1979.

48b. Wigger-Alberti, W., Elsner, P. and Wüthrich, B., Immediate-type allergy to hair dye Basic Blue 99 in a hairdresser, *Allergy,* 51, 64, 1996.

48c. Jagtman, B., Urticaria and contact urticaria due to Basic Blue 99 in a hair dye, *Contact Dermatitis,* 35, 52, 1996.

49a. Frosch, P. J. and Hausen, B. M., Allergische Reaktionen vom Soforttyp auf das Haarfärbemittel Henna, *Allergologie,* 9(8), 351, 1986.

49b. Majoie, I. M. L. and Bruynzeel, D., Occupational immediate-type hypersensitivity to henna in a hairdresser, *Am. J. Contact Dermatitis,* 7, 38, 1996.

50. Starr, J. C., Yunginger, J. and Brasher, G. W., Immediate type I asthmatic response to henna following occupational exposure in hairdressers, *Ann. Allergy,* 48, 98, 1982.

51. Helin, T. and Mäkinen-Kiljunen, S., Occupational asthma and rhinoconjunktivitis caused by senna, *Allergy,* in press.

52. Frosch, P., Burrows, D., Camarasa, J. G., Dooms-Goossens, A., Ducombs, G., Lahti, A., Menne, T., Rycroft, R. J., Shaw, S., White, I. R. and Wilkinson, J. D., Allergic reactions to a hairdressers' series: results from nine European centres, *Contact Dermatitis,* 28, 180,1993.

53. Lang, G., Hairstyling preparations, in *Ullmann's Encyclopedia of Industrial Chemistry,* 5th ed., Elvers, B., Hawkins, S., Ravenscroft, M., Rounsville, J. F. and Schulz, G., Eds., VCH Publishers, New York, 1989, 580.

54. Fisher, A. A., *Contact Dermatitis,* 2nd ed., Lea & Febiger, Philadelphia, 1973, 284.

55. Rivers, J. K. and Rycroft, R. J., Occupational allergic contact urticaria from colophony, *Contact Dermatitis,* 17, 181, 1987.

56. De Groot, A. C., Weyland, J. and Nater, J. D., The contact urticaria syndrome, in *Unwanted Effects of Cosmetics and Drugs Used in Dermatology,* Elsevier, Amsterdam, 1994, Chap. 7.

57. Mikkelsen, F. and Thomsen, K., Occupational contact dermatitis to human hair, *Contact Dermatitis,* 4, 165, 1978.

58. Freeman, S., Woman allergic to husband's sweat and semen, *Contact Dermatitis,* 14, 110, 1985.

59. Yu, B., Sawai, T. and Uehara, M., Immediate hypersensitivity skin reactions to human dander in atopic dermatitis, *Arch. Dermatol.,* 124, 1530, 1988.

60. Adachi, J. and Aoki, T., IgE antibody to sweat in atopic dermatitis, *Acta Derm. Venereol. (Stockh),* 144 (Suppl.), 83, 1989.

61. Adachi, J., Aoki, T. and Yamatodani, A., Demonstration of sweat allergy in cholinergic urticaria, *J. Dermatol. Sci.,* 7, 142, 1994.

62. Jensen-Jarolim, E., Poulsen, L. K., With, H., Kieffer, M., Ottevanger, V. and Skov, P. S., Atopic dermatitis of the face, scalp, and neck: Type I reaction to the yeast Pityrosporum ovale?, *J. Allergy Clin. Immunol.,* 89, 45, 1992.

63. Shuster, S. and Blatchford, N., Seborrhoeic dermatitis and dandruff — a fungal disease, *R. Soc. Med. Serv.,* 132, 1, 1988.

64. Leino, T., Nordman, H. and Kanerva L., Human dandruff as a cause for occupational allergy?, in *Abstracts of the 44. Nordic Work Environment Meeting*, Naantali, Finnish Institute of Occupational Health, 1995, 224.

65. Dalquist, I., Fregert, S. and Gruvberger, B., Release of nickel from plated utensils in permanent wave liquids, *Contact Dermatitis*, 5, 52, 1979.

66. Valsecchi, R. and Canelli, T., Contact urticaria from nickel, *Contact Dermatitis,* 17, 187, 1987.

67. Estlander, T., Kanerva, L., Tupasela, O., Keskinen, H. and Jolanki, R., Immediate and delayed allergy to nickel with contact urticaria, rhinitis, asthma, and contact dermatitis, *Clin. Exp. Allergy*, 23, 306, 1993.

68. Smith, J. D., Odom R. B. and Maibach, H. I., Contact urticaria from cobalt chloride, *Arch. Dermatol.*, 11, 1610, 1975.

69. Bergqvist-Karlsson, A, Delayed and immediate-type hypersensitivity to chlorhexidine, *Contact Dermatitis*, 18, 84, 1988.

70. Wong, W. K., Goh C. L. and Chan K. W., Contact urticaria from chlorhexidine, *Contact Dermatitis*, 22, 52, 1990.

71. Lahti, A., Immediate contact reactions, in *Textbook of Contact Dermatitis*, Rycroft, R. J. G., Menné, T., Frosch, P. J. and Benezra, C., Eds., Springer-Verlag, Berlin, 1992, 62.

72. Zajonz, C. and Frosch, P. J., Ursachen von Kontakturtikaria unter besonderer Berücksichtigung von Arbeitsstoffen, *Hausarzt*, 45, 65, 1994.

18

Contact Urticaria from Latex Gloves

Kristiina Turjanmaa

CONTENTS

18.1   INTRODUCTION

Rubber allergy has been known for decades as a cause of eczema among glove users.[1] It has also been a marked occupational disorder among workers in different fields who want to protect their hands from irritative and sensitizing chemicals.[2] Little was known about the more far-reaching consequences of rubber allergy before 1979, when Nutter reported his first case of immediate contact urticaria in hands after use of household gloves.[3] It soon became evident that contact urticaria from gloves not only causes itching but can even give rise to life-threatening symptoms.[4-6] Förström fixed attention on the occupational nature of this allergy in a nurse who wore surgical gloves.[7] The "old" rubber allergy represents a type IV sensitization to the chemicals used in rubber manufacture; the "new" one is an immediate, type I, IgE-mediated allergy to proteins originating from cytoplasm of specialized cells situated beneath of the bark of rubber tree (Hevea brasiliensis) and which still are present in products made from natural rubber latex (NRL).[8-10] The symptoms of IgE-mediated allergy cover the whole spectrum of contact urticaria syndrom extending from contact urticaria and eczema to generalized urticaria, conjunctivitis, rhinitis, asthma, and anaphylaxis; even lethal cases have been described.[11-13] They can be elicited from all NRL products such as pacifiers, balloons, toys, condoms, and medical devices, but surgical and protective gloves are the most important cause of symptoms (Table 18.1).[14] It is a major occupational hazard among health care workers, but another group of people especially at danger are sensitized but undiagnosed persons who come into contact with different kinds of NRL products as patients in the health care sector.[15-25]

TABLE 18.1   NRL Products Giving Symptoms in 57 Health Care Workers and in 67 Adults of Other Professions with NRL Allergy, Diagnosed at the Department of Dermatology, Tampere University Hospital

Product	Health care workers	Others
Household gloves	14 (25%)	57 (85%)
Surgical gloves	54 (95%)	4 (6%)
Balloons	4 (7%)	18 (27%)
Condoms	9 (16%)	6 (9%)
Rubber bands	3 (5%)	5 (7%)
Medical intervention	5 (9%)	8 (12%)
Aerogen	9 (16%)	5 (7%)

18.2   CONTACT URTICARIA SYNDROME

Natural rubber latex allergy is a typical example of immunologic contact urticaria, with a positive Prausnitz-Küstner test verifying its IgE-mediated mechanism.[8-9] The distribution of the symptoms elicited by NRL gloves was analyzed in a material comprising 42 subjects: no local skin symptoms were seen in 2%; redness, itching, or exacerbation of hand eczema in 10%; CUS stage 1 in 40%; stage 2 in 17%;

stage 3 in 21%; and stage 4 in 10%.[11] Division of the symptoms of CU into four different stages seems to be clinically justified. In the case of allergy to NRL gloves, conjunctivitis might be classified as stage 1, since the symptoms often appear after touching the eye with an ungloved hand after gloves have been worn and the symptom is consequently one-sided. Rhinitis may also be caused by direct mucosal contact with airborne NRL-contaminated particles of the corn starch powder used in the manufacture of latex gloves.[26-27] Gastrointestinal symptoms may also be related to direct mucosal contact with allergens eluted from gloves when eating food, e.g., sandwiches, prepared by a person wearing gloves.[28]

18.3 DIAGNOSIS

Since clinical history does not identify all persons with NRL allergy, reliable tests should be available. The American Academy of Allergy and Immunology has published a committee report: Task Force on Allergic Reactions to Latex,[29] and the American College of Allergy, Asthma and Immunology published a position paper: Latex allergy — an emerging healthcare problem,[30] giving quidelines on management of latex allergic persons. Sussman and Beezhold published a very comprehensive and practical overview on the identification and management of persons with NRL allergy.[31] Skin prick tests (SPT), serological tests, and use tests have proved useful in diagnosis of NRL allergy, but no test is 100% sensitive and specific. SPT may even be unsafe when too strong of allergens or intradermal techniques are used.[32-34]

18.3.1 Skin Prick Test

Rubber end-products like gloves and natural rubber latex with or without ammonia as a preservative have been used as test materials. The choice of methods is considerable: open patch test, rub test, scratch and scratch chamber test, and SPT.[7-9,35-38] Nonstandardized allergenic preparations have been compared in prick testing and a good correlation was found between the glove eluates, nonammoniated latex, and crushed rubber-tree leaves.[39] Several types of lancets and needles can be used for the skin prick or puncture tests. An 1-mm one peaked lancet (ALK, Allergologisk Laboratorium A/S, Denmark, and Stallergpoint, Stallergènes, S.A., France) with shoulders to prevent deeper penetration can be recommended as a safe tool for SPT both in adults and children.

At the moment, there is a new standardized, commercially available SPT latex allergen on the European market (Stallergènes, S.A., France).[40] In addition to that, there are several nonstandardized SPT allergens on the European market and one in Canada (Bencard, Mississuaga, Ontario, Canada).[41] The allergens of Stallergènes, ALK, and Bencard were compared with an allergenic glove eluate (1:5 w/v, Triflex, Baxter, lot 06 92L12DPGN 12/92) by testing a group of 110 patients with earlier diagnosed NRL allergy. The sensitivity was 88% for Stallergènes, 54% for ALK, 92% for Bencard, and 92% for the reference glove.[42] The specificity of all test materials was 100% in 200 control patients with no NRL allergy. Glove eluates have been widely used earlier in Europe for diagnosing NRL allergy. Using 1:5 w/v eluates, no adverse reactions have been described, but because the allergenicity of gloves differs from each other and even earlier high allergenic gloves tend to be made less allergenic recently, the selection of a good test glove can become difficult.[43-44] The investigator using this kind of self-made eluates should be aware of the allergenicity of the test material to avoid false negative test results. In addition, the use of the gloves as a test material has been criticized, because they may also contain other water-soluble elements causing type I reactions in the skin.[45-46] In our laboratory, 80 patients with NRL allergy have been retested concomitantly with glove eluates and dilutions of nonammoniated, nonthiuram-containing latex. The results were 100% concordant. When LATZ is used for SPT, it is possible to get reactions from thiurams, because LATZ stands for low-ammonia-tetramethylthiuramdisulphide-zinc oxide. Type I reactions to rubber chemicals are still questionable, because the test materials are in petrolatum, and the solubility of rubber chemicals from that substance is badly controlled.[47]

18.3.2 RAST

NRL-specific IgE-antibodies in the patient´s serum can be measured with the radioallergosorbent test (RAST) or more recently with the CAP RAST system (Pharmacia, Uppsala, Sweden). The sensitivity with RAST so far has been only 60–65%.[11,15] CAP RAST has been described to give more positive test results, but the clinical significance could not always be estimated.[24,48-51] In patients with previous anaphylactic reactions, the sensitivity is higher, but not 100%. Even anaphylactic reactions are described in patients with negative RAST.[52] Another serological test is used today in the U.S. (AlaSTAT, Diagnostic Products Corporation, Los Angeles, CA).[53] In 1000 otherwise healthy blood donors, it revealed NRL allergy in 6.5%.[54] In other studies, the AlaSTAT method has been found to give false positivity in atopic people but in nonatopics sensitivity was 80% and specificity 100%.[55] IgE-antibodies to NRL can also be evaluated with immunoblotting, immunoelectrophoretic methods such as crossed radioimmunoelectrophoresis, solid phase radioimmunoassay, and enzyme immunoassay.[56-59] In addition, the histamine-release test has been found to be a sensitive *in vitro* study.[60] However, all these methods are expensive and time consuming and less well suitable for routine use in the diagnosis of NRL allergy.

18.3.3 Use Test

The use test with a rubber latex glove should always be performed when there is some discrepancy between positive SPT and/or RAST results and negative clinical history and also in cases where the person is convinced about being allergic to NRL and the skin and serological tests remain negative.[24,31] It is not recommended for patients with a history of NRL-related anaphylaxis when SPT and/or RAST are positive. The use test should always be started with one finger of a glove on a wet skin because the whole-hand use test on eczematous skin has been observed to cause anaphylaxis.[14,61] If there are some wheals after 15 min, the test is judged as positive and stopped. If not, the test is continued with the whole glove on the wetted hand

TABLE 18.2   Symptoms Caused by NRL Products in 57 Health Care Workers and in 67 Adults of Other Professions with Verified Immediate Allergy to NRL

Symptom	Health care workers	Others
Contact urticaria	79%	72%
Hand eczema	42%	64%
Conjunctivitis	28%	16%
Rhinitis	16%	13%
Facial edema	14%	28%
Asthma	2%	4%
Generalized urticaria	9%	13%
Anaphylaxis	7%	10%

for another 15 min, always keeping a vinyl glove on the other hand as a negative control to exclude dermographism. If negative, the test should be prolonged up to 1 week using an allergenic latex glove and a vinyl glove as a control for at least 2 hours a day to exclude mild NRL allergy or delayed-type NRL allergy (protein contact dermatitis). In milk allergic persons (especially in atopic children), the use test may give false positive results because of casein used as stabilizer in some latex gloves.[62]

Patients with suspicion of NRL-related rhinitis or asthma should be challenged on nasal or bronchial mucosa especially when verification is needed for insurance or other authorities in occupational cases.[27,63]

18.4 SYMPTOMS

The most typical symptom from type I allergy to latex gloves is contact urticaria, i.e., wheal-and-flare reaction at the site of contact.[11] The thinner skin of the dorsal side of hands and fingers reacts more easily, as do the wrists. The symptoms begin in a few to 30 min after contact and disappear without treatment in 1–2 hours. Some people experience only itching and redness, and some develop eczema. Since eczema on hands often looks the same, whether caused by irritation, type IV allergy to rubber chemicals, or type I protein contact dermatitis from latex gloves, it always needs to be examined for all these possibilities.[64]

With regard to CU from gloves, there are always two types of sensitized recipients: the one wearing the gloves and the other being touched with gloves worn by others, e.g., nursing personnel. Both can contract the whole variety of CUS. The different symptoms are described in Table 18.2.[24]

In 70 German patients, all (100%) had contact urticaria; 51% rhinitis; 44% conjunctivitis; 31% dyspnea; 24% systemic symptoms; and 6% severe systemic reactions during surgery.[63] Contact urticaria begins by definition on the place of contact: in the case of using a balloon, swelling of lips and facial edema are common, and by using condoms, the symptoms are mostly on genitals or in the vagina first.

Fingers can be contaminated by touching NRL products and the allergens can be transferred to more distant places.[65]

NRL allergens are verified to become airborne and thus to cause rhinitis and asthma.[26,66-69] In a Belgian study, 13 of 273 hospital workers were SPT positive (4.7%) to NRL, and in 2.5% occupational asthma due to NRL was diagnosed.[27] Latex extract has been included in the routine series for airborne allergens since 1988 at the Department of Dermatology, Tampere University Hospital, and the series is used for testing of all patients suspected for atopy and also for everybody who is going to be patch tested (Table 18.3). Testing latex routinely shows that health care workers remain the largest single occupation with work related sensitization, but all together there are more representatives of other occupations among the sensitized persons (Table 18.4). Hadjiliadis and co-workers have included latex allergen (Bencard) recently in the series of 13 common aeroallergens by testing newly referred adult asthma and allergy patients. Of a total of 224 patients, 10 (4.5%) had a positive SPT response to latex. They confirmed that NRL allergy can be diagnosed in patients who have not been referred because of suspicion of NRL allergy and recommend addition of latex allergen to a routine battery of skin tests in allergy practice.[25]

TABLE 18.3 Cause of Referral to Allergy Testing in 124 Adult Patients with Verified NRL Allergy Including 57 Health Care Workers and 67 of Other Professions

Symptom	Health care workers	Others
Hand eczema	27 (47%)	22 (33%)
Atopic eczema	12 (21%)	26 (39%)
Intraoperative anaphylaxis	3 (5%)	7 (10%)
Routine hospital screening	15 (26%)	0
Facial eczema	0	4 (6%)
Rhinitis	0	5 (7%)
Urticaria	0	2 (3%)
Other dermatoses	0	1 (2%)

TABLE 18.4 Professions of 49/57 (86%) Health Care Workers and of 17/67 (25%) Nonmedical Workers with Work Related Allergy to NRL

Health care workers		Other occupations	
Physicians	14	Farmers wives	2
Nurses	17	Kitchen workers	3
Dental nurses	6	Cleaners	3
Laboratory nurses	4	Textile workers	2
Physiotherapists	1	Workers in rubber band plant	3
Workers in a medical plant	3	Paper mill worker	1
Other medical occupations	4	Dairy workers	1
		Departmental secretary	1
		Private caretaker	1

18.5 FREQUENCY

Since the first report of Nutter in 1979, there have been several hundreds of case reports on immediate allergy to NRL, mostly in connection with the use of gloves.[11,14,15,70-73] The incidence seems to be increasing but many of the diagnosed cases have had symptoms for years — for up to 20 years in some cohorts.[74] It may be only the increasing awareness and the better diagnostic facilities that reflect the rising number of diagnosed cases. On the other hand, the use of both surgical latex gloves and, particularly, of examination gloves has increased immensely since the outbreak of hepatitis and HIV infection. Exposure to other NRL products such as protecting gloves and balloons and condoms is also increasing. There are, however, no exact numbers on the incidence and prevalence of the NRL allergy, and the comparison between different published materials is difficult because of diversity of diagnostic tools. In different cohorts of operating room personnel, 2.5–10.7% of the tested workers have been diagnosed as having immediate allergy to NRL.[24,27,48,49,74-79] In a small cohort (n = 77) tested by Cormio, 99% of the workers in an operating room were skin prick tested with three different latex glove eluates.[80] All solitary weak positive reactions (in size at least half of that of histamine dihydrochloride 10 mg/ml) were controlled by a use test. They all turned out to be false SPT positive: all suspected persons wore for 90 min the same glove brand as that which had given the weak positive SPT reaction. All four (5.2%) persons with at least histamine size reactions to 2–3 different glove brands showed relevant immediate NRL glove allergy. These results demonstrate the importance of the use test in judging the relevancy of weak skin test reactions.

In Tampere, Finland, 4708 patients were consecutively tested for atopy and 0.85% were positive to latex by skin prick testing. 804 patients were prick tested preoperatively for latex allergy and one patient (0.12%) was found to be latex allergic.[24] In 1993, 1140 new work-related skin diseases were reported to the Finnish Register for Occupational Diseases.[81] Delayed type allergy to rubber chemicals was seen in 82(7.2%) subjects and allergy to natural rubber latex in 59(5.2%) subjects. These numbers are probably too low because health care workers especially are known to avoid registers of this kind.

18.6 RISK FACTORS

In various studies, atopy and hand eczema have frequently been connected with type I allergy to NRL.[11,14,15] In the material of 124 adult persons presented in Tables 18.1–18.4, 75% of the health care workers and 81% of the people in other occupations had a personal history of atopy and, in the same frequency, hand eczema, but not always in the same person at the same time. Rysted´s studies confirm that chronic hand eczema is often a complication of atopic dermatitis in childhood, so the concomitant occurrence of the two risk factors is easy to explain.[82] Also, exposure to rubber gloves is enhanced in patients with hand eczema and dry skin because they try to protect their skin. Spina bifida patients as well as other patient populations frequently operated on and using catheters on a regular basis constitute another big group of risk persons.[83] More recently, atopic infants with food allergy have proved to be another important risk group. Simultaneously occurring allergy to several foods makes the diagnosis especially difficult. A use test is difficult in milk allergic infants because of nondeclared occurrence of casein in many gloves.[84]

18.7 CONCOMITANT TYPE IV AND TYPE I ALLERGY TO RUBBER PRODUCTS

Concomitant sensitization both to rubber chemicals and to NRL has been reported. In an earlier study: 1 of 18 patients with delayed type allergy to rubber chemicals showed concomitant sensitization to NRL and, vice versa, of 35 patients with NRL allergy, 5 showed positive patch tests to thiurams.[47]

In the material presented in Tables 18.1–18.4, 83 of 124 patients were patch tested either only with the European Contact Dermatitis Research Group standard series including different rubber mixes or also with a rubber series including individual rubber chemicals. Of these, 11/83 (13%) showed positive patch test reactions to some rubber chemical or mixes, while 7/11 were positive for thiurams only, and 2/11 tested positive to both thiurams and carbamates.[24] Type IV allergy to NRL has also been reported recently, but the patch tests were performed with LATZ containing thiurams. Consequently, thiuram allergy as a cause of the reaction cannot be fully excluded without retesting with pure material.[85] Heese has pointed to the possible allergies caused by other ingredients included in rubber gloves, but so far in addition to casein the only verified type I reaction to glove ingredients is that caused by ethylene oxide which was earlier used for sterilization of latex gloves.[46,86]

18.8 RUBBER PROTEIN ALLERGENS

In freshly collected latex, 240 different polypeptides have been demonstrated by 2-dimensional immunoblotting and at least 57 of them can be considered as allergens because of their capability to bind IgE antibodies from NRL-allergic patient sera.[59] It has been demonstrated that several proteins in NRL are capable of causing immediate hypersensitivity reactions in NRL-allergic patients.[87] Many of these proteins have recently been characterized at the primary structure level. The most significant allergens known at present include 20 kD prohevein, 14 kD hevein C-domain, 14.6 kD rubber elongation factor (REF), with a 36 kD protein being presumably a rubber tree endo-1,3-beta-glucosidase, and previously uncharacterized NRL proteins with apparent molecular weights of 27, 45, and 75 kD.[88-92] At present, there is increasing evidence that some low molecular weight peptides, carrying the responsible allergen epitopes, may play a crucial role in this respect. In one highly allergenic latex glove, the majority of IgE-binding ability was attributable to hevein (a 43-amino acid *N*-terminal fragment of prohevein with molecular mass of 4719 d) molecules, suggesting that these peptides can be significant sensitizers in NRL allergy.[93] Recent investigations have revealed common allergens in fruit such as banana and avocado and NRL. It has not yet been satisfactorily established whether infants showing positive SPR reactions to banana and NRL at the same time but without any symptoms from using pacifiers are really sensitized to NRL or if it is only because they are allergic to bananas.[94-97]

18.9 PROPHYLACTICS

The best prophylactic method is to eliminate the allergens from latex gloves. The proteins are, however, needed to some extent in the manufacture of gloves. Comparison of the allergenicity of different latex gloves by the SPT method showed great variation suggesting that it is possible to manufacture rubber latex gloves with so small amounts of allergens that even most of the sensitized persons can use them.[43,74] At the moment we lack a reliable worldwide available method to estimate *in vitro* allergenicity of NRL products, but once we have it, the latex gloves should be labeled accordingly. Although all proteins in gloves are not allergens, a relatively good correlation has been found between allergens and proteins by using a modified Lowry microassay procedure.[98] Therefore, protein content may be useful for labeling of the latex glove packages as long as better methods are not available.

NRL allergens are known to get airborne by contaminated glove powder. Use of powder-free gloves by all workers at the same place has been found to enable latex allergic patients to continue working in their own profession.[99,100] In Finland, the Finnish National Research and Development Centre for Welfare and Health provided for study 20 brands of international surgical and examination gloves commonly used in the country in 1994 and covering over 90% of the market. The allergenicity was investigated using the skin prick test, RAST inhibition, and ELISA inhibition simultaneously.[101] The correlation between the methods was highly significant (r = 0.94–0.96). Differences of more than 1000-fold in the allergenicity of the latex gloves studied were demonstrated. Glove marketing companies and glove purchasing personnel in hospitals and health care centers were informed of the observed variation in the allergenicity of the gloves. It appears that this information has already had a clear impact of glove purchasing policies in Finland. The study has been repeated with gloves on the market in 1995 and will be extended to condoms as well.

PVC gloves are good for people not working in the health care sector, where the larger amount of pin holes is not acceptable because of the risk of infections. Totally latex free surgical gloves (Dermapren, Ansell International, Melbourne; Neolon, Deseret Medical Inc., Sandy, Utah, U.S.; Tactylon, Smart Practice, Phoenix, Arizona, U.S.; Elastyren, Danpren Gloves A/S, Albertslund, Denmark; Allergard, J&J, U.S.) are needed when operating on or examining latex allergic patients or when the health care worker does not tolerate even the less allergenic or powder free latex gloves.

The other part of prophylactics is diagnosing sensitized persons in time to prevent exposure to latex material. The method of choice is to include latex allergen in SPT series for aeroallergens and foods and to use these series for testing of atopic allergy (atopic eczema, allergic rhinitis, asthma) and food allergy in children and in addition to patch tests for patients with hand dermatitis.[24,25,84]

18.10 CONCLUSIONS

Contact urticaria from rubber latex gloves is an increasing problem both in the health care sector and among people using different kinds of protecting gloves, not to forget housewives using household gloves. Because the symptoms are variable, the sensitized persons consult doctors from different specialties. Besides allergologists, all doctors, but at least dermatologists, otorhinolaryngologists, pulmonists, gynecologists, and surgeons should be aware of the symptoms, diagnostic possibilities, and prophylactics. All health care workers and people using protecting gloves should be increasingly informed to understand the importance of using either non-powder or low-allergenic gloves if one co-worker suffers from NRL allergy. The accurate information of big populations is difficult; therefore, the manufacturers of rubber latex gloves and other NRL products should produce better quality as regards type I allergenicity, and their products should bear adequate labeling. In addition to information concerning allergenic proteins in NRL products, the rubber chemicals used should be indicated on the label.

REFERENCES

1. Downing, J. G., Dermatitis from rubber gloves, *N. Engl. J. Med.,* 208, 196, 1933.
2. Cronin, E., *Contact dermatitis,* Churchill Livingstone, Edinburgh, 1980, 714.
3. Nutter, A. F., Contact urticaria to rubber, *Br. J. Dermatol.,* 101, 597, 1979.
4. Axelsson, I. G. K., Eriksson, M., and Wrangsjö, K., Anaphylaxis and angioedema due to rubber allergy in children, *Acta Pediatr. Scand.,* 77, 314, 1988.
5. Turjanmaa, K., Reunala, T., Tuimala, R., and Kärkkäinen, T., Allergy to latex gloves: unusual complication during delivery, *Br. Med. J.,* 297, 1029, 1988.
6. Pecquet, C., Leynadier, F., and Dry, J., Contact urticaria and anaphylaxis to natural latex, *J. Am. Acad. Dermatol.,* 22, 631, 1990.
7. Förström, L., Contact urticaria from latex surgical gloves, *Contact Dermatitis,* 6, 33, 1980.
8. Köpman, A. and Hannuksela, M., Contact urticaria to rubber, *Duodecim,* 3, 39, 1983.
9. Turjanmaa, K., Reunala, T., Tuimala, R., and Kärkkäinen, T., Severe IgE-mediated allergy to surgical gloves (Abstract), *Allergy,* 39, 35, 1984.
10. Frosch, P. J., Wahl, R., Bahmer, F. A., and Maasch, H. J., Contact urticaria to rubber gloves is IgE-mediated, *Contact Dermatitis,* 14, 241, 1986.
11. Turjanmaa, K., Latex glove contact urticaria, Thesis, *Acta Universitatis Tamperensis,* Ser A, Vol 254, University of Tampere, 1988.
12. Feczko, P. J., Simms, S. M., and Bakirci, N., Fatal hypersensitivity reaction during a barium enema, *Am. J. Roentgenol.* 153, 275, 1989.
13. Ownby, D. R., Tomlanovich, M., Sammons, N., and McCullough, J., Anaphylaxis associated with latex allergy during barium enema examinations, *Am. J. Roentgenol.,* 156, 903, 1991.
14. Wrangsjö, K., Wahlberg, J. E., and Axelsson, I. G. K., IgE-mediated allergy to natural rubber in 30 patients with contact urticaria, *Contact Dermatitis,* 19, 264, 1988.
15. Levy, D. A., Charpin, D., Pecquet, C., Leynadier, F., and Vervloet, D., Allergy to latex, *Allergy,* 47, 579, 1992.

16. Fisher, A. A., Allergic contact reactions in health care personnel, *J. Allergy Clin. Immunol.*, 90, 729, 1992.
17. Tomazic, V. J., Withrow, T. J., Fisher, B. J., and Dillard, S. F., Latex-associated allergies and anaphylactic reactions, *Clin. Immunol. Immunopathol.* 64, 89, 1992.
18. Weiss, M. E. and Hirshman, C. A., Latex allergy, *Can. J. Anaesth.*, 39, 528, 1992.
19. Taylor, J. S., Latex allergy, *Am. J. Contact Dermatitis*, 4, 114, 1993.
20. Hamann, C. P., Natural rubber latex protein sensitivity in review, *Am. J. Contact Dermatitis*, 4, 4, 1993.
21. Pumphrey, R. S. H., Allergy to Hevea latex, *Clin. Exp. Immunol.*, 98, 358, 1994.
22. Slater, J. E., Latex allergy, *J. Allergy Clin. Immunol.*, 94, 139,1994.
23. Charous, B. L., Hamilton, R. G., and Yunginger, J. W., Occupational latex exposure: characteristics of contact and systemic reactions in 47 workers, *J. Allergy Clin. Immunol.*, 94, 12, 1994.
24. Turjanmaa, K., Mäkinen-Kiljunen, S., Reunala, T., Alenius, H., and Palosuo, T., Natural rubber latex allergy, the European experienxe, *Immunol. Allergy Clin. N. Am.*, 15, 71, 1995.
25. Hadjiliadis, D., Khan, K., and Tarlo, S. M., Skin test responses to latex in an allergy and asthma clinic, *J. Allergy Clin. Immunol.*, 96, 431, 1995.
26. Vandenplas, O., Occupational asthma caused by natural rubber latex, *Eur. Respir. J.*, 8, 1957, 1995.
27. Vandenplas, O., Delwiche, J-P., Evrard, G., Aimont, P., van der Brempt, X., Jamart, J., and Delaunois, L., Prevalence of occupational asthma due to latex among hospital personnel, *Am. J. Respir. Crit. Care Med.*, 151, 54, 1995.
28. Schwartz, H. J., Latex: a potential hidden "food" allergen in fast food restaurants, *J. Allergy Clin. Immunol.*, 95, 139, 1995.
29. AAAI Task Force on Allergic Reactions to Latex, Committee report, *J. Allergy Clin. Immunol.*, 92, 16, 1993.
30. American College of Allergy, Asthma & Immunology position statement, Latex allergy — an emerging healthcare problem, *Annals of Allergy, Asthma, & Immunlogy*, 75, 19, 1995.
31. Sussman, G. L. and Beezhold, D. H., Allergy to latex rubber, *Ann. Intern. Med.*, 122, 43, 1995.
32. Kelly, K. J., Kurup, V., Zacharisen, M., Resnick, A., and Fink, J. N., Skin and serologic testing in the diagnosis of latex allergy. *J. Allergy Clin. Immunol.*, 91, 1140, 1993.
33. Bonnekoh, B. and Merk, H. F., Safety of latex prick skin testing in allergic patients, *J. Am. Med. Assoc.*, 267, 2603, 1992.
34. Sussman, G. L., In reply to Bonnekoh, *J. Am. Med. Assoc.*, 267, 2603, 1992.
35. Kleinhans, D., Contact urticaria to rubber gloves, *Contact Dermatitis*, 10, 124, 1984.
36. Wrangsjö, K., Mellström, G., and Axelsson, G., Discomfort from rubber gloves indicating contact urticaria, *Contact Dermatitis*, 15, 79, 1986.
37. Carrillo, T., Cuevas, M., Munoz, T., Hinojosa, M., and Moneo, I., Contact urticaria and rhinitis from latex surgical gloves, *Contact Dermatitis*, 15, 69, 1986.
38. Estlander, T., Jolanki, R., and Kanerva, L., Dermatitis and urticaria from rubber and plastic gloves, *Contact Dermatitis*, 14, 20, 1986.
39. Turjanmaa, K., Reunala, T., and Räsänen, L., Comparison of diagnostic methods in latex surgical glove contact urticaria, *Contact Dermatitis*, 19, 241, 1988.
40. Turjanmaa, K., Palosuo, T., Alenius, H., Leynadier, F., Autegarden, J-E., André, C., Sicard, H., Hrabina, M., and Tran, X. T., Latex allergy diagnosis: *in vivo and in vitro* standardization of a natural rubber latex extract, *Allergy*, 41, 52, 1997.

41. Sussman, G. L., Latex allergy: Its importance in clinical practice, *Allergy Proc.*, 13, 67, 1992.
42. Turjanmaa, K., Alenius, H., Mäkinen-Kiljunen, S., Palosuo, T., and Reunala, T., Commercial skin prick test preparations in the diagnosis of rubber latex allergy (Abstract), *J. Allergy Clin. Immunol.*, 93, 299, 1994.
43. Turjanmaa, K., Laurila, K., Mäkinen-Kiljunen, S., and Reunala, T., Rubber contact urticaria. Allergenic properties of 19 brands of latex gloves, *Contact Dermatitis*, 19, 362, 1988.
44. Yunginger, J. W., Jones, R. T., Fransway, A. F., Kelso, J. M., Warner, M. A., and Hunt, L. W., Extractable latex allergens and proteins in disposable medical gloves and other rubber products, *J. Allergy Clin. Immunol.*, 93, 836,1994.
45. Mäkinen-Kiljunen, S., Reunala, T., Alenius, H., Turjanmaa, K., Palosuo, T., and Cacioli, P., Non-latex allergens as a cause for positive use test with gloves (Abstract), *J. Allergy Clin. Immunol.*, 93, 284, 1994.
46. Heese, A., v.Hintzenstern, J., Peters, K., Koch, H.U., and Hornstein, O.P., Allergic and irritant reactions to rubber gloves in medical health services, *J. Am. Acad. Dermatol.*, 25, 831, 1991.
47. Turjanmaa, K. and Reunala, T., Latex contact urticaria associated with delayed allergy to rubber chemicals, in *Current Topics in Contact Dermatitis*, Frosch, P. J., Dooms-Goossens, A., Lachapelle, J.-M., Rycroft, R. J. G., and Scheper, R. J., Eds., Springer-Verlag, Heidelberg, 1989, 460.
48. Mäkinen-Kiljunen, S., Alenius, H., Palosuo, T., Reunala, T., and Turjanmaa, K., Measurement of latex IgE and IgG antibodies with RAST, *Program and Proceedings*, International Latex Conference: Sensitivity to Latex in Medical Devices, Baltimore 1992, p. 39.
49. Lagier, F., Vervloet, D., Lhermet, I. et al., Prevalence of latex allergy in operating room nurses, *J. Allergy Clin. Immunol.*, 90, 319, 1992.
50. Wrangsjö, K., Osterman, K., and van Hage-Hamsten, M., Glove-related skin symptoms among operating theatre and dental care unit personnel. II. Clinical examination, tests and laboratory findings indicating latex allergy, *Contact Dermatitis*, 30, 139, 1994.
51. Sorva, R., Mäkinen-Kiljunen, S., Suvilehto, K., Juntunen-Backman, K., and Haahtela, T., Latex allergy in children with no known risk factor for latex sensitization, *Pediatr. Allergy Immunol.*, 6, 36, 1995.
52. Leynadier, F. and Dry, J., Allergy to latex, *Clin. Rev. Allergy*, 9, 371, 1991.
53. Ownby, D. R. and McCullough, J., Testing for latex allergy, *Journal of Clinical Immunoassay*, 16, 109, 1993.
54. Ownby, D. R., Ownby, H. E., McCullough, J. A., and Shafer, A. W., The prevalence of anti-latex IgE antibodies in 1000 volunteer blood donors (Abstract), *J. Allergy Clin. Immunol*, 93, 282, 1994.
55. Turjanmaa, K. and Mäkinen-Kiljunen, S., AlaSTAT latex specific IgE measured in three patient populations. Annual meeting of the European academy of allergy and clinical immunology Stockholm 1994, *Abstracts*, 493 (Abstract 1806).
56. Hamilton, R. G., Charous, B. L., Adkinson, N. F., and Yunginger, J. W., Serologic methods in the laboratory diagnosis of latex rubber allergy: Study of nonammoniated, ammoniated latex, and glove (end-product) extracts as allergen reagent sources, *J. Lab. Clin. Med.*, 123, 594, 1994.
57. Alemohammad, M. M., Malki, J., and Foley, T. J., Detection of IgE antibodies to latex allergens in human serum, *Contact Dermatitis*, 32, 298, 1995.

58. Alenius, H., Palosuo, T., Kelly, K., Kurup, V., Reunala, T., Mäkinen-Kiljunen, S., Turjanmaa, K., and Fink, J., IgE reactivity to 14-kD and 27-kD natural rubber proteins in latex-allergic children with spina bifida and other congenital anomalies, *Int. Arch. Allergy Immunol,* 102, 61, 1993.

59. Alenius, H., Kurup, V., Kelly, K., Palosuo, T., Turjanmaa, K., and Fink, J., Latex allergy: Frequent occurrence of IgE antibodies to a cluster of 11 latex proteins in patients with spina bifida and histories of anaphylaxis, *J. Lab. Clin. Med.,* 123, 712, 1994.

60. Turjanmaa, K., Räsänen, L., Lehto, M., Mäkinen-Kiljunen, S., and Reunala, T., Basophil histamine release and lymphocyte proliferation tests in latex contact urticaria, *Allergy,* 44, 181, 1989.

61. Turjanmaa, K. and Reunala, T., Contact urticaria from rubber gloves, *Dermatologic Clinincs,* 6, 47, 1988.

62. Mäkinen-Kiljunen, S., Reunala, T., and Turjanmaa, K. et al., Is cow´s milk casein an allergen in latex rubber gloves? *Lancet,* 342, 863, 1993.

63. Jaeger, D., Kleinhans, D., Czuppon, A. B., and Baur, X., Latex-specific proteins causing immediate-type cutaneous, nasal, bronchial and systemic reactions, *J. Allergy. Clin. Immunol.,* 89, 759, 1992.

64. Cronin, E., Clinical patterns of hand eczema in women, *Contact Dermatitis,* 13, 153, 1985.

65. Beezhold, D. H., Measurement of latex protein by chemical and immunological methods. Conference on Latex protein allergy: the present position, Amsterdam, 1993, p. 25.

66. Turjanmaa, K., Reunala, T., Alenius, H., Brummer-Korvenkontio, H., and Palosuo, T., Allergens in latex surgical gloves and glove powder (letter), *Lancet,* 336, 1588, 1990.

67. Beezhold, D. and Beck, W. C., Surgical glove powders bind latex antigens, Arch. Surg., 127, 1354, 1992.

68. Tomazic, V. J., Shampaine, E. L., Lamanna, A., Withrow, T. J., and Adkinson, N. F., Cornstarch powder on latex products is an allergen carrier, *J. Allergy Clin. Immunol.,* 93, 751, 1994.

69. Swanson, M. C., Bubak, M. E., Hunt, L., Yunginger, J. M., Warner, M. A., and Reed, C. E., Quantification of occupational latex aeroallergens in a medical center, *J. Allergy Clin. Immunol.,* 94, 445, 1994.

70. Maso, M. J. and Goldberg, D. J., Contact dermatoses from disposable glove use: A review, *J. Am. Acad. Dermatol.,* 23, 733, 1990.

71. Fuchs, T. and Wahl, R., Immediate reactions to rubber products, *Allergy Proc.,* 13, 61, 1992.

72. Belsito, D. V., Contact urticaria caused by rubber. Analysis of seven cases, *Dermatologic Clinics,* 8, 61, 1990.

73. Dooms-Goossens, A., Contact urticaria caused by rubber gloves (letter), *J. Am. Acad. Dermatol.,* 18, 1360, 1988.

74. Turjanmaa, K., Incidence of immediate allergy to latex gloves in hospital personnel, *Contact Dermatitis,* 17, 270, 1987.

75. Beaudouin, E., Pupil, P., Jacson, F., Laxenaire, M. C., and Moneret-Vautrin, D. A., Allergie professionelle au latex. Enquete prospective sur 907 sujets du milieu hospitalier, *Rev. fr. Allergol.,* 30, 157, 1990.

76. Turjanmaa, K., Cacioli, P., Thompson, R. L., Simlote, P., and Lopez, M., Frequency of natural rubber latex allergy among US operating room nurses using skin prick testing (Abstract), *J. Allergy Clin. Immunol.,* 95, 214, 1995.

77. Akasawa, A., Matsumoto, K., Saito, H., Sakaguchi, N., Tanaka, K.,Obata, T., Tsubaki, T., Uchiyama, H., Matsunaga, T., Kurosaka, K., and Iikura, Y., Incidence of latex allergy in atopic children and hospital workers in Japan, *Int. Arch. Allergy Immunol.,* 101, 177, 1993.

78. Salkie, M. L., The prevalence of atopy and hypersensitivity to latex in medical laboratory technologists, *Arch. Pathol. Lab. Med.,* 117, 897, 1993.

79. Wrangsjö, K., Osterman, K., and van Hage-Hamsten, M., Glove-related skin symptoms among operating theatre and dental care unit personnel. I. Interview investigation, *Contact Dermatitis,* 30, 102, 1994.

80. Cormio, L., Turjanmaa, K., Talja, M. T., Andersson, L. C., and Ruutu, M., Biocompability of surgical gloves, *Program and Proceedings,* p. 26, International Latex Conference: Sensitivity to Latex in Medical Devices, Baltimore, 1992.

81. Toikkanen, J., Kauppinen, T., Vaaranen, V., Vasama, M., and Jolanki, R., Occupational diseases in Finland in 1993. Finnish Institute of Occupational Health, Helsinki, 1994.

82. Rystedt, I., Factors influencing the occurrence of hand eczema in adults with a history of atopic dermatitis in childhood, *Contact Dermatitis,* 12, 185, 1985.

83. Slater, J. E., Mostello, L. A., and Shaer, C., Rubber-specific IgE in children with spina bifida, *J. Urol.,* 146, 578, 1991.

84. Ylitalo, L. Turjanmaa, K., and Reunala, T., Natural rubber latex (NRL) allergy in food allergic children (Abstract), *J. Allergy Clin. Immunol.,* 97, 321, 1996.

85. Lezaun, A., Marcos, C., Martin, J. A., Quirce, S., and Gomez, M. L. D., Contact dermatitis from natural latex, *Contact Dermatitis,* 27, 334, 1992.

86. Moneret-Vautrin, D. A., Laxenaire, M. C., and Bavoux, F., Allergic shock to latex and ethylene oxide during surgery for spina bifida, *Anesthesiology,* 73, 556, 1990.

87. Alenius, H., Turjanmaa, K., Mäkinen-Kiljunen, S., Reunala, T., and Palosuo, T., IgE immune response to rubber proteins in adult patients with latex allergy (Abstract), *J. Allergy Clin. Immunol.,* 93, 859, 1994.

88. Czuppon, A. B., Chen, Z., Rennert, S. et al. The rubber elongation factor of rubber trees (Hevea brasiliensis) is the major allergen in latex, *J. Allergy Clin. Immunol.,* 92, 690, 1993.

89. Beezhold, D., Sussman, G., Kostyal, D., and Chang, C-S., Identification of a 46-kD latex protein allergen in health care workers, *Clin. Exp. Immunol.,* 98, 408, 1994.

90. Alenius, H., Kalkkinen, N., Lukka, M., Turjanmaa, K., Reunala, T., Mäkinen-Kiljunen, S., and Palosuo, T., Purification and partial amino acid sequencing of a 27 kD natural rubber allergen recognized by latex-allergic children with spina bifida, *Int. Arch. Allergy Immunol.,* 106, 258, 1995.

91. Alenius, H., Kalkkinen, N., Lukka, M., Reunala, T., Turjanmaa, K., Yip, E., and Palosuo, T., Prohevein from rubber tree (Hevea brasiliensis) is a major latex allergen, *Clin. Exp. Allergy,* 25, 659, 1995.

92. Alenius, H., Kalkkinen, N., Yip, E., Hasmin, H., Turjanmaa, K., Mäkinen-Kiljunen, S., Reunala, T., and Palosuo, T., Significance of the rubber elongation factor as a latex allergen, *Int. Arch. Allergy Immunol.,* 109, 362, 1996.

93. Alenius, H., Kalkkinen, N., Reunala, T., Turjanmaa, K., and Palosuo, T., The main IgE binding epitope of a major latex allergen, prohevein, is present in its N-terminal amino acid fragment, hevein, *The Journal of Immunology,* 156, 1618, 1996.

94. Ross, B. D., McCullough, J., and Ownby, D. R., Partial cross-reactivity between latex and banana allergens, *J. Allergy Clin. Immunol.,* 90, 409, 1992.

95. M'Raihi, L., Charpin, D., Pons, A., Bongrand, P., and Vervloet, D., Cross-reactivity between latex and banana, *J. Allergy Clin. Immunol.,* 87, 129, 1991.

96. Lavaud, F., Cossart, C., Reiter, V., Bernard, J., Deltour, G., and Holmquist, I., Latex allergy in patient with allergy to fruit, *Lancet,* 339, 492, 1992.

97. Mäkinen-Kiljunen, S., Banana allergy in patients with immediate hypersensitivity to natural rubber latex: Characterization of cross-reacting antibodies and allergens, *J. Allergy Clin. Immunol.,* 93, 990, 1994.

98. Yip, E., Turjanmaa, K., Ng, K. P., and Mok, K. L., Allergic responses and levels of extractable proteins in NR latex gloves and dry rubber products, *J. Nat. Rubb. Res.,* 9, 79, 1994.

99. Tarlo, S. M., Sussman, G., Contala, A., and Swanson, M. C., Control of airborne latex by use of powder-free latex gloves, *J. Allergy Clin. Immunol.,* 93, 985, 1994.

100. Vandenplas, O., Delwiche, J-P., Depelchin, S., Sibille, Y., Vande Weyer, R., and Delaunois, L., Latex gloves with a low protein content reduce bronchial reactions in subjects with occupational asthma by latex, *Am. J. Respir. Crit. Care Med.,* 151, 887, 1995.

101. Turjanmaa, K., Mäkinen-Kiljunen, S., Alenius, H., Reunala, T., and Palosuo, T., *In vivo* and *in vitro* evaluation of allergenicity of natural rubber latex (NRL) gloves used in health care: a nation-wide study (Abstract), *J. Allergy Clin. Immunol.,* Jan., 1996.

19

Metals

Jurij J. Hostýnek

CONTENTS

ABBREVIATIONS

RIST   Radioimmunosorbent Test for Total IgE Concentration
RAST   Radioallergosorbent Test for Specific IgE Concentration
ACD   Allergic Contact Dermatitis
ICU   Immunological Contact Urticaria
CUS   Contact Urticaria Syndrome
PCA   Passive Cutaneous Anaphylaxis
P-K   Prausnitz-Küstner Test
QSAR   Quantitative Structure Activity Relationships

19.1   INTRODUCTION AND PERSPECTIVE

According to our present understanding of structure and function of the skin, percutaneous absorption of environmental agents is governed by their physicochemical parameters. Intuitively, we anticipate easy penetration there by lipophilic compounds. Biophysically, this is explained by the nature of the outermost and rate-determining layer of the skin, the stratum corneum, which consists of densely packed corneocytes cemented in a lipid matrix, the latter believed to provide the principal route of transit for exogenous agents through the membrane. Also, metals can form lipophilic compounds, e.g., the organometallics, where the metal is bound covalently to carbon, principally represented by alkyl and aryl derivatives of several elements, as well as chelates and complexes, where the electrophilic electropositive atom of a metal and nucleophilic atoms of peptides, usually nitrogen, oxygen, or sulfur, form stable structures. These also show skin-penetrating characteristics comparable to other small-molecular weight nonelectrolytes. It is rather counter-intuitive, however, that electrolytes, e.g., water soluble metal salts and their ionic complexes, should also be able to penetrate the skin. For many hydrophilic compounds, and most metal compounds, this is indeed the case, although the process was shown to proceed at an average of one or two orders of magnitude slower than the penetration of small molecular weight, lipophilic nonelectrolytes. For a number of metals, this process of passive diffusion has been measured in quantitative terms,[1] and their presence at various depths of the epidermal and dermal tissue has been visualized using ultrastructural localization methods, e.g., X-ray microanalysis.[2,3] In the process of diffusion, metals follow all paths available: intra- or inter-cellularly through the stratum corneum membrane, as well as appendageal pores, the mode of transit being determined by the physical parameters of the individual permeant. Prima facie evidence of such skin penetration by metals in their various states of oxidation is the adverse effect they have in the skin, whether such reactions are immunologically or nonimmunologically mediated.

With the possible exception of mercury, metals do not penetrate the stratum corneum in the elemental state, but as ions and complexes. When focusing on the immunological factors which determine adverse reactions to metals and their compounds, it is useful to visualize the process that leads to antigenicity. Most metal ions are incomplete antigens, i.e., too small to stimulate an immune response (e.g.,

0.72 Å for Cu^{+2}; 0.69 Å for Ni^{+2}). Due to the electrophilic character of their mostly cationic state, upon tissue penetration they will bind as ligands to the nucleophilic sites (O, S or N) encountered on a host protein or other macromolecule to form a hapten conjugate. For their part, endogenous proteins possess not only a primary, chemical structure, but also higher order structures of spatial orientation, a prerequisite for their biological activity. Their reaction and interaction with metals can then result in chemical as well as physical alteration. The net effect of such change is denaturation and loss of their intended biological activity, which renders them foreign and therefore potentially toxic to the host organism. It is the metal-protein (hapten-carrier) conjugate thus formed which is immunogenic, capable of stimulating either T-lymphocyte proliferation or the production of antibodies. So far, specific IgE antibody to metal ions themselves has been identified in exceptional cases only: platinum,[4] cobalt,[5] nickel,[6] and chromium.[6] For other metals, positive identification of metal-specific reaginic antibody by RAST assay requires a preformed hapten conjugate, mostly with human serum albumin.

In a discussion of allergic skin reactions, it is also useful to bring ACD into perspective with ICU, particularly since recent insights gained in the pathogenesis of allergic disease reveal that the two expressions of hypersensitivity have more in common than had formerly been suspected. Of the two, ACD is clearly the more frequent and easily recognized skin reaction, and familiar ground for the dermatologist; witness the frequency of world-wide symposia convoking specialists in the field and the sheer volume of literature dealing with that altered state. Since Jadassohn first used the patch test to diagnose allergic reactions to mercury and published his work on contact dermatitis in 1896,[7] literature addressing ACD has grown to fill entire shelves in libraries and practitioners' offices. Not only are several animal models available for prospective testing of compounds as to their contact sensitization potential, but also QSAR approaches have been developed which allow facile and accurate prediction of immunogenic potential based on clinical experience.[8]

Inhalation appears to be the major route of exposure to exogenous antigens, which causes contact CUS, an array of signs and symptoms, most notably acute or chronic respiratory problems with potentially fatal outcome. Accordingly, asthmology has evolved into a specialty in its own right. Dermatological problems associated with CUS, on the other hand, rate lower priority and attention because of the relative lack of severity in clinical symptoms, and also due to the complexities involved in obtaining unambiguous proof of the nature of disease. In earlier years, only the significant frequency of asthma and dermatological problems due to platinoids, nickel, and chromium occurring in the metals refining and construction industries, and the magnitude of socioeconomic problems they comport, seemed to justify the relatively complex testing procedure necessary to establish an unambiguous diagnosis of ICU: the P-K test in humans, or the PCA test in animals. After all, formation, structure, and function of antibody molecules was only described in the late 1950s and early 1960s by R.R. Porter, G.M. Edelman, and A. Nisonoff, and the role played by IgE specifically in initiating the cascade of events leading to immediate-type hypersensitivity and anaphilactoid reactions in 1966 by K. Ishizaka.[9] In the years that followed then, testing for specific antibody (IgE) against the causative agent in a patient's serum by the RAST technique as proof of immunological hypersensitivity became part of the dermatologists' instrumentarium.[10,11] Up to that time, ICU diagnosis relied mainly on symptoms, attaching a certain degree of doubt to their validity. Also, only in recent years has a stepwise protocol of skin tests specifically designed for recognition of immediate-type reactions been proposed as a diagnostic tool.[12,13]

These are some of the factors that help explain why involvement of the skin in Type I reactions has remained relegated to a level of secondary importance. Even to date, immunological contact urticaria is discussed as a chapter in toxicology and dermatology texts, but is most often addressed in individual papers only, which until recently have been published in occupational health journals. An animal model for prospective testing of sensitization potential is not yet available, and a QSAR approach is in its initial stages only, hampered by the paucity and ambiguity of clinical data that deal with urticaria and the scarcity of epidemiology in this field.

19.2 UPDATING IMMUNOLOGICAL CONTACT URTICARIA

Traditionally, the literature dealing with causative agents for CUS has featured primarily large-molecular weight compounds: glycoproteins and polysaccharides of animal, vegetable, or microbial origin. More recently and increasingly, small molecular weight chemicals are becoming part of such reviews, including fragrances, medicaments, pesticides, and preservatives; but even in that category, metals are still a minor sub-item. Even most recent textbooks identify only copper, nickel, platinum, and rhodium as agents likely to cause immunologically mediated contact reactivity,[14,15] or examples of professional correspondence, citing literature review, also restrict such etiology to cobalt chloride, nickel, phenyl mercuric propionate, and platinum salts, demonstrating the limits in current awareness.[16] Only recently have occupational medicine, and dermatologists in particular, come to appreciate the full extent to which even the intact skin and mucous membranes are permeable to metals, inorganic (ionized), as well as organometallics, moving them into the limelight of immunology. As a consequence, metal compounds are now becoming part of the standard diagnostic test tray in the allergologist's office. At least in part, this awareness stems from investigation of the immune state among dental professionals and patients.[17,18] Up to that time, as is generally true for human perception, the allergologist also only saw what he looked for. Thus, awareness is rapidly growing of the role metals play in the etiology of CUS, also as it involves the skin, regardless of route of entry: cutaneous, oral-mucosal, or systemic (gastro-intestinal, respiratory or parenteral) in the everyday environment and, most importantly, from occupational exposure. In medicine, CUS may be the consequence of novel prosthetic and medicinal uses of alloys and injectables, in orthodontry, joint replacement, or anti-inflammatory therapy. Metals such as palladium, gold, and even cobalt, tin, and zinc are increasingly brought to the attention of the allergist, supporting the widely held view that the increase in allergies in the general public is indeed due to anthropogenic causes.

Paralleling the upgrading of the role of small-molecular weight chemicals in the etiology of immunologically mediated disease, the desire to understand the mechanisms involved in such pathology has grown appreciably among molecular biologists, as they realize that the straightforward compartmentalization of hypersensitivity into 4 distinct types as originally defined by Coombs and Gell[19] is no longer adequate. Distinctions are becoming less and less clear, especially between Types I and IV hypersensitivity.[20-23] As a consequence, experimental immunologists strive for better insight into the regulatory phenomena which determine the course of allergic responses, in order to explain the commonality or cross-over point in the two pathways leading to divergent immune reactions in particular.[24-28] Such interdependence is consistent with the observation resulting from this synopsis: all metals so far recognized to give rise to allergy without exception also cause eczema, sometimes even in the same patient.[24-28]

From the perspective of the dermatologist, signs and symptoms thereby become more difficult to interpret and classify, as correlation of cause and effect no longer are self-evident. Dermal exposure can lead to systemic effects, as dietary sensitization also results in cutaneous manifestation, late-phase reactions can occur as consequence of parenteral or dermal challenge, in Type I as well as Type IV hypersensitivity,[13,29,30] and exposure to one and the same agent can give rise to divergent reactions, both immediate and delayed. Thus, the process of anamnesis and interpretation of diagnostic tests requires ever increasing acumen and refinement.

19.3 LIMITS OF EPIDEMIOLOGY

A comprehensive and meaningful epidemiology of CUS as caused by metals is difficult to establish at present. As entries under the individual hapten sections illustrate, for the most part data are fragmentary, resulting in a composite picture which consists mostly of industrial case reports, and few if any exposures from the general public. Limited industry-internal surveys cover relatively small samples, which in most countries are not subject to mandatory reporting, thus representing clusters inadequate for statistical evaluation.

With the exception of platinum, cobalt, and nickel, reports of CUS to individual metals are sparse and for some, more unique than rare. This, at least in part, may be attributed to underreporting due to unawareness of their disease-causing potential.

An accurate historical perspective is not yet possible, also due to a lack of widely established, reliable diagnostic procedures allowing definite correlation of cause and effect. See also the late introduction of the RAST, mentioned earlier.

Reactivity to extrinsic allergens is determined by genetic factors,[31] and immunological contact urticaria is considered more prevailing in atopic patients than in nonatopics.[32] Genetic variability of defense mechanisms (polymorphism) thus accounts for idiosyncratic toxicity, a confounding factor for any epidemiological intent, making meaningful correlations from surveys difficult. This is manifest in the occurrence of subclinical or asymptomatic sensitization, i.e., the fact that RAST positive individuals do not necessarily develop allergic disease.[33]

Conversely, although the generally accepted criterion indicative of immediate immunologic mechanism is the presence of antigen-specific IgE, urticaria and asthma may also be caused through pathways not involving reagins,[34-36] i.e., not all individuals with asthma also have detectable specific IgE antibody.

19.4 CONCLUSIONS

The science addressing ICU in the skin as part of CUS is young and in a dynamic state of growth, due in large part to impulses emanating from the rapid evolution of technology and materials science, which introduces increasingly exotic composites into the daily life of everyman, and exposes him to immunogenic agents previously not encountered. Increased general awareness of the role small-molecular weight chemicals play in the etiology of CUS and the growing list of immunogenic metals in particular are the measurable expressions of the immunologists' heightened acumen. Although these recent additions to the spectrum of allergens hardly warrant the concern of health officials or industrial chemists due to the low incidence of disease they elicit, they certainly fire the interest of immunologists who feel challenged to deepen their understanding of the pathogenic process induced by a burgeoning array of immunogenic agents. Insight gained as to the interdependence of reaction pathways leading to divergent clinical manifestations ultimately furthers the understanding of type I reactions as they also involve the skin.

The growing body of accurately interpreted data promises to bring the development of predictive QSAR models within reach. Structure-activity hypotheses designed for CUS or ICU are already being proposed for a wide range of chemicals, but that approach is still in its infancy.[37] A larger database of human evidence relating reliable qualitative and quantitative measures of exposure to unambiguous interpretation of effects on the human immune system is required first, before predicting ICU by QSAR will reach the degree of accuracy already seen in the prediction of ACD.

Exposure to a significant number of metals is seen to give rise to immediate hypersensitivity, regardless of exposure route, and to most of them specific IgE immunoglobulin has been detected; either to the metal itself, or to the metal-protein conjugate. All of them cause delayed-type hypersensitivity reactions as well. It appears that this list of metals will grow as the use of alloys diversifies further, and human exposure to them increases in all aspects of activity — domestic, professional, and industrial. At this point, it is not yet possible to discern a pattern in the immunogenic activity of metals based solely on their relative arrangement in the periodic table of elements, because those so far recognized to have the potential for sensitization belong to the groups of transition elements, the heavy metals, and possibly some metalloids as well. In addition, investigation on a molecular level of the particular pathway leading to immunogenic activity by individual metals reveals that they can follow individual and diverse modes of peptide binding.[38]

The bulk of the literature reviewed here consists of individual case reports and investigations into occupational asthma within relatively small industrial cohorts. Even for metals causing important incidence of CUS or occupational asthma in particular, epidemiology is still insufficient to determine prevalence and incidence rates. Literature sporadically made available from the former Soviet Union has implicated most of the Group VIII metals in the etiology of CUS, reaching well beyond platinum and palladium. Yet, epidemiological and bibliographic studies carried out by such authors as Dueva[39] are still only available as sweeping statements in summary form, published by supranational organizations such as the WHO. They fail to give a closer definition of exposure, signs, symptoms, and methods of diagnosis, and only with time may such research documentation become available in all the details necessary for a correlation of cause and effect.

19.5 IMMEDIATE IMMUNOLOGICAL REACTIONS DUE TO METALS

For the purpose of concise tabulation under individual headings, the term asthma is used to describe all signs and symptoms associated with mucosal and respiratory involvement due to metal exposure.

19.5.1 Antimony

Injection of antimonials as it was practiced formerly for the treatment of cutaneous leishmaniasis, urogenital schistosomiasis, etc., can result in anaphylactoid response, characterized by urticarial weals; fatal cases of anaphylaxis, preceded by hemolytic anemia (HA), have also been reported. In some cases, such HA was demonstrated by a positive Coombs test, a technique used to detect erythrocyte-bound immunoglobulin.[40-42] Occupational exposure to irritating antimony dust in metal fabrication can result in lichenoid and eczematous eruptions, and cases of dermatitis have recently been confirmed as immunological in nature (Table 19.1).[43,44]

TABLE 19.1   CUS Due to Antimony

Etiology	Symptoms	Diagnostic Test	Ref.
Parenteral stibophen	Hemolytic anemia	Coombs, PCA[a]	40
Parenteral stibophen	Anaphylaxis, hemolytic anemia	Coombs	41
Parenteral antimonials	Anaphylaxis, gen. urticaria		42

[a] Passive cutaneous anaphylaxis.

19.5.2 Chromium

Although metallic chromium is not reported to be an allergen,[45] in contact with the skin its alloys are easily oxidized, and the derivative chromium salts can cause immediate, anaphylactoid type sensitization, with specific IgE antibody confirmed by a positive RAST,[6] as well as the delayed-type,[46] sometimes granulomatous hypersensitivity.[47] Patients suffering from chromium dermatitis also reacted with urticaria on intradermal testing with chromium chloride and its human serum albumin conjugate.[48] It is notable that a patient giving a positive RAST result did not react with urticaria on prick testing with chromate.[6] Chronic inhalation exposure to chromium-containing dust can result in systemic sensitization, and recall dermatitis was noted on dermal re-exposure of sensitized patients.[49] Inhalation exposure to chromate fumes, which are generated in industrial activities such as welding, is known to cause asthma by an immunologically mediated mechanism, rather than being a direct toxic effect on the airways.[50-53]

Of the several forms of chromium ion known, skin contact with the hexavalent form, as it occurs in chromate in alkaline solution $\{(CrO_4)^{2-}\}$, is believed to present the greatest skin sensitizing potential.[54] Chromate or dichromate anion, however, does not complex with protein and must first be reduced to its trivalent, cationic form. Immunological methods have shown that Cr^{3+} is the true hapten responsible for the induction of ACD, as it tightly binds to sulfhydryl groups present in tissue protein, to form a complete antigen. In fact, in animals sensitized with dichromate, only antibody to trivalent chromium were demonstrated by the PCA technique, and none against hexavalent chromium.[55-58] *In vitro* studies have shown that cystine, cysteine, and methionine have the capacity to reduce Cr^{6+} to Cr^{3+} (Table 19.2).[54,59,60]

TABLE 19.2   CUS Due to Chromium

Etiology	Symptoms	Diagnostic Test	Challenge/Reaction	Ref.
Dermal; chromic acid	Asthma	ID[a]	Dichromate/weal and flare	51
Inhalation; chromate	Asthma	ID	Dichromate/asthma, generalized rash	144
Chromate ACD	ACD[b] to chromium	ID, patch	Chromium chloride and Cr-HSA[c]/urticaria, eczema	48
Inhalation; chromate	Asthma	RAST, BPT[d]	Chromium sulfate/asthma	6
Dermal; chromate	Generalized urticaria, eczema	Patch	Chromate/urticaria, eczema	16
Denture prosthesis	Urticaria, eczema	Patch	Chromium metal/gen. urticaria, eczema	113

[a] Intradermal.

[b] Allergic contact dermatitis.

[c] Chromate-human serum albumin conjugate.

[d] Bronchial provocation.

19.5.3   Cobalt

Cobalt metal as respirable dust or in its water-soluble ionized salt form in aerosols is an industrial risk factor, expressing primarily as bronchospastic reactions in the metal-cutting and diamond polishing industries, described as hard metal asthma.[5,61,62] Hard metal is an alloy consisting primarily of a tungsten carbide and cobalt matrix, but other metals such as nickel, vanadium, and chromium can also be present. Cobalt dust is allergenic[5,63,64] as well as photoallergenic,[65,66] shown to cause immediate and delayed type skin sensitization, sometimes observed in the same patient.[64,67] IgE and IgG antibodies specific to cobalt have been demonstrated.[5,63] A number of patients allergic to cobalt showed a positive intradermal test reaction to both cobalt chloride and cobalt bound to human serum albumin, suggesting that the latter sensitivity is caused by cobalt-denatured protein.[48] Hard metal disease is due to reactions in the lung parenchyma, potentially leading to end-stage pulmonary fibrosis. It is presumed to comport an immunological component, long assumed to be in synergism with concomitant exposure to tungsten carbide. Bronchial provocation tests performed separately with cobalt and tungsten powder, however, demonstrated that only cobalt provoked asthma in workers with hard metal disease.[68]

The first case of occupational asthma in workers exposed to hard metal dust was described in 1967.[69] Since then, numerous studies conducted in industry have analyzed and confirmed the risks comported by cobalt containing alloys, and in the tabulation of cobalt-related allergic disease presented here citations are limited to the most recent and representative prevalence studies published (Table 19.3).

TABLE 19.3   CUS Due to Cobalt

Etiology	Symptoms	Diagnostic Test	Challenge/Reaction	Ref.
Hard metal inhalation	Asthma	BPT,[a] RAST, patch, eos.,[b] IgE	Cobalt chloride/asthma, (dual onset), divergent response	142
Hard metal inhalation	Asthma	BPT	Cobalt sulfate/asthma, (dual onset)	143
Hard metal inhalation	Asthma	BPT	Cobalt chloride/asthma	100
Hard metal inhalation	Asthma	BPT, RAST, patch, eos., IgE, ID[c]	Cobalt chloride, Co-HSA[d]/asthma (dual onset), divergent response	5
Denture prosthesis	Urticaria, eczema	Patch	Cobalt metal/generalized urticaria, eczema	113
Hard metal inhalation	Asthma	BPT, patch, ID	Cobalt sulfate/Asthma (dual onset), divergent response	64

[a] Bronchial provocation.

[b] Eosinophilia.

[c] Intradermal.

[d] Human serum albumin.

19.5.4   Copper

Although rarely causing hypersensitivity, and that mostly from occupational exposure, systemic as well as topical exposure to copper has caused both immediate[70-73] and delayed-type sensitization.[74-84]

A positive skin reaction to copper acetyl acetonate was observed at 40 minutes after open-patch testing in a case of sensitization attributed to that antimicrobial agent present in self-adhesive pads. The patient also reacted to patch tests with the reagent at 24, 48, and 72 hours.[73] Copper-containing IUDs release measurable amounts of metal ion, also believed capable of causing immediate-type hypersensitivity. One such reaction was diagnosed as ICU by scratch test using 1% copper sulfate solution.[71] Another case of ICU attributed to the presence of a copper IUD was characterized as occult sensitivity to copper on testing. While a patch with metallic copper elicited no response, punctate weals developed at the test sites when injected with acetyl choline in subthreshold concentration. That cholinergic urticaria reaction is attributed to a collaborative effect of acetylcholine and copper on mast cell membranes inducing degranulation, a clinical response which an antibody-antigen reaction on the mast cell surface alone could not produce (Table 19.4).[72]

TABLE 19.4   CUS Due to Copper

Etiology	Symptoms	Diagnostic Test	Challenge/Reaction	Ref.
Copper IUD	Generalized urticaria	Scratch	Copper sulfate/erythema	71
Copper IUD	Urticaria, flushing, pruritus	Copper+acetyl choline	Punctate wheals	72
Adhesive	Urticaria, eczema	Open+ closed patch	Copper acetyl acetonate/urticaria, eczema	73
Denture prosthesis	Urticaria, eczema	Patch	Copper metal/ generalized urticaria, eczema	113

19.5.5   Gold

Gold in the metallic form and also its salts can be the cause of contact urticaria syndrome, as well as delayed-type, cell-mediated sensitization. Demonstrating the latter, gold-specific T-cell clones were isolated from peripheral blood mononuclear cells of patients with gold contact dermatitis.[85] In addition, based on the observed occurrence of nephropathy in patients receiving parenteral gold therapy for the treatment of adult rheumatoid arthritis, it is also suspected to give rise to circulating immune complexes (type III hypersensitivity).[86,87] The most prevalent cause of sensitization to gold in fact is such systemic administration of soluble gold salts for therapeutic purposes (Table 19.5).

TABLE 19.5   CUS Due to Gold

Etiology	Symptoms	Diagnostic Test	Challenge/Reaction	Ref.
Gold RA[a] therapy	Rash, pruritus	IgE, RAST, Eosinophilia	Eosinophilia, IgE, rash, pruritus	88
Gold RA therapy	Rash, pruritus	IgE, RAST, Eosinophilia	Eosinophilia, IgE, rash, pruritus	33
Gold RA therapy	Rash, pruritus	RAST		6

[a] Rheumatoid arthritis.

Serial monitoring of eosinophil counts and IgE levels by RAST in 47 nonatopic patients on gold therapy demonstrated that cutaneous side effects and eosinophil count as well as IgE levels rose and fell repeatedly, in concordance with therapy onset and cessation.[33] Elevated IgE levels were also noted there in patients without symptoms of allergy. While this is suggestive of type I hypersensitivity, 2 of 12 patients with hematological side effects to gold also had positive lymphocyte transformation responses, indicative of a delayed (type IV) hypersensitivity reaction.[88] One patient on chrysotherapy showing symptoms of hypersensitivity had a specific RAST score ten times higher than control values.[6]

19.5.6 Nickel

Although only a moderate sensitizer,[89] characteristic properties and occurrence of nickel serve to explain the fact that it is by far the most common allergen among the metals: it is present in articles of everyday use, dissolves in sweat,[90] accumulates in the stratum corneum,[91] occurs widely in foodstuffs,[92] and is suspended as respirable particulate, especially in urban air.[93] Unlike cobalt or platinum, hypersensitivity to nickel is not primarily an occupational hazard. Although more often found to be an allergen among women than in men, due primarily to practices more prevalent in that gender, cases of sensitization reported in the literature represent diverse etiologies: work-related inhalation, prosthetic inplants, diet, incidental skin contact with metal accessories, or voluntarily inflicted injury for the sake of embellishment. Such exposure and contacts give rise to CUS and ACD, or both in the same individuals, and once the organism is sensitized, this state is likely to remain a lifetime condition, because re-exposure in the industrialized environment and lifestyle is virtually unavoidable. Inhalation in particular represents an occupational hazard.[53,94,95] Demonstrating ACD to the metal, nickel-specific T-cell clones were isolated from peripheral blood mononuclear cells of patients with nickel contact dermatitis.[96] Nickel-reactive IgE antibodies as well as elevated levels of the IgG, IgA, and IgM types have actually been identified in sera of asthmatics exposed to emissions containing the metal,[6,95,97-101] eliciting both immediate and late-phase reactions. Also P-K tests have been performed successfully to confirm the presence of antibody in sensitized patients (Table 19.6).[102]

19.5.7 Mercury

Immunotoxicity of mercury becomes manifest in symptoms of autoimmunity[103,104] and hypersensitivity, both of the cell-mediated[105] and humoral type.[106,107] The ability of mercuric chloride to enhance specific and total IgE production has been confirmed in animal studies.[108] Both type I and IV reactions have been noted in the same patient after topical application of mercurials,[107,109] as well as the gradual transition from urticaria to eczema on the same test site (Table 19.7).[110] Severe cases of anaphylactic shock ending in death following parenteral administration of mercurials for diuretic purposes have been recorded.[111] In the work environment in particular, under conditions of chronic exposure, mercury vapor was seen to cause type III or Arthus reactions,

TABLE 19.6 CUS Due to Nickel

Etiology	Symptoms	Diagnostic Test	Challenge/Reaction	Ref.
Metal dust; inhalation	Asthma	BPT[a]	Nickel sulfate/asthma	100
Dental prostheses	Urticaria	ID,[b] patch	Syst. nickel sulfate/gen. urticaria, eczema	145
Inhalation; nickel	Asthma	RAST, BPT	Nickel sulfate/asthma	6
Inhalation; hard metal	Asthma	RAST, IgE, BPT, SPT,[c] patch	Nickel sulfate/dual and divergent response	95
Inhalation; hard metal	Asthma	RAST, BPT, IgE, ID, patch	Ni-HSA/eczema	101
Dental prostheses	Urticaria, eczema	Patch	Nickel metal/gen. urticaria, eczema	113
Inhalation; nickel	Urticaria, asthma, ACD	ID, patch, RAST, BPT, IgE	Nickel sulfate/gen. urticaria, eczema	146

[a] Bronchial provocation.

[b] Intradermal.

[c] Skin prick.

TABLE 19.7 CUS Due to Mercury

Etiology	Symptoms	Diagnostic Test	Challenge/Reaction	Ref.
Dermal. amm. mercury[a]	Generalized urticaria	Patch	Amm. mercury/urticaria	147
Dermal phenyl mercurial	Asthma, urticaria, angioedema	PK,[b] SPT,[c] BPT,[d] patch	Mercurials/weal and flare, asthma	148
Dermal mercurochrome	Anaphyl. shock	PK, ID,[e] IgE, SPT, patch	Mercurochrome; mercuric chloride	107
Dermal mercurial	Asthma	IgE, eos.,[f] patch	Mercurials/urticaria and eczema	110
Dermal merbrominum	Urticaria and eczema	SPT, patch	Mercurials/urticaria and eczema	21
Dermal phenyl mercurial	Asthma	IgE, eos., patch	Urticaria and asthma	106
Dermal mercurochrome	Gen. urticaria, anaphylaxis	SPT, PK, ID, patch	Mercurials/urticaria and eczema	109

[a] Ammoniated mercury ($HgNH_2Cl$).

[b] Prausnitz-Küstner.

[c] Skin prick.

[d] Bronchial provocation.

[e] Intradermal.

[f] Eosinophilia.

involving antigen-antibody complexes deposited in the vascular endothelium and leading to destructive inflammatory reactions, specifically causing glomerulonephritis.[112]

19.5.8 Molybdenum

Incidence of molybdenum sensitivity in humans occurs in consequence of occupational exposure in molybdenum refining, where exposure to dust can result in IgE-dependent sensitization,[113] as well as delayed-type hypersensitivity, verified by a positive patch test to aqueous ammonium paramolybdate (Table 19.8).[114]

TABLE 19.8 CAS Due to Molybdenum

Etiology	Symptoms	Diagnostic Test	Challenge/Reaction	Ref.
Dermal; dust	Pruritus, urticaria and eczema	ID,[a] IgE, patch	Ammonium molybdate/ urticaria and eczema	39
Denture	Urticaria	Epicut. metal patch	Metal patch/generalized urticaria	113

[a] Intradermal.

19.5.9 Palladium

Evaluation of workers exposed to palladium and other platinum group metal salts in the metals refining industry mostly identified the occurrence of delayed-type hypersensitivity, but cases of type I reactions have also been described, showing positive PCA immune responses to palladium in the monkey.[115] As part of the group VIII metals, the palladium ion by its size, charge, and protein reactivity can also be expected to form conjugates with endogenous proteins *in vivo*, apt to induce antibody formation and hypersensitivity, in analogy with platinum. It is not definitely established whether such reactivity is to be ascribed to a palladium-specific response, or to cross-reactivity to platinum, since sensitization has not been noted to palladium alone. Several cases showed presence of concomitant specific antibody to platinum and palladium (Table 19.9).[116]

Several reports from the former Soviet Union confirm induction of both immediate and delayed-type hypersensitivity by palladium. In a number of animal experiments,

TABLE 19.9 CUS Due to Palladium

Etiology	Symptoms	Diagnostic Test	Challenge/Reaction	Ref.
Metal dust; inhalation	Asthma	PCA[a]		115
Metal dust; inhalation	Asthma	IgE, IgG, PCA		116
Metal dust; inhalation		IgE, SPT,[b] RAST	Ammoniumtetrachloro-palladite/wheal and flare	130

[a] Passive cutaneous anaphylaxis.

[b] Skin prick.

mast cell histamine releasing action and both immediate and delayed skin hypersensitivity were noted, as induced by various both group VIII metal and group III metalloid salts, but primarily by intercutaneous injection of palladium salts. Such induction of hypersensitivity did not require prior conjugation with an exogenous high molecular weight carrier.[117-121]

19.5.10   Platinum

Platinum is a renowned sensitizer, primarily in the salt form, as ammonium tetrachloroplatinate and hexachloroplatinate, through inhalation in the work environment. While delayed type allergic reactions to platinum jewelry are rare, long-term contact with the metal has occasionally resulted in contact hypersensitivity also, probably due to dissolution of trace amounts of platinum by skin fatty acids.[122] Such potential of platinum salts to induce cell-mediated hypersensitivity was confirmed by the murine ear swelling test.[123] Type-I hypersensitivity, which gives rise to urticaria, rhinoconjunctivitis, bronchial asthma, and anaphylactic reactions was confirmed through identification of platinum-specific antibody in sensitized patients.[116,124,125] Prolonged dermal or inhalation exposure to complex platinum salts, such as tetra- and hexa-chloro platinates, can result in severe skin and disabling respiratory conditions, such as urticaria and contact dermatitis, allergic conjunctivitis, rhinitis, and asthma, conditions termed collectively as "platinosis"[126,127] or platinum salt sensitivity (PSS).[128] Early surveys in the precious metals refining industry reported a prevalence of sensitization among workers with symptoms as high as 73%;[129] with time, these figures decreased to the more recent levels of 12%.[130] A definite association between PSS and smoking was documented in a study estimating risk as eight times greater in smokers than in nonsmokers.[128] Sensitized individuals give a positive P-K reaction[131] and PCA test,[116] exhibit allergic symptoms upon subsequent re-exposure, and may demonstrate positive direct skin tests to platinum independent of the time interval between exposures.[116,124,126] Diagnostic scratch or intradermal testing can be life-threatening to sensitized individuals; concentrations of 1 mg/ml $KPtCl_6$ have caused anaphylactic reactions.[131] Thus, in testing for platinum hypersensitivity, the least invasive procedure, the skin prick test, is recommended. With a typical delivery of 3×10^{-15} g of platinum compound, it is sufficient to elicit a positive reaction in a sensitized individual.[132]

The earliest significant survey of occupational asthma in workers exposed to platinum salts and metal dust was described in 1945. While recording the occurrence of both erythematous dermatitis and urticarial rash in those sensitized, the authors also noted that even massive exposure to platinum in its elemental form as respirable dust does not comport the risk of sensitization, or provoke reactions in sensitized individuals. Since then, numerous studies conducted in industry have analyzed and described the risks comported by inhalation and dermal exposure to these agents, and in the tabulation of PSS presented here citations are limited to the most recent and representative prevalence studies published (Table 19.10).

TABLE 19.10 CUS Due to Platinum

Etiology	Symptoms	Diagnostic Test	Challenge/Reaction	Ref.
Dermal, inhalation; Pt salts	Asthma	SPT,[a] IgE, RAST, PCA[b]	Diammonium hexachloroplatinate	116
Dermal, inhalation; Pt salts		SPT, IgE, RAST,	Hexachloroplatinates, Pt-HSA/weal and flare	130
Dermal, inhalation; Pt salts	Asthma, dermatitis	SPT, IgE	Hexachloroplatinates	124
Dermal, inhalation; Pt salts	Asthma, urticaria	SPT, open patch	Chloroplatinate/Asthma, urticaria	149
Dermal, inhalation; Pt salts	Asthma	SPT, IgE, RAST	Potassium hexachloroplatinate	125

[a] Skin prick.

[b] Passive cutaneous anaphylaxis.

19.5.11 Tin

Significant accidental cutaneous exposure to triphenyltin acetate of the arms resulted in long-term elevated tin levels in plasma, and equally protracted generalized urticaria accompanied by elevated circulating IgE levels (Table 19.11).[133]

TABLE 19.11 CUS Due to Tin

Etiology	Symptoms	Diagnostic Test	Ref.
Organotin	Generalized urticaria	IgE	133

Several reports also document contact dermatitis due to occupational exposure, as well as to presence of the metal in prosthetic materials.[44,83,134,135]

19.5.12 Vanadium

As a minor component in hard-metal alloys, vanadium was also shown to contribute to so-called hard metal asthma, as subjects undergoing provocation tests with vanadium displayed positive reactions.[150] Elevated total IgE and eosinophilia were reported, but not detection of specific antibodies to vanadium (Table 19.12).[100] Delayed-type allergic responses have been recorded following industrial exposure to vanadium pentoxide.[136]

TABLE 19.12 CUS Due to Vanadium

Etiology	Symptoms	Diagnostic Test	Challenge/Reaction	Ref.
Metal dust inhalation	Asthma	IgE, eosin.[a]	Metal dust/asthma	150
Metal dust inhalation	Asthma	BPT[b]	Sodium vanadate/asthma	100

[a] Eosinophilia.

[b] Bronchial provocation.

19.5.13 Zinc

For the general population, neither zinc nor its salts are known to be allergens. In the industrial environment, however, zinc organo-compounds, such as zinc pyrithione (also a widely used antidandruff agent) and zinc dimethyl- and diethyldithiocarbamate, chemicals used in the manufacture of rubber, in rare cases have been reported to cause ACD or CUS.[83,137,138]

Occupational exposure to zinc vapor, occurring at elevated temperatures generated in galvanization processes and in work with soldering fluxes containing zinc salts, was also reported to result in asthma: positive skin tests for immediate-type sensitization confirm hypersensitivity, although specific IgE could not be demonstrated.[139-141] One case of immediate-type reaction was recorded to zinc diethyldithiocarbamate, used in the manufacture of rubber gloves (Table 19.13).[138]

TABLE 19.13   CUS Due to Zinc

Etiology	Symptoms	Diagnostic Test	Challenge/Reaction	Ref.
Dermal. ZDC[a]	Wealing, oedema	Scratch chamber	ZDC/weal	138
Inh. zinc oxide	Urticaria, asthma	BPT;[b] IgE	Welding fumes/immediate and delayed angioedema and urticaria	139
Inh. zinc chloride	Asthma	BPT; IgE	Soldering fumes/asthma	140
Inh. zinc oxide	Asthma	SPT;[c] BPT	Zinc sulfate/weal, asthma	141

[a] Zinc diethyldithiocarbamate.

[b] Bronchial provocation.

[c] Skin prick.

ACKNOWLEDGMENTS

Thanks go to Gerald J. Gleich, M.D. (Mayo Clinic) for discussion of the manuscript.
This research was supported by the U.S. Air Force Office of Scientific Research (94NL023), the U.S. Environmental Protection Agency (CR-816785), and the U.S. National Institutes of Health (ES06825).

REFERENCES

1. Hostýnek, J. J., Hinz, R. S., Lorence, C. R., Price, M. and Guy, R. H., Metals and the skin, *Crit. Rev. Toxicol.*, 23, 171, 1993.
2. Forslind, B., Grundin, T. G., Lindberg, M., Roomans, G. M. and Werner, Y., Recent advances in X-ray microanalysis in dermatology, *Scanning Electron Microscopy*, part 2, 687, 1985.
3. Silberberg, I., Ultrastructural identification of mercury in epidermis after one topical application of mercuric chloride, *Clin. Res.*, 19, 365, 1971.

4. Pepys, J., Parish, W. E., Cromwell, O. and Hughes, E. G., Specific IgE and IgG antibodies to platinum salts in sensitized workers, *Monogr. Allergy,* 14, 142, 1979.

5. Shirakawa, T., Kusaka, Y., Fujimura, N., Goto, S. and Morimoto, K., The existence of specific antibodies to cobalt in hard metal asthma, *Clin. Allergy,* 18, 451, 1988.

6. Novey, H. S., Habib, M. and Wells, I. D., Asthma and IgE antibodies induced by chromium and nickel salts, *J. Allergy Clin. Immunol.,* 72, 407, 1983.

7. Jadassohn, J., Zur Kenntnis der medicamentösen Dermatosen, *Verhandlungen der Deutschen Dermatologischen Gesellschaft, V. Congress. Wien (1895),* 103, 1896.

8. Magee, P. S., Hostynek, J. J. and Maibach, H. I., A classification model for allergic contact dermatitis, *Quantitative Structure-Activity Relationships,* 13, 22, 1994.

9. Ishizaka, K., Ishizaka, T. and Hornbrook, M. M., Physicochemical properties of reaginic antibody V. Correlation of reaginic activity with gamma E-globulin antibody, *J. Immunol.,* 97, 840, 1966.

10. Wide, L., Bennich, H. and Johansson, S. G. O., Diagnosis of allergy by an *in vitro* test for allergen antibodies, *Lancet,* 2, 1105, 1967.

11. Wide, L., Radioimmunoassays employing immunosorbents, *Acta Endocrinologica,* 142, 207, 1969.

12. Tanglertsampan, C. and Maibach, H. I., Contact urticaria, in *Occupational Skin Disorders,* Hogan, D. J., Ed., Igaku-Shoin, New York, 1994, 81.

13. Kanerva, L., Estlander, T. and Jolanki, R., Skin testing for immediate hypersensitivity in occupational allergology, in *Metal Toxicology,* Goyer, R. A., Klaassen, C. D. and Waalkes, M. P., Eds., Academic Press, New York, 1995, 104.

14. Fisher, A. A., Contact urticaria, in *Contact Dermatitis,* 4th ed., Rietschel, R. L. and Fowler, J. F., Eds., Williams & Wilkins, Baltimore, 1995, 778.

15. Lahti, A., Immediate contact reactions, *Textbook of Contact Dermatitis,* 2nd ed., Roycroft, R. J. G., Menné, T. and Frosch, P. J., Eds., Springer Verlag, New York, 1995, 62.

16. Pizzino, J., Possible chromate-associated urticaria, *J. Occup. Med.,* 35, 96, 1993.

17. Kanerva, L., Estlander, T. and Jolanki, R., Occupational skin allergy in the dental profession, *Dermatol. Clin.,* 12, 517, 1994.

18. Kanerva, L., Estlander, T. and Jolanki, R., Dental problems, in *Practical Contact Dermatitis,* Guin, J. D., Ed., McGraw-Hill, Inc., New York, 1995, 397.

19. Coombs, R. R. A. and Gell, P. G. H., *Classification of Allergic Reactions Responsible for Hypersensitivity and Clinical Disease,* 3rd ed., Blackwell, London, 1975.

20. Keskinen, H., Kalliomäki, P.-L. and Alanko, K., Occupational asthma due to stainless steel welding fumes, *Clin. Allergy,* 10, 151, 1980.

21. Barranco-Sanz, B., Martin Munoz, F., López Serrano, C. and Martín Esteban, M., Hypersensitivity to mercuric fluorescein compounds, *Allergologia et Immunopathologia,* 17, 219, 1989.

22. Dearman, R. J. and Kimber, I., Differential stimulation of immune function by respiratory and contact chemical allergens, *Immunology,* 72, 563, 1991.

23. Ophaswongse, S. and Maibach, H. I., Alcohol dermatitis: allergic contact dermatitis and contact urticaria syndrome, *Contact Dermatitis,* 30, 1, 1994.

24. Thomas, W. R., Vardinon, N., Watkins, M. C. and Asherson, G. L., Antigen-specific mast cell degranulation in contact sensitivity to picryl chloride. An early event, *Immunology,* 39, 331, 1980.

25. van Loveren, H., Meade, R. and Askenase, P. W., An early component of delayed-type hypersensitivity mediated by T-cells and mast cells, *J. Exp. Med.,* 157, 1604, 1983.

26. Dearman, R. J., Mitchell, N., Basketter, D. A. and Kimber, I., Differential ability of occupational chemical contact and respiratory allergens to cause immediate and delayed dermal hypersensitivity reactions in mice, *Intern. Arch. Allergy Immunol.*, 97, 315, 1992.

27. Dearman, R. J., Basketter, D. A., Coleman, J. W. and Kimber, I., The cellular and molecular basis for divergent allergic reponses to chemicals, *Chemico-Biological Interactions*, 84, 1, 1992.

28. Kimber, I. and Dearman, R. J., Immune responses to contact and respiratory allergens, in *Immunotoxicology and Immunopharmacology*, 2nd ed., Dean, J. H., Luster, M. I., Munson, A. E. and Kimber, I., Eds., Raven Press, Ltd., New York, 1994, 663.

29. Aro, T., Kanerva, L., Hayrinenimmonen, R. and Silvennoinenkassinen, S., Long-lasting allergic patch test reaction caused by gold, *Contact Dermatitis*, 28, 276, 1993.

30. Bruze, M., Hedman, H., Björkner, B. and Öller, H., The development and course of test reactions to gold sodium thiosulfate, *Contact Dermatitis*, 33, 386, 1995.

31. Polak, L., Barnes, J. M. and Turk, J. L., The genetic control of contact sensitization to inorganic metal compounds in guinea-pigs, *Immunology*, 14, 707, 1968.

32. Fisher, A. A., Presence of mercury compound in plants, *Am. J. Contact Derm.*, 1, 208, 1990.

33. Davis, P. and Hughes, G. R. V., A serial study of eosinophilia and raised IgE antibodies during gold therapy, *Ann. Rheum. Dis.*, 34, 203, 1975.

34. Chan-Yeung, M. and Lam, S., State of the art: occupational asthma, *Am. Rev. Resp. Dis.*, 133, 686, 1986.

35. Karol, M. H., Predictive testing for respiratory allergy, in *Allergic Hypersensitivities Induced by Chemicals*, Vos, J. G., Younes, M. and Smith, E., Eds., CRC Press, Boca Raton, 1996, 125.

36. Karol, M. H., Graham, C., Gealy, R., Macina, O. T., Sussmen, N. and Rosenkranz, H. S., Structure-activity relationships and computer-assisted analysis of respiratory sensitization potential, in *Toxicology Letters*, 86, 187, 1996.

37. Agius, R. M., Nee, J., McGovern, B. and Robertson, A., Structure activity hypotheses in occupational asthma caused by low molecular weight substances, *Ann. Occup. Hygiene*, 35, 129, 1991.

38. Sinigaglia, F., The molecular basis of metal recognition by T cells, *J. Invest. Dermatol.*, 102, 398, 1994.

39. Dueva, L. A., Kogan, V. J., Suvorov, S. V., and Sterengarts, R. J., *Industrial Allergens*, United Nations Environment Programme, Centre for International Projects, Moscow, 1989 (English Edition 1994).

40. Harris, J. W., Studies on the mechanism of a drug-induced hemolytic anemia, *J. Lab. Clin. Med.*, 47, 760, 1956.

41. de Torregrosa, V., Rodriguez Rosado, A. L. and Montilla, E., Hemolytic anemia secondary to stibophen therapy, *J. Am. Med. Assoc.*, 186, 598, 1963.

42. Davis, A., Comparative trials of antimonial drugs in urinary schistosomiasis, *Bull. W.H.O.*, 38, 197, 1968.

43. Motolese, A., Truzzi, M., Giannini, A. and Seidenari, S., Contact dermatitis and contact sensitization among enamellers and decorators in the ceramics industry, *Contact Dermatitis*, 28, 59, 1993.

44. Hayashi, Y. and Nakamura, S., Clinical application of energy dispersive X-ray microanalysis for nondestructively confirming dental metal allergens, *Oral Surgery, Oral Medicine, Oral Pathology*, 77, 623, 1994.

45. Walsh, E. N., Chromate hazards in industry, *J. Am. Med. Assoc.*, 153, 1305, 1953.

46. Cavelier, C. and Foussereau, J., Kontaktallergie gegen Metalle und deren Salze, *Dermatosen,* 43, 100, 1995.

47. Epstein, W. L., Cutaneous granulomas as a toxicologic problem, in *Dermatotoxicology and Pharmacology,* Marzulli, F. N. and Maibach, H. I., Eds., John Wiley & Sons, New York, 1977, 465.

48. Cohen, H. A., The role of carrier in sensitivity to chromium and cobalt, *Arch. Dermatol.,* 112, 37, 1976.

49. el Sayed, F. and Bazex, J., Airborne contact dermatitis from chromate in cement with recall dermatitis on patch testing, *Contact Dermatitis,* 30, 58, 1994.

50. Smith, A. R., Chrome poisoning with manifestations of sensitization, *J. Am. Med. Assoc.,* 97, 95, 1931.

51. Joules, H., Asthma from sensitisation to chromium, *Lancet,* 2, 182, 1932.

52. Royle, H., Toxicity of chromium acid in the chromium plating industry, *Environ. Res.,* 10, 141, 1975.

53. Menné, T. and Maibach, H. I., Reactions to systemic exposure to contact allergens: systemic contact allergy reactions (SCAR), *Immunol. Allergy Prac.,* 9, 373, 1987.

54. Polak, L., Immunology of chromium, in *Chromium: Metabolism and Toxicity,* Burrows, D., Ed., CRC Press, Boca Raton, 1973, 51.

55. Cohen, H. A., Experimental production of circulating antibodies to chromium, *J. Invest. Dermatol.,* 38, 13, 1962.

56. Mali, J. W. H., Van Kooten, W. J. and Van Neer, F. C. J., Some aspects of the behavior of chromium compounds in the skin, *J. Invest. Dermatol.,* 41, 111, 1963.

57. Mali, J. W. H., Malten, K. and Van Neer, F. C. J., Allergy to chromium, *Arch. Dermatol.,* 93, 41, 1966.

58. Polak, L., Turk, J. L. and Frey, J. R., Studies on contact hypersensitivity to chromium compounds, *Progress in Allergy,* 17, 145, 1973.

59. Samitz, M. H. and Katz, S., Preliminary studies on the reduction and binding of chromium with skin, *Arch. Dermatol.,* 88, 816, 1963.

60. Samitz, M. H. and Katz, S., A study of the chemical reactions between chromium and skin, *J. Invest. Dermatol.,* 43, 35, 1964.

61. Cronin, E., Metals, *Cobalt,* Churchill Livingstone, Edinburgh, 1980.

62. Gawkrodger, D. J. and Lewis, F. M., Isolated cobalt sensitivity in an etcher, *Contact Dermatitis,* 28, 46, 1993.

63. Cirla, A. M., Cobalt-related asthma: clinical and immunological aspects, *Sci. Total Environ.,* 150, 85, 1994.

64. Pisati, G. and Zedda, S., Outcome of occupational asthma due to cobalt hypersensitivity, *Sci. Total Environ.,* 150, 167, 1994.

65. Camarasa, J. G. and Alomar, A., Photosensitization to cobalt in a bricklayer, *Contact Dermatitis,* 7, 154, 1981.

66. Romaguera, C., Lecha, M., Grimalt, F., Muniesa, A. M. and Mascaro, J. M., Photocontact dermatitis to cobalt salts, *Contact Dermatitis,* 8, 383, 1982.

67. Lauwerys, R. and Lison, D., Health risks associated with cobalt exposure-an overview, *Sci. Total Environ.,* 150, 1, 1994.

68. Davison, A. G., Haslam, P. L., Corrin, B., Cotts, I. I., Dewar, A., Riding, W. D., Studdy, P. R. and Newman-Taylor, A. J., Interstitial lung disease and asthma in hard metal workers: bronchoalveolar lavage, ultrastructural, and analytical findings and results of bronchial provocation tests, *Thorax,* 38, 119, 1983.

69. Bruckner, H. C., Extrinsic asthma in a tungsten carbide worker, *J. Occ. Med.,* 9, 918, 1967.

70. Reid, D. J., Allergic reaction to copper cement, *Br. Dental J.,* 124, 92, 1968.
71. Barkoff, J. R., Urticaria secondary to a copper intrauterine device, *Int. J. Dermatol.,* 15, 594, 1976.
72. Shelley, W. B., Shelley, E. D. and Ho, A. K. S., Cholinergic urticaria: acetylcholine-receptor-dependent immediate-type hypersensitivity reaction to copper, *Lancet,* 1, 843, 1983.
73. Sterry, W. and Schmoll, M., Contact urticaria and dermatitis from self-adhesive pads, *Contact Dermatitis,* 13, 284, 1985.
74. Romaguera, C. and Grimalt, F., Contact dermatitis from a copper-containing intrauterine contraceptive device, *Contact Dermatitis,* 7, 163, 1981.
75. Gaul, L. E., Metal sensitivity in eczema of the hands, *Ann. Allergy,* 11, 758, 1953.
76. Gaul, L. E., Incidence of sensitivity to chromium, nickel, gold, silver, and copper compared to reactions to their aqueous salts including cobalt sulfate, *Ann. Allergy,* 12, 429, 1954.
77. Saltzer, E. I. and Wilson, J. W., Allergic contact dermatitis due to copper, *Arch. Dermatol.,* 98, 375, 1968.
78. Barranco, V. P., Eczematous dermatitis caused by internal exposure to copper, *Arch. Dermatol.,* 106, 386, 1972.
79. Jirasek, L. and Kalensky, J., Hypersensitivity to platinum, rhodium, gold, copper, antimony and other precious metals and occupational dermatitis caused by selenium, *Ceskoslovenska Dermatologie,* 50, 361, 1975.
80. Jouppila, P., Niinimäki, A. and Mikkonen, M., Copper allergy and copper IUD, *Contraception,* 19, 631, 1979.
81. Karlberg, A. T., Boman, A. and Wahlberg, J. E., Copper — a rare sensitizer, *Contact Dermatitis,* 9, 134, 1983.
82. van Joost, T., Habets, J. M. W., Stolz, E. and Naafs, B., The meaning of positive patch tests to copper sulphate in nickel allergy, *Contact Dermatitis,* 18, 101, 1988.
83. Namikoshi, T., Yoshimatsu, T., Suga, K., Fujii, H. and Yasuda, K., The prevalence of sensitivity to constituents of dental alloys, *J. Oral Rehab.,* 17, 377, 1990.
84. Kawahara, D., Oshima, H., Kosugi, H., Nakamura, M., Sugai, T. and Tamaki, T., Further epidemiologic study of occupational contact dermatitis in the dental clinic, *Contact Dermatitis,* 28, 114, 1993.
85. Romagnoli, P., Spinas, G. A. and Sinigaglia, F., Gold-specific T cells in rheumatoid arthritis patients treated with gold, *J. Clin. Invest.,* 89, 254, 1992.
86. Palosuo, T., Provost, T. T. and Milgrom, F., Gold nephropathy: serologic data suggesting an immune complex disease, *Clin. Exp. Immunol.,* 25, 311, 1976.
87. Kazantzis, G., The role of hypersensitivity and the immune response in influencing susceptibility to metal toxicity, *Environ. Health Persp.,* 25, 111, 1978.
88. Davis, P., Ezeoke, A., Munro, J., Hobbs, J. R. and Hughes, G. R. V., Immunological studies on the mechanism of gold hypersensitivity reactions, *Br. Med. J.,* 3, 676, 1973.
89. Wahlberg, J. E., Nickel: animal sensitization assays, in *Nickel and the Skin: Immunology and Toxicology,* Maibach, H. I. and Menné, T., Eds., CRC Press, Boca Raton, 1989, 65.
90. Hemingway, J. D. and Molokhia, M. M., The dissolution of metallic nickel in artificial sweat, *Contact Dermatitis,* 16, 99, 1987.
91. Menczel, E., Bucks, D. A. W., Wester, R. C. and Maibach, H. I., Skin binding during percutaneous penetration, in *Percutaneous Absorption. Mechanisms, Methodology, Drug Delivery,* Bronaugh, R. I. and Maibach, H. I., Eds., Marcel Dekker, New York, 1985, 43.

92. Ellen, G., van den Bosch-Tibbesma, G. and Douma, F. F., Nickel content of various Dutch foodstuffs, *Zeitschrift fur Lebensmittel-Untersuchung und -Forschung,* 166, 145, 1978.

93. Schroeder, H. A., A sensible look at air pollution by metals, *Arch. Environ. Health,* 21, 798, 1970.

94. Block, G. T. and Yeung, M., Asthma induced by nickel, *J. Am. Med. Assoc.,* 247, 1600, 1982.

95. Shirakawa, T., Kusaka, Y., Fujimura, N., Kato, M., Heki, S. and Morimoto, K., Hard metal asthma: cross immunological and respiratory reactivity between cobalt and nickel?, *Thorax,* 45, 267, 1990.

96. Sinigaglia, F., Scheidegger, D., Garotta, G., Scheper, R., Pletscher, M. and Lanzavecchia, A., Isolation and characterization of Ni-specific T cell clones from patients with Ni-contact dermatitis, *J. Immunol.,* 135, 3929, 1985.

97. Malo, J. L., Cartier, A., Doepner, M., Nieboer, E., Evans, S. and Dolovich, J., Occupational asthma caused by nickel sulfate, *J. Allergy Clin. Immunol.,* 69, 55, 1982.

98. Dolovich, J., Evans, S. L. and Nieboer, E., Occupational asthma from nickel sensitivity: I. Human serum albumin in the antigenic determinant, *Br. J. Ind. Med.,* 41, 51, 1984.

99. Nieboer, E., Evans, S. L. and Dolovich, J., Occupational asthma from nickel sensitivity, 2. Factors influencing the interaction of Ni2+, HSA, and serum antibodies with nickel related specificity, *Br. J. Ind. Med.,* 41, 56, 1984.

100. Shirakawa, T., Kusaka, Y., Fujimura, M., Kato, M., Heki, S., Goto, S. and Izumi, T., Positive bronchoprovocation with cobalt and nickel in hard metal asthma, *Am. Rev. Resp. Dis.,* 135, 233, 1987.

101. Shirakawa, T., Kusaka, Y. and Morimoto, K., Specific IgE antibodies to nickel in workers with known reactivity to cobalt, *Clin. Exp. Allergy,* 22, 213, 1992.

102. McKenzie, A. W. and Aitken, C. V. E., Urticaria after insertion of Smith-Petersen Vitallium nail, *Br. Med. J.,* 4, 36, 1967.

103. Pelletier, L., Pasquier, R., Rossert, J., Vial, M. C., Mandet, C. and Druet, P., Autoreactive T cells in mercury-induced autoimmunity. Ability to induce the autoimmune disease, *J. Immunol.,* 140, 750, 1988.

104. Pelletier, L., Castedo, M., Bellon, B. and Druet, P., Mercury and autoimmunity, in *Immunotoxicology and Immunopharmacology,* 2nd ed., Dean, J. H., Luster, M. I., Munson, A. E., and Kimber, I., Eds., Raven Press, New York, 1994, 539.

105. Vena, G., C., F., Grandolfo, M. and Angelini, G., Mercury Exanthem, *Contact Dermatitis,* 31, 214, 1994.

106. Torresani, C., Caprari, E. and Manara, G. C., Contact urticaria syndrome due to phenylmercuric acetate, *Contact Dermatitis,* 29, 282, 1993.

107. Corrales Torres, J. L. and De Corres, F., Anaphylactic hypersensitivity to mercurochrome (merbrominum), *Ann. Allergy,* 54, 230, 1985.

108. Prouvost-Danon, A., Abadie, A., Sapin, C., Bazin, H. and Druet, P., Induction of IgE synthesis and potentiation of anti-ovalbumin IgE antibody response by HgCl2 in the rat, *J. Immunol.,* 126, 699, 1981.

109. Hernández, A. P., Aznar, J. V. B., Martinez, G. J., Puchades, A. R. and Baixauli, E. B., Mercurochrome allergy: concurrence of 2 hypersensitivity mechanisms in the same patient, *Contact Dermatitis,* 30, 48, 1994.

110. Temesvári, E. and Daróczy, J., Histological examination of immediate and delayed contact allergy provoked by mercuric chloride, *Contact Dermatitis,* 21, 271, 1989.

111. Gottlieb, P. M., Sensitivity to mercurial diuretics, *Ann. Allergy,* 6, 518, 1948.

112. Zelikoff, J. T., Smialowicz, R., Bigazzi, P. E., Goyer, R. A., Lawrence, D. A., Maibach, H. I. and Gardner, D., Immunomodulation by metals, *Fund. Appl. Toxicol.*, 22, 1, 1994.

113. Bezzon, O. L., Allergic sensitivity to several base metals: a clinical report, *J. Prosthetic Dentistry*, 69, 243, 1993.

114. Dueva, L. A. and Stepanian, S. S., Clinico-immunologic characteristics and prevention of occupational allergic dermatoses due to molybdenum exposure, *Vestnik Dermatologii I Venerologii*, 1989, 47, 1989.

115. Biagini, R. E., Clark, J. C., Gallagher, J. S., Bernstein, I. L. and Moorman, W. M., Passive transfer in the monkey of human immediate hypersensitivity to complex salts of platinum and palladium, *Fed. Proc.*, 41, 827, 1982.

116. Biagini, R. E., Bernstein, L., Gallagher, J. S., Moorman, W. J., Brooks, S. and Gann, P. H., The diversity of reaginic immune responses to platinum and palladium metallic salts, *J. Allergy Clin. Immunol.*, 76, 794, 1985.

117. Tomilets, V. A. and Zakharova, I. A., Anaphilactic and anaphilactoid properties of complex palladium compounds, *Farmakologiia i Toksikologiia*, 42, 170, 1979.

118. Tomilets, V. A., Dontsov, V. I. and Zakharova, I. A., Experimental allergic reactions of the immediate and delayed type to compounds of group VIII metals, *Fiziologicheskii Zhurnal*, 25, 653, 1979.

119. Tomilets, V. A., Dontsov, V. I., Zakharova, I. A. and Klevtsov, A. V., Histamine releasing and histamine binding action of platinum and palladium compounds, *Archivum Immunologiae et Therapiae Experimentalis*, 28, 953, 1980.

120. Tomilets, V. A., Dontsov, V. I., Ado, V. A. and Zakharova, I. A., Toxic, anaphylactoid and sensitizing properties of mercaptoquinolinates, metals of the 8th and 3rd group, *Biulleten Eksperimentalnoi Biologii i Meditsiny*, 89, 328, 1980.

121. Tomilets, V. A., Zakharova, I. A., Dontsov, V. I. and Ado, V. A., Comparative study of the toxic, anaphylactoid and sensitizing properties of 5-sulfo-8-mercaptoquinolinates of metals of the 8th and 3rd groups of the periodic table, *Biulleten Eksperimentalnoi Biologii i Meditsiny*, 89, 463, 1980.

122. Sheard, C., Contact dermatitis from platinum and related metals. Report of a case, *Am. Med. Assoc. Arch. Dermatol.*, 71, 357, 1955.

123. Schuppe, H.-C., Lerchenmüller, C., Kulig, J., Huch, J., Goerz, G., Gleichmann, E. and Kind, P., Contact hypersensitivity to halide salts of platinum in mice, *J. Invest. Dermatol.*, 100, 475, 1993.

124. Baker, D. B., Gann, P. H., Brooks, S. M., Gallagher, J. and Bernstein, I. L., Cross-sectional study of platinum salts sensitization among precious metals refinery workers, *Am. J. Ind. Med.*, 18, 653, 1990.

125. Bolm-Audorff, U., Bienfait, H. G., Burkhard, J., Bury, A. H., Merget, R., Pressel, G. and Schultze-Werninghaus, G., Prevalence of respiratory allergy in a platinum refinery, *Int. Arch. Occ. Environ. Health*, 64, 257, 1992.

126. Roberts, A. E., Platinosis. A five year study of the effects of soluble platinum salts on employees in a platinum laboratory and refinery, *Am. Med. Assoc. Arch. Ind. Hyg. Occup. Med.*, 4, 549, 1951.

127. Levene, G. M. and Calnan, C. D., Platinum sensitivity: treatment by specific hyposensitization, *Clin. Allergy*, 1, 75, 1971.

128. Calverley, A. E., Rees, D., Dowdeswell, R. J., Linnett, P. J. and Kielkowski, D., Platinum salt sensitivity in refinery workers: incidence and effects of smoking and exposure, *Occup. Environ. Med.*, 52, 661, 1995.

129. Hunter, D., Milton, R. and Perry, K. M. A., Asthma caused by the complex salts of platinum, *Br. J. Ind. Med.*, 2, 1945.

130. Murdoch, R. D., Pepys, J. and Hughes, E. G., IgE antibody responses to platinum group metals: a large scale refinery survey, *Br. J. Ind. Med.*, 43, 37, 1986.

131. Freedman, S. O. and Krupey, J., Respiratory allergy caused by platinum salts, *J. Allergy*, 42, 233, 1968.

132. Pepys, J., Pickering, C. A. C. and Hughes, E. G., Asthma due to inhaled chemical agents — Complex salts of platinum, *Clin. Allergy*, 2, 391, 1972.

133. Colosio, C., Tomasini, M., Cairoli, S., Foa, V., Minoia, C., Marinovich, M. and Galli, C. L., Occupational triphenyltin acetate poisonong: a case report, *Br. J. Ind. Med.*, 48, 136, 1991.

134. Menné, T., Andersen, K. E., Kaaber, K., Osmundsen, P. E., Andersen, J. R., Yding, F. and Valeur, G., Tin: an overlooked contact sensitizer?, *Contact Dermatitis*, 16, 9, 1987.

135. de Fine Olivarius, F., Balslev, E. and Menné, T., Skin reactivity to tin chloride and metallic tin, *Contact Dermatitis*, 29, 110, 1993.

136. Roshchin, A. V., Taranenko, L. A. and Muratova, N. Z., Sensitizing properties of indium, palladium, and vanadium, *Gigiena Truda I Professional'nye Zabolevanija*, 2, 5, 1982.

137. Jordaan, H. F. and Sandler, M., Zinc-induced granuloma — a unique complication of insulin therapy, *Clin. Exp. Dermatol.*, 14, 227, 1989.

138. Helander, I. and Mäkelä, A., Contact uticaria to zinc diethyldithiocarbamate, *Contact Dermatitis*, 9, 327, 1983.

139. Farrell, F. J., Angioedema and urticaria as acute and late phase reactions to zinc fume exposure, with associated metal fume fever-like symptoms, *Am. J. Ind. Med.*, 12, 331, 1987.

140. Weir, D. C., Robertson, A. S., Jones, S. and Sherwood Burge, P., Occupational asthma due to soft corrosive soldering fluxes containing zinc chloride and ammonium chloride, *Thorax*, 44, 220, 1989.

141. Malo, J. L., Cartier, A. and Dolovich, J., Occupational asthma due to zinc, *Eur. Resp. J.*, 6, 447, 1993.

142. Kusaka, Y., Yokoyama, K., Sera, Y., Yamamoto, S., Sone, S., Kyono, H., Shirakawa, T. and Goto, S., Respiratory diseases in hard metal workers: an occupational hygiene study in a factory, *Br. J. Ind. Med.*, 43, 474, 1986.

143. Pisati, G., Bernabeo, F. and Cirla, A. M., A bronchial challenge test for cobalt in the diagnosis of asthma due to inhalation of hard metal dust, *Medicina del Lavoro*, 77, 1986.

144. Card, W. I., A case of asthma sensitivity to chromates, *Lancet*, 1348, 1935.

145. España, A., Alonso, M. L., Soria, C., Guimaraens, D. and Ledo, A., Chronic urticaria after implantation of 2 nickel-containing dental prosthesis in a nickel-allergic patient, *Contact Dermatitis*, 21, 204, 1989.

146. Kanerva, L., Komulainen, M., Estlander, T. and Jolanki, R., Occupational allergic contact dermatitis from mercury, *Contact Dermatitis*, 28, 26, 1993.

147. Urbach, E. and Gottlieb, P. M., *Allergy*, Grune & Stratton, New York, 1946.

148. Mathews, K. P., Immediate type hypersensitivity to phenylmercuric compounds, *Am. J. Med.*, 44, 310, 1968.

149. Conde-Salazar, L., Cannavo, A., Meza, B., Guimaraens, D. and Yus, E. S., Occupational argyrosis and platinosis, *Am. J. Contact Derm.*, 3, 44, 1992.

150. Musk, A. W. and Tees, J. G., Asthma caused by occupational exposure to vanadium compounds, *Med. J. Austr.*, 1, 183, 1982.

20

Contact Urticaria Syndrome by Milk and Milk Products

Flora B. de Waard-van der Spek and Arnold P. Oranje

CONTENTS

20.1   INTRODUCTION

Cow's milk allergy affects 2–8% of infants.[1] Together with egg white, it is the most common food allergen. The clinical presentation is very variable. One distinguishes milk-induced pulmonary disease, allergic gastroenteropathy, iron-losing enteropathy, neonatal thrombopenia, and milk-induced colitis in infancy. Hill mentioned as dermatological symptoms urticaria, angioedema, circumoral lesions, morbilliform eruptions, eczema, and perianal eruptions, but did not include milk-induced contact urticaria. Contact urticaria is common in infants and toddlers with atopic dermatitis

(AD) and food allergy[15] (see Chapter 25). A reason for the variability of food allergy symptoms is not clear.

20.2 DEFINITION

Milk-induced contact urticaria is a wheal and flare reaction elicited after cutaneous exposure to cow's milk or cow's milk products such as cheese, yogurt, and others. Contact urticaria can be immune mediated, nonimmunological, or of unknown origin.[2,3] Cow's milk induced CUS is always immune-mediated.

20.3 DIAGNOSIS

Children with AD and milk allergy can present with immune mediated contact urticaria.[4,5] Based on the mechanisms of the contact urticaria syndrome (CUS), several provocation tests, such as open application test, SAFT, and RUB test, have been described.[4-6]

20.4 MILK AND MILK PRODUCTS

20.4.1 Allergens in Milk Protein

Cow's milk contains more than 25 proteins. Casein is the most prominent protein in cow's milk but is not as important in allergy as beta-lactoglobulin, which is only 10% of the total protein.[7] Allergens in cow's milk listed are beta-lactoglobulin, and then casein, lactalbumin, and bovine serum albumin.[7] Human milk contains mainly beta-lactoglobulin.[8]

20.4.2 Incidence and Course

The prevalence of CUS by cow's milk is unknown. About half of the children with AD and food allergy also suffer from CUS. Allergens such as milk can penetrate the skin easily and cause urticarial reactions in sensitized individuals. A 12-month-old boy had been reported, who had a strong history of cow's milk allergy, and developed two episodes of anaphylaxis following cutaneous application of a casein containing ointment to an inflamed diaper area.[9] In our out-patient clinic, a manifest food allergy and CUS were observed in 20% of the children with atopic dermatitis.[10] The most common allergens are cow's milk, egg, and peanut. CUS by cow's milk is decreasing after the age of 2 years. At the age of 4 years, 75% of all the cases has been cleared. A probable explanation is the role of the inadequate immune system in young allergic children.[11] It concerns especially the immaturity of the gastrointestinal tract. Cow's milk allergy seldom develops in adulthood.

20.5 DIETARY INTERVENTIONS

Children with cow's milk allergy need intensive nutritional counseling and regular monitoring of growth. A 4-year-old boy was reported who had rickets, thought to be the result of dietary calcium deficiency caused by the prolonged elimination from his diet of cow's milk and milk products because of allergy. Adequate intake of calcium resulted in rapid improvement.[12] Milk substitutes are largely used in children with cow's milk allergy. Protein hydrolysates are being used. There are reports that some children develop intolerance to protein hydrolysates. Polypeptides of protein hydrolysates may induce an IgE antibody response or crossreact with IgE antibodies against determinants of cow milk proteins.[13] Sensitization or cross-reactivity to protein hydrolysates may occur and may be associated with poor response to an exclusion diet based on protein hydrolysates.[14]

20.6 PRACTICAL CONSEQUENCES

Contact urticaria syndrome is often not difficult to recognize, if you consider it. The most important symptoms of food allergy with the skin as the most prominent target are food refusal and redness on hands and round the mouth. In infancy, especially, cow's milk is the most common allergen.

In case of cow's milk allergy, one has to evaluate the allergy again after the age of 2 years, because in most children the cow's milk allergy disappears. Children with cow's milk allergy need intensive nutritional counseling and regular monitoring of growth. Sensitization or cross-reactivity to protein hydrolysates may occur, and should be kept in mind. Contact urticaria to big particulated hydrolysates has been described and also observed by us.

REFERENCES

1. Hill, D.J., Clinical recognition of the child with food allergy. In: Harms, H.K., Wahn, U., *Food Allergy in Infancy and Childhood.* Springer Verlag, Berlin 1989; 61-9.
2. Von Krogh, G., Maibach, H.I., The contact urticaria syndrome — an updated review. *J. Am. Acad. Dermatol.,* 1981; 5: 328-42.
3. Von Krogh, G., Maibach, H.I. The contact urticaria syndrome — 1982. *Sem. Dermatol.* 1982;1: 59-66.
4. Salo, O.P., Mäkinen-Kiljunen, S., Juntunen, K. Milk causes a rapid urticarial reaction on the skin of children with atopic dermatitis and milk allergy. *Acta Derm. Venereol.* 1986;66: 438-42.
5. Oranje, A.P., Aarsen, R.S.R., Liefaard, G. Immediate contact reactions to cow's milk and egg in atopic children. *Acta Dermatovenereol* (Stockholm) 1991;71: 263-6.
6. Gronemeyer, W., Fuchs, E., Bandilla, K. 'Reibtest' und RAST. *Z. Hautkr.* 1979;54: 205-12.
7. Aas, K. Biochemical characteristics of food allergens. In: Harms, H.K., Wahn, U. *Food Allergy in Infancy and Childhood.* Springer Verlag, Berlin 1989: 1-12.
8. Jakobsson. Food antigens in human milk. In: Harms, H.K., Wahn, U. *Food Allergy in Infancy and Childhood.* Springer Verlag, Berlin 1989: 47-52.
9. Jarmoc, L.M., Primack, W.A. Anaphylaxis to cutaneous exposure to milk protein in a diaper rash ointment. *Clin. Pediatr.* 1987;26: 154-5.
10. Aarden, J.M., Mulder, P.G.H., Oranje, A.P. Vijfjaars na-onderzoek bij kindereczeem. [Five-years follow up in childhood eczema]. *Tijdschr. Kindergeneeskd* 1994;62: 269-72.

11. Baert, M.R.M., Koning, H., Neijens, H.J. et al. Role of the immune system in allergic children. *Pediatr. Allergy Immunol.* 1995; 6 (s7): 27-30.
12. Davidovits, M., Levis, Y., Avramovitz, T. et al. Calcium-deficiency rickets in a four-year-old boy with milk allergy. *A. Pediatr.* 1993;122: 249-51.
13. Businco, L., Cantani, A., Longhi, M.A. Anaphylactic reactions to a cow's milk whey protein hydrolysate in infants wityh cow milk allergy. *Ann. Allergy* 1989;62: 333.
14. Plebani, A., Albertini, A., Scotta, S. et al. IgE antibodies to hydrolysates of cow milk proteins in children with cow milk allergy. *Ann. Allergy* 1990;64: 279-80.

21

Skin Allergy Caused by Organic Acid Anhydrides

Riitta Jolanki, Lasse Kanerva, Tuula Estlander, and Kyllikki Tarvainen

CONTENTS

21.1   INTRODUCTION

Organic acid anhydrides form a group of industrially important, reactive chemicals with a low molecular weight (MW) (100–300 Da). They are widely used in the chemical industry, especially in the manufacture of plastics. The workers are exposed to anhydrides either during their production or when they are used in the production of polymers.

21.2   CHEMISTRY AND USE

Phthalic anhydride (PA; CAS 85-44-9)

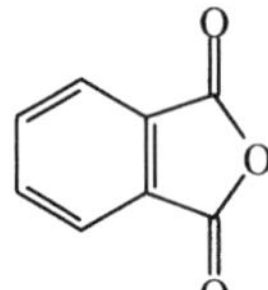

Properties: White, crystalline needles; mild odor; MW 148.12; melting point (mp) 131.16°C; boiling point (bp) 285°C; soluble in alcohol, carbon disulfide, and hot water; combustible; skin, eye, and respiratory irritant.[1-2]

Use: Alkyl resins, plasticizers, hardener for resins, polyesters, synthesis of phenolphthalein and other phthaleins, many other dyes, chlorinated products, pharmaceutical intermediates, insecticides, diethyl phthalate, dimethyl phthalate, and laboratory reagent, vulcanizing retarder.[1-3]

Trimellitic anhydride (TMA; 1,2,4-benzenetricarboxylic acid-1,2-anhydride; CAS 552-30-7)

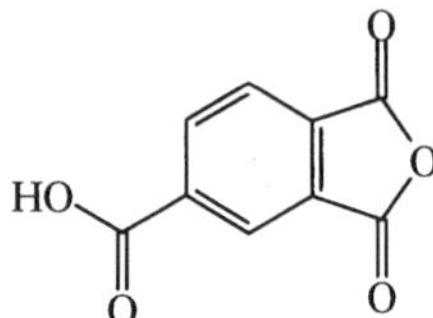

Properties: Solid; MW 192.12; mp 164–166°C; combustible.[1]

Use: Plasticizer for polyvinyl chloride, alkyd coating resins, high-temperature plastics, wire insulation, gaskets, automotive upholstery.[1]

Tetrachlorophthalic anhydride (TCPA; CAS 117-08-8)

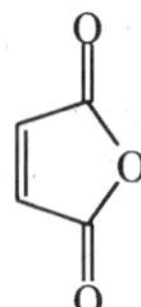

Properties: White, odorless, free-flowing, nonhygroscopic powder; MW 285.88; mp 254–255°C; bp 371°C; slightly soluble in water.[1]

Use: Intermediate in dyes, pharmaceuticals, plasticizers, and other organic materials, flame-retardant in epoxy resins.[1]

Maleic anhydride (MA; 2,5-furandione; CAS 108-31-6)

Properties: Colorless needles; MW 98.06; mp 53°C; bp 200°C; soluble in water, acetone, alcohol, and dioxane; partially soluble in chloroform and benzene; skin, eye, and respiratory irritant.[1-2]

Use: Polyester resins, alkyd coating resins, fumaric and tartaric acid manufacture, pesticides, preservative for oils and fats, permanent-press resins (textiles), Diels-Alder reactions, plasticizers and pharmaceuticals, vulcanizing retarder.[1,3,4]

Pyromellitic dianhydride (PMDA; CAS 89-32-7)

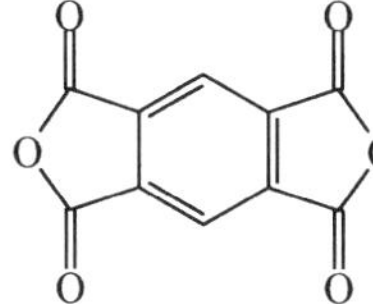

Properties: White powder; MW 218.12; mp 286°C; bp 397–400°C; soluble in some organic solvents; hydrolyzes to the acid when exposed to moisture; skin irritant.[1]

Use: Curing agent for epoxy resins used in high temperature laminates, molds, and coatings; cross-linking agent for epoxy plasticizers in vinyls, alkyd resins; intermediate for pyromellitic acid.[1]

Hexahydrophthalic anhydride (HHPA; 1,2-cyclohexandicarboxylic anhydride; CAS 85-42-7)

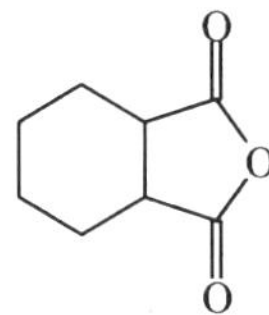

Properties: Clear, colorless, viscous liquid which becomes a glossy solid at 35–36°C; bp 158°C, MW 154.17; miscible with benzene, toluene, acetone, carbon tetrachloride, chloroform, ethanol, and ethyl acetate; slightly soluble in petroleum ether; strong irritant to eyes and skin.[1]

Use: Intermediate for alkyds, plasticizers, insect repellents, and rust inhibitors; hardener in epoxy resins.[1]

Himic anhydride (HA; 3,6-endomethylene-Δ^4-tetrahydrophthalic anhydride)[5]

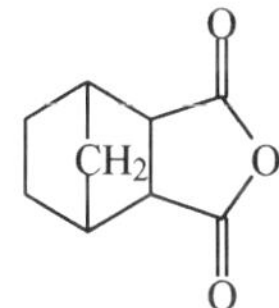

Properties: MW 166.19
Use: Production of brominated fire retardants.[5]

Methylhexahydrophthalic anhydride (MHHPA; 4-methylcyclohexyl-1,6-dicarboxylic anhhydride; CAS 19438-60-9)

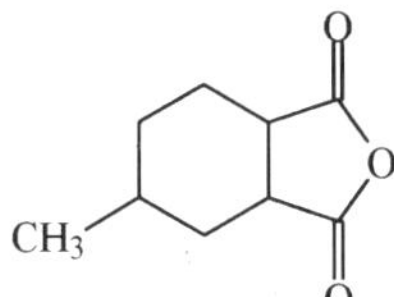

Properties: Oily liquid; MW 168.19; bp 120°C
Use: Hardener in epoxy resins.[4]

Tetrahydrophthalic anhydride (THPA; CAS 85-43-8)

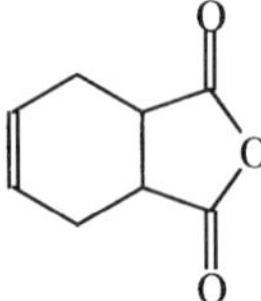

Properties: White, crystalline powder; MW 152.15; solidification point 90–101°C; slightly soluble in petroleum ether and ethyl ether, soluble in benzene; combustible.[1]

Use: Chemical intermediate for light-colored alkyds, polyesters, plasticizers, and adhesives; intermediate for pesticides; hardener for resins.[1]

Methyltetrahydrophthalic anhydride (MTHPA; CAS 26590-20-5)

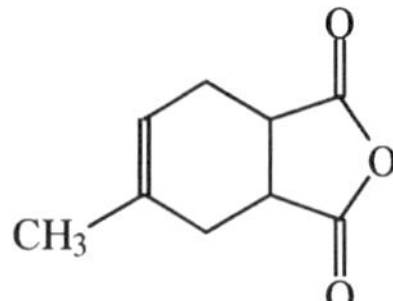

Properties: MW 166.18

Use: Hardener in epoxy resins.[4]

Succinic anhydride (2,5-diketotetrahydrofurane; succinyl oxide; butanedoic anhydride CAS 108-30-5)

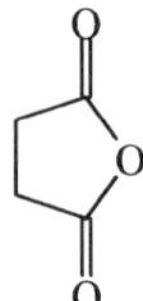

Properties: Colorless or light-colored needles or flakes; MW 100.08; mp 120°C; bp 261°C; soluble in alcohol and chloroform, insoluble in water, sublimes at 115°C; combustible.[1]

Use: Manufacture of chemicals, pharmaceuticals, esters; hardener of resins, starch modifier in foods.[1]

Dodecenylsuccinic anhydride (DDS; CAS 25377-7)

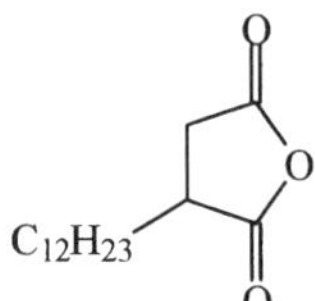

Properties: Light yellow, clear, viscous oil; bp 180–182°C.[1]

Use: Alkyd, epoxy and other resins, anticorrosive agents, plasticizers, wetting agents for bituminous compounds, pharmaceuticals.[1,4]

21.3   ALLERGIC CONTACT DERMATITIS

Organic acid anhydrides are well-known occupational respiratory allergens,[6] but only a few cases of allergic-type dermatoses due to the anhydrides have been reported. Allergic contact dermatitis from epoxy hardener dodecenyl succinic anhydride was reported by Göransson[7] in a female laboratory technician preparing tissues for electron microscopy for several hours each week. The embedding material consisted of an epoxy resin, two hardeners, one of which was dodecenyl succinic anhydride, and additional chemicals. After 2 months, she developed a bullous dermatitis on her fingers which had been contaminated with embedding material. Three other laboratory technicians doing the same work had no dermatitis. Patch tests including epoxy resin and embedding material components were negative, except for patch tests with dodecenyl succinic anhydride at 0.5 and 1% in acetone, which were strongly positive. Fifteen controls were negative. Skin tests for immediate allergy were not performed.

Kanerva et al.[8] reported on a horizontal boring machine worker who developed allergic contact dermatitis as well as rhinitis from MHHPA. Patch testing with a dilution series of MHHPA in petrolatum elicited strong allergic reactions at 2, 1, and 0.5% in petrolatum, and weak allergic reactions at 0.25 and 0.125%. An immunohistochemical and electron microscopic study indicated that the patch test reactions were conventional delayed allergic reactions. Prick testing with human serum albumin conjugated MHHPA gave a strong allergic reaction. Conjugated HHPA, MTHPA, and MA also gave the patient allergic reactions, but that of PA and TMA gave negative results. Total IgE was normal, and the radioallergosorbent test (RAST) to all of the above anhydrides was negative. A respiratory challenge test with MHHPA was negative, but provoked skin symptoms within 15 minutes on the upper arms and the sites of the patient's previous dermatitis, still persisting 24 hours later. A diagnosis of probable occupational rhinitis was based on the history (work-related nasal symptoms) and the sensitization to MHHPA verified by prick tests.

21.4 CONTACT URTICARIA

Menschick[9] and Baader[10] reported on urticarial reactions in workers in the manufacture of PA. The first case reports on contact urticaria from acid anhydrides describe two patients investigated at the Finnish Institute of Occupational Health (FIOH).[11-12] The patients worked in the same electrical factory where condensers were manufactured. The first patient's work was to fill the condensers with a slightly warmed uncured mixture of an epoxy resin, MHHPA hardener, accelerator, and a colorant.[11] Within 2 months, she developed urticarial eruptions on her face, neck, chest, and arms. After changing her job, the skin eruptions disappeared. All patch tests were negative, but open tests with complete filling mixture and undiluted MHHPA on the antecubital area of the arm were positive (small urticas on test area). The test with all the other components, both mixed and separately applied, were negative. Skin prick tests or RAST to MHHPA were not performed. Open tests with the undiluted MHHPA in 12 control patients were negative. The other patient was a maintenance worker.[12] After 10 months' work at the factory, he developed symptoms of contact urticaria on the forehead, and also symptoms of rhinitis. Patch tests were negative, but MHHPA at 1% in petrolatum showed considerable irritation. An open test with 100% MHHPA caused a urticarial reaction in 5 minutes, which enlarged and became more indurant during the first hour, and persisted for 8 hours. 1% MHHPA caused a similar (but less intense) reaction in 40 minutes. A scratch chamber test with MHHPA (1%) caused a strong wheal (9 mm diameter) with pseudopodia (histamine hydrochloride 10 mg/ml, 5 mm), and the RAST to MHHPA was positive, but scratch chamber and RASTs to PA, TMA, and MA were negative. Occupational rhinitis from MHHPA obliged the patient to change his worksite to an isolated building, whereupon the symptoms of urticaria and rhinitis disappeared.

Tarvainen et al.[13] reported on two patients who developed contact urticaria from MHHPA and MTHPA from airborne exposure. One patient had fixed caps onto ski poles with a two-component glue based on unsaturated polyester resin. Epoxy resin, reinforced with fiberglass and hardened by MTHPA, was used in the manufacture of the ski poles. The patient had no contact with liquid epoxy resin or hardener, but her worksite was situated in a large industrial hall where epoxy resin and hardener mixture were cured in ovens. She was exposed to MTHPA fumes escaping during opening of the ovens, and also fumes from drying ski poles. She was also exposed to dust that was formed during cutting or sawing of the poles. The other patient worked as a winder in a plant producing electrical machines. He insulated conducting wires with tape containing novolak-epoxy resin. In the plant, MHHPA was used as epoxy hardener in another process. The patient did not handle MHHPA hardener as such, but was exposed to fumes of anhydride during his working day. Both of the patients contracted hives and itching on uncovered skin after 2 months of exposure to MTHPA and MHHPA, to which they had airborne exposure. Later, the patients also developed conjunctivitis, rhinitis, sore throat, cough, or asthma. Both patients' immediate allergy to MTHPA and MHHPA was verified by positive prick tests to MTHPA and MHHPA, conjugated with human serum albumin, and positive RASTs to these anhydrides. On prick testing, both patients also reacted to a PA-conjugate, and the first patient to polyester resin conjugate. Specific immediate allergy to polyester resin was shown by RAST. RAST inhibition with MTHPA, MHHPA, and polyester resin conjugates confirmed IgE-mediated allergy and cross-reactivity between anhydrides. The PA present in the polyester resin was possibly responsible for the immediate reaction of the skin.

21.5 OTHER ALLERGIC REACTIONS AND SKIN EFFECTS

Occupational asthma caused by an organic acid anhydride was first reported by Kern in 1939.[14] During the past 15 years, a growing number of asthma cases due to the anhydrides has been reported. Up to 1990, the cases have been reviewed in detail by Keskinen; thereafter still more cases have been reported.[15-23] In addition, nasal and bronchial irritation, presenting as sneezing, coughing, and dyspnea, are common features in patients exposed to acid anhydrides.[9,10,24]

Acid anhydrides such as PA and MA, when cold, are not very harmful to dry skin, but hot compounds may cause severe chemical burns. On sweating skin, anhydrides are hydrated to the corresponding acids and can cause caustic dermatitis and burns.[9,25]

Kanerva et al.[26] have described three patients who developed strong long-lasting IgE-mediated reactions in skin prick testing with MHHPA and MTHPA. Two of the patients had been exposed to MTHPA and one to MHHPA. The reactions were negative in 20 controls.

21.6   CONCLUSION

Acid anhydrides are well-known respiratory allergens. They have the ability to induce specific IgE-mediated sensitization. Only a few cases of immediate type contact urticaria or delayed type contact allergy have been reported. Anhydrides should nevertheless be regarded as potential causes of the contact urticaria syndrome.

REFERENCES

1. Lewis, R. J., *Hawley's Condensed Chemical Dictionary*, 12th ed., Van Nostrand Reinhold, New York, 1993.
2. Council Directive 67/548/EEC, Annex 1: *Index of Dangerous Substances for which Harmonized Classification and Labeling have been agreed at Community Level.*
3. Fuchs, T., *Gummi und Allergie*, Dustri-verlag Dr. Karl Feistle, München-Deisenhofen, 1995.
4. Ministry of Labour, *Register of Chemical Products*, Finland, February 1996.
5. Rosenman, K. D., Bernstein, D. I., O'Leary, K., Gallagher, J. S., D'Souza, L., and Bernstein, I. L., Occupational asthma caused by himic anhydride, *Scand. J. Work Environ. Health*, 13, 150, 1987.
6. Keskinen, H., Organic acid anhydrides, in Criteria Documents from the Nordic Expert Group 1990. Arbetsmiljöinstitutet, *Arbete och Hälsa*, 2, 129, 1991.
7. Göransson, K., Allergic contact dermatitis to an epoxy hardener: dodecenyl-succinic anhydride, *Contact Dermatitis*, 3, 277, 1977.
8. Kanerva, L., Hyry, H., Jolanki, R., Hytönen, M., and Estlander, T., Delayed and immediate allergy caused by methylhexahydrophthalic anhydride, *Contact Dermatitis*, 36, 34, 1997.
9. Menschnik, H., Gesundheitliche Gefahren bei der Herstellung von Phthalsäureanhydrid, *Arch. Gewerbepathol. Gewerbehyg.*, 183, 454, 1955.
10. Baader, E. W., Erkrankungen durch Phthalsäure und ihre Verbindungen, *Arch. Gewerbepathol. Gewerbehyg.*, 13, 419, 1995.
11. Jolanki, R., Estlander, T., and Kanerva, L., Occupational contact dermatitis and contact urticaria caused by epoxy resins, *Acta Dermatol.Venereol.*, Suppl. 134, 90, 1987.
12. Jolanki, R., Kanerva, L., Estlander, T., Tarvainen, K., Keskinen, H., and Henriks-Eckerman, M.-L., Occupational dermatoses from epoxy resin compounds, *Contact Dermatitis*, 23, 172, 1990.
13. Tarvainen, K., Jolanki, R., Estlander, T., Tupasela, O., Pfäffli, P., and Kanerva, L., Immunologic contact urticaria due to airborne methylhexahydrophthalic and methyltetrahydrophthalic anhydride, *Contact Dermatitis*, 32, 204, 1995.
14. Kern, R. A., Asthma and allergic rhinitis due to sensitization to phthalic anhydride, *J. Allergy*, 10, 164, 1939.
15. Baur, X., Czuppon, A. B., Rauluk, I., Zimmermann, F. B., Schmitt, B., Egen-Korthaus, M., Tenkhoff, N., and Degens, P. O., A clinical and immunological study on 92 workers occupationally exposed to anhydrides, *Int. Arch. Occup. Environ. Health*, 67, 395, 1995.
16. Grammer, L. C., Shaughnessy, M. A., Henderson, J., Zeiss, C. R., Kavich, D. E., Collins, M. J., Pecis, K. M., and Kenamore, B. D., A clinical and immunologic study of workers with trimellitic-anhydride-induced immunologic lung disease after transfer to low exposure jobs, *Am. Rev. Respir. Dis.*, 148, 54, 1993.

17. Grammer, L. C., Shaughnessy, M. A., Hogan, M. B., Lowenthal, M., Yarnold, P. R., Watkins, D. M., and Berggruen, S. M., Study of employees with anhydride-induced respiratory disease after removal from exposure, *J. Occup. Environ. Med.,* 37, 820, 1995.

18. Liss, G. M., Bernstein, D., Genesove, L., Roos, J. O., and Lim, J., *J. Allergy Clin. Immunol.,* 92, 237, 1993.

19. Nielsen, J., Bensryd, I., Almquist, H., Dahlqvist, M., Welinder, H., Alexandersson, R., and Skerfving, S., Serum IgE and lung function in workers exposed to phthalic anhydride, *Int. Arch. Occup. Environ. Health,* 63, 199, 1991.

20. Nielsen, J., Welinder, H., Horstmann, V., and Skerfving, S., Allergy to methyltetrahydrophthalic anhydride in epoxy resin workers, *Br. J. Ind. Med.,* 49, 769, 1992.

21. Venables, K. M. and Newman Taylor, A. J., Exposure-response relationships in asthma caused by tetrachlorophthalic anhydride, *J. Allergy Clin. Immunol.,* 85, 55, 1990.

22. Welinder, H. and Nielsen, I., Immunologic tests of specific antibodies to organic anhydrides, *Allergy,* 46, 601, 1991.

23. Zeiss, C. R., Reactive chemicals in industrial asthma, *J. Allergy Clin. Immunol.,* 87, 755, 1991.

24. Nielsen, J., Welinder, H., Schütz, A., and Skerfving, S., Specific serum antibodies against phthalic anhydride in occupationally exposed subjects, *J. Allergy Clin. Immunol.,* 82, 126, 1988.

25. Malten, K. and Zielhuis, R., Polyester resins, in *Industrial Toxicology and Dermatology in the Production and Processing of Plastics,* Elsevier Publishing Company, Amsterdam, London, New York, 1964, 71.

26. Kanerva, L., Tupasela, O., Jolanki, R., Tarvainen, K., and Estlander, T., Histopathology and electron microscopy of long-lasting IgE-mediated skin prick test reaction caused by methyltetrahydrophthalic anhydride and methylhexahydrophthalic anhydride, in *Immunological and Pharmacological Aspects of Atopic and Contact Eczema. Pharmacol. Skin,* Czernielewski, J. M., Karger, Basel, 4, 106, 1991.

22

Reactive Dyes in Textiles

Tuula Estlander, Riitta Jolanki, and Lasse Kanerva

CONTENTS

22.1   INTRODUCTION

Reactive dyes have been used since the beginning of the 1950s for dyeing textile fibers. The first dyes were for wool and entered the market under the trade names Remalan® (Hoechst) and Cibalan® (Ciba-Geigy). In 1956, Imperial Chemical Industries Ltd. (ICI) introduced its Procion® dyes for cellulose fibers, and they were followed by the appearance of other dyes for the same purpose, including Remazol® (Hoechst), Cibacron® (Ciba-Geigy), Levafix® (Bayer), and Drimaren® (Sandoz) dyes. The Procinyl® dyes (ICI) were the first used for polyamide fibers. New reactive dyes with one, two, or more reactive groups have continuously been developed and manufactured under different commercial names by the aforementioned companies and several other manufacturers, including BASF, Sumimoto, Coloni, DyStar (Hoechst-Bayer), and Ehwa. The world demand for reactive dyes reached about 97,000 metric tons in 1990.[1-3]

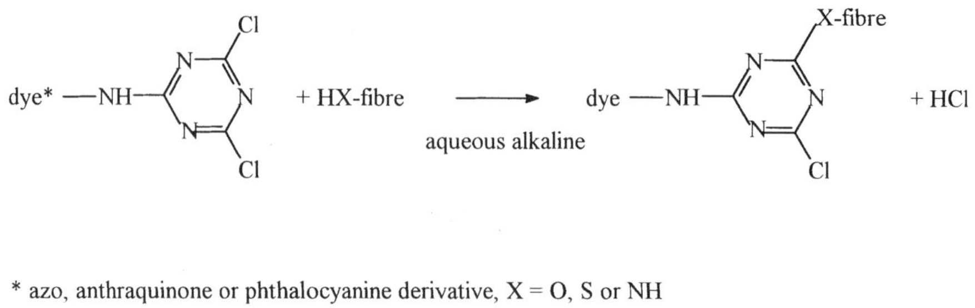

dye* —NH— (triazine ring with Cl, Cl substituents) + HX-fibre $\longrightarrow$ dye —NH— (triazine ring with X-fibre, Cl substituents) + HCl

aqueous alkaline

* azo, anthraquinone or phthalocyanine derivative, X = O, S or NH

FIGURE 22.1 An example of the dyeing reaction with reactive dyes.

22.2 USE AND APPLICATION OF REACTIVE DYES

Water-soluble reactive dyes are extensively used because they produce bright colors, their application is fast, and their fixation is permanent in both natural and synthetic fibers. In the past, they were marketed mainly as powders, but nowadays they are sold as liquids, granules, and finished powders in order to minimize the industrial hygiene problems connected with dusty unfinished powders. Their chief application is in the dyeing of cellulose, wool, and polyamide fibers, but they can also be used to color silk, furs, and leather. Apart from professional use for textile dyeing and printing in industry and in artists' shops, reactive dyes can also be used for home dyeing.[1,3,4]

Reactive dyes have molecular weights of 0.5–1 kD. They are distinguished from other textile dyes in that they form covalent bonds with cellulose, protein, polyamide, and other synthetic fibers (Figure 22.1). The dye molecules contain both a color-forming component (chromophore) and a fiber-reactive component. They also have hydrophilic groups to improve their water solubility. The color forming dye component can be an azo, anthraquinone, phthalocyanine, triphenodioxazine or formazan dye, but most reactive dyes fall into the category of azo dyes. Covalent bonds are brought about by a chemical reaction between the reactive component and hydroxyl (-OH), sulfhydryl (-SH), or amino (-NH2) groups of textile fibers. Apart from dye molecules, commercial reactive dyestuffs contain many other ingredients to improve their dyeing properties. In addition to a reactive dye, the dye pastes applied to cellulose fibers during textile printing contain several other components, including a thickening agent (an alginate), urea, alkali, and an oxidant.[3,5-7]

22.3 ALLERGIC REACTIONS

22.3.1 Types of Reactions and Associated Dyes

As extremely reactive chemical compounds, reactive dyes are capable of reacting with proteins of the body, as well as with textile fibers, and are thus also capable of evoking allergic reactions. Immediate reactions[1-2,6,8-15] are the most frequent and usually appear as rhinitis and asthma, but skin symptoms can also occur. Atopics

$$NaO_3SOCH_2CH_2O_2S \text{—} \bigcirc \text{—} N{=}N \text{—} [\text{naphthalene: } OH, NH_2, NaO_3S, SO_3Na] \text{—} N{=}N \text{—} \bigcirc \text{—} SO_2CH_2CH_2OSO_3Na$$

FIGURE 22.2 CI Reactive Black 5.

generally have a greater tendency to develop side effects, but also nonatopics have developed allergy. Pre-employment determinations of total IgE or skin prick tests with common environmental allergens do not seem to be good predictors of type I allergy to reactive dyes.[15] Delayed or type IV allergic reactions with contact eczema have been reported on a few occasions only.[1,8,16,17] Positive patch test reactions without contact eczema[4,9] have also been described for patients having asthma due to reactive dyes. Very little is known about the mechanisms of asthma caused by chemical haptens, but some recent reports suggest that type IV allergy might also be involved in respiratory and conjunctival symptoms.[18-20]

Sensitization to reactive dyes has taken place from occupational exposure to the dyes during textile dyeing and printing processes, as well as during the manufacturing process.[1,2,4,15] The dyed textiles have good wet and light-fastness. They can be considered safe to users and textile workers handling the fabrics, that is, if the dyeing process is not faulty and the textile fibers are of good quality, complete dye fixation thus being ensured in the fibers.[1] Recently, sensitization to reactive dyes has also been reported in contact dermatitis patients, but in none of the patients could the relevance of positive patch test reactions to the dyes clearly be proved.[17]

In the literature published up until 1996, about 90 reactive dyes have been reported to be associated with allergic reactions in humans.[2,4,15,17] Of these dyes, 17 have at least two commercial names, but have the same Color Index (CI) name, and thus represent similar dyes. One dye, Reactive Black 5 has several commercial names (i.e., Remazol Schwarz B, Remazol Black B, Remazol Black GF, Remazol B, Drimarene Black K3B, Levafix Black EB, Black Remazol B gran, and Rifazol Black GR).[1,2,4,17,21]

Reactive Black 5 (Figure 22.2) has been considered to be the most frequent sensitizer of the reactive dyes. It causes both type I and type IV allergic reactions.[1,2,4,6,8-15,17] It is also one of the most commonly used black dyes. It is manufactured by several companies throughout the world and marketed under more than 10 commercial names. Nowadays in Finland textile dye houses use 150 metric tons of reactive dyes a year, the proportion of Reactive Black (CI) dyes being 50–60 tons.

Pure dye compounds are not available, and suspected commercial reactive dyes have been used in investigations of exposed employees. The component(s) responsible for the allergic reactions induced by these dyes have not been defined. Dye compounds, auxiliaries, intermediates, or other impurities[1,15] are possible causes of the allergic reactions. According to the manufacturer, Remazol Schwarz powder is, for instance, 60% one dye compound with other components (an antidusting agent, salts) accounting for the remaining 40%. Thin-layer chromatography of the dye showed that it contains at least 10 different chemical substances.[1] In addition, chemical construction (CI number) of commercial dyes has not always been given in the Color Index, but radioallergosorbent (RAST) inhibition test and patch test results indicate that cross-reactions occur between some reactive dyes.[1,2,15,26] Thus, a sensitized person may be at risk experiencing symptoms of allergy when exposed to other reactive dyes. Several commercial dyes are used in workplaces, and in individual cases not all of the allergenic substances are necessarily known. Therefore, sensitized workers are often obliged to change jobs.

22.3.2 Contact Urticaria

The respiratory tract seems to be especially susceptile to reactive dyes, but urticaria, contact urticaria, and dermatitis are also well described manifestations of exposure to dyes.[1,2,4,6,8,15,21-23] The skin symptoms are usually associated with respiratory symptoms, and the same patient may have both type I and type IV allergic dermatosis.[1] Already in the 1950s the containers of Procion M® dye marketed by ICI warned that reactive dyes might cause respiratory allergy,[24] but it was not until about 20 years later, in 1978, that the first cases of asthma and rhinitis were reported from the Finnish Institute of Occupational Health (FIOH).[6] Since then, several reports of asthma and rhinitis in relation to direct,[1,2,4,6,8,15,21-23] and even indirect (airborne), exposure in factories in the neighborhood of a dye factory[25] have been published.

The first two reports describing urticaria in association with asthma caused by reactive dyes in workers of textile industry were published in 1985.[21,22] Dermatoses are, however, much less frequent than respiratory symptoms among exposed workers. In a study consisting of 309 employees in a Korean factory producing reactive dyes, 8 of 107 symptomatic workers had urticaria and pruritus.[2] In one of them, the skin symptoms were the only manifestation of type I allergy confirmed by a positive prick test and RAST. Of the workers, 78 (25.2%) had lower respiratory symptoms with or without other symptoms, including eye symptoms and urticaria and pruritus, 26 (8.7%) had nasal symptoms, and 1 worker experienced eye symptoms only. In a survey conducted at 15 textile plants with dyehouses in western Sweden, 162 of 1142 workers were exposed to reactive dyes,[15] 17 reported work-related respiratory or skin symptoms, and 15 cases were individually investigated. Type I allergy to reactive dyes could be confirmed with prick tests in five of them and four also showed a positive RAST to one dye, Reactive Black 5 (Remazol Black B, Remazol Black GF). Ten of the patients had upper or lower respiratory symptoms and ten had skin symptoms. Seven had work-related contact dermatitis, and three had urticaria or Quincke edema. All except two were weighers or dyers. None of the employees who had work-related dermatitis was patch test positive to the nine reactive dyes tested, but one was positive to a monoazo dye, Basic Red 46. Only for one urticaria patient were reactive dyes the cause of the symptoms. Positive prick tests to reactive dyes and also postive RASTs to five different dyes (i.e., Reactive Blue 203, Reactive Black 5, Reactive Yellow 107 and 160, Reactive Orange 82) under six commercial names confirmed the sensitization. However, RAST inhibition suggested cross-allergy between some of the dyes.

At FIOH, we have detected seven cases of occupational allergic dermatoses from reactive dyes.[1,16] Five patients were dyers or dye mixers in textile plants or dye houses and had been exposed to reactive dyes for 8 months to 4 years before they developed symptoms. Two of the five patients (patients 3 and 5) had a history of contact urticaria. A local urticaria reaction as a result of an accidental splash of a reactive dye solution was seen on one of them by the plant doctor. Both also had rhinitis and asthma. Type I allergy to reactive dyes was verified by a positive scratch or prick test and RAST. In addition, one of the two urticaria patients had eczema and was both patch and prick test positive to the same dye, Drimaren Schlarlach K 2G (Reactive Red 123). He was also RAST positive to four other commercial reactive dyes: Drimaren BR Yellow K 3GL and Levafix BR Yellow E 3G (both Reactive Yellow 25), Drimaren BR Blue K BL (Reactive Blue 114), and Cibacron BR Scarlet 3B (CI name unknown). Bronchial challenge with Drimaren Scharlach K 2G also provoked generalized urticaria consistent with his history. One other patient had eczema and rhinitis (patient 1) and three others (patients 2, 4, and 6) had only eczema. The sixth patient was an artist who had developed persistent hand dermatitis after 16 years of textile printing with pigment dyes and of 6 years with reactive dyes. In patch testing, she had allergic reactions to 2 of the 13 reactive dyes tested, namely, Reactive Black 5 and Reactive Blue 21. She was also allergic to formaldehyde which proved to be a component of the pigment paste. The seventh patient was a textile teacher who had had atopic dermatitis without any mucosal symptoms since her childhood. After 8 years of periodically handling textile dyes, including many reactive dyes of different colors, she developed work-related rhinitis, and her hand dermatitis persistently worsened. Patch tests with the series of organic dyes (Chemotechnique Diagnostics AB, Malmö, Sweden) and other relevant series were negative. Patch and prick tests with five "own" dyes including an undefined black Levafix® reactive dye and Remazol Schwarz B were also negative. A positive RAST to Remazol Schwarz B and a positive nasal challenge with the same dye suggested, however, that type I sensitization to the dye could be the cause of her work-related symptoms.

Only two of seven patients were able to continue their jobs after they stopped using the dyes to which they were sensitized. They had allergic contact eczema without any other symptoms.

22.3.3 Examinations

When type I allergy is suspected, the examinations should include skin prick tests with the suspected dyes. Unconjugated dyes can be used for the tests;[1,15] a 1% dilution of a commercial dye in distilled water or a dye diluted in saline-glycerol to a concentration of 2 mg/ml seems to be suitable for screening for type I allergy to reactive dyes. For the confirmation of type I sensitization and possible cross-allergy between the suspected dyes RAST and RAST inhibition tests are needed. In the RAST, it is necessary to use an optimized preparation of a dye-human serum protein (HSA) conjugate to elicit reliable results.[13,15]

Patch tests are needed in cases of contact eczema, but they can also be considered in some cases of respiratory or conjunctival symptoms. The study of the workers in the Korean reactive dye factory, for instance, suggests that in addition to IgE-mediated sensitization, other immunological or nonimmunological mechanisms may be involved in reactive dye asthma.[2] A 1–5% concentration of a commercial dye in petrolatum is suitable for patch testing with reactive dyes.[1,17] When respiratory symptoms are suspected, nasal or bronchial challenges may be necessary to confirm the positive relation between the reactive dye exposure and the symptoms.[1,2,6] Because pure dye compounds are not available, it would be useful to know the proportion of dye compound(s) in commercial dyes before any test preparations are made.[1]

Reactive dyes are dangerous sensitizers inducing both type I and type IV allergic reactions. A lethal asthma attack has even been described.[22] The potential risk of anaphylactic reactions with reactive dyes should be emphasized. The risk of an anaphylactic reaction is even associated with skin testing. One patient with reactive dye asthma experienced cough, chest tightness, and wheezing, as well as generalized urticaria from a scratch chamber test with an undiluted commercial reactive dye powder.[26] In a short chamber inhalation provocation with a very low provoking dose, another asthma patient allergic to Lanasol Yellow 4G developed a severe immediate obstructive ventilatory defect followed by hypotension and urticaria.[4] Extreme care is necessary during bronchial challenge tests, which should be performed only in specialist clinics and under strict supervision.[1,4,6]

22.4 CONSUMER RISK

Reactive dyes have not given side effects from dyed fabrics because they are covalently bound in the fibers, and no dye compounds with reactive groups remain free in the fabrics. Accordingly, reactive dyes display an occupational problem. A recent study of contact dermatitis patients also suggests, however, sensitization to reactive dyes in consumers, but further investigations are necessary to clarify the real importance of reactive dyes in textile dye dermatitis.[17]

REFERENCES

1. Estlander, T., Allergic dermatoses and respiratory disease from reactive dyes, *Contact Dermatitis,* 18, 290, 1988.
2. Park, H. S., Lee, M. K., Kim, B. O., Lee, K. J., Roh, J. H., Moon, Y. H. and Hong, C-S., Clinical and immunologic evaluations of reactive dye-exposed workers, *J. Allergy Clin. Immunol.,* 87, 639, 1991.
3. Tappe, H., Helmling, W., Mischke, P., Rebramen, K., Russ, W., Schläfer, L. and Vervehren, P., Reactive dyes, in *Ullmann's Encyclopedia of Industrial Chemistry,* Vol A22, VCH Publishers, Inc., 1993, 651.
4. Romano, C., Sulotto, F., Pavan, I., Chiesa, A. and Scansetti G., A new case of occupational asthma from reactive dyes with severe anaphylactic response to the specific challenge, *Am. J. Ind. Med.,* 21, 209, 1992.
5. Abrahart, E. N., *Dyes and Their Intermediates,* Edward Arnold Ltd., London, 1977, 185.
6. Alanko, K., Keskinen, H., Björksten, F. and Ojanen, S., Immediate-type hypersensitivity to reactive dyes, *Clin. Allergy,* 8, 25, 1978.

7. Park, H. S. and Hong C-S., The significance of specific IgG and IgG4 antibodies to a reactive dye in exposed workers, *Clin. Exp. All.*, 21, 357, 1991.

8. Hagmar, L., Welinder, H. and Dahlqvist I., Immunoglobin E antibodies against a reactive dye — a case report, *Scand. J. Work Environ. Health*, 12, 221, 1986.

9. Thoren, K., Meding, B., Nordlinder, R. and Belin, L., Contact dermatitis and asthma from reactive dyes, *Contact Dermatitis*, 15, 186, 1986.

10. Docker, A., Wattie, J. M., Topping, M. D., Luzynska, C. M., Newman Taylor, A. J., Pickering, C. A. C., Thomas, P. and Compertz, D., Clinical and immunological investigations of respiratory disease in workers using reactive dyes, *Br. J. Ind. Med.*, 44, 534, 1987.

11. Topping, M. D., Forster, H. W., Ide, C, W., Kennedy, F. M., Leach, A. M. and Sorkin, S., Respiratory allergy and specific immunoglobin E and immunoglobin G antibodies to reactive dyes used in the wool industry, *J. Occup. Med.*, 31, 857, 1989.

12. Park, H. S., Lee, M. K. and Hong, C-S., Occupational asthma and IgE antibodies to reactive dyes, *Yonsei Med. J.*, 30, 298, 1989.

13. Wass, U., Nilsson, R., Nordlinder, R. and Belin, L., An optimized assay of specific IgE antibodies to reactive dyes and studies of immunologic responses in exposed workers, *J. All. Clin. Immunol.*, 85, 642, 1990.

14. Hong, C-S. and Park, H. S., Heterogeneity of IgE antibody response to reactive dye in sera from four different sensitized workers, *Clin. Exp. Allergy*, 23, 606, 1992.

15. Nilsson, R., Nordlinder, R., Wass, U., Meding, B. and Belin, L., Asthma, Rhinitis, and dermatitis in workers exposed to reactive dyes, *Br. J. Ind. Med.*, 50, 65, 1993.

16. Estlander, T., Jolanki, R., Kanerva, L. and Plosila, M., An artist's allergy to reactive dyes and formaldehyde, *Contact Dermatitis*, 23, 303, 1990.

17. Manzini, B., Motolese, A., Conti, A., Ferdani, G. and Seidenari, S., Sensitization to reactive dyes in patients with contact dermatitis, *Contact Dermatitis*, 34, 172, 1996.

18. Kanerva, L., Estlander, T., Jolanki, R. and Pekkarinen, E., Occupational pharyngitis associated with allergic patch test reactions from acrylics, *Allergy*, 47, 571, 1992.

19. Estlander, T., Kari, O., Kanerva, L. and Jolanki, R., Occupational blepharoconjunctivitis and contact dermatitis from gold, *JEADV*, Abstracts, the 4th Congress of the European Academy of Dermatology and Venereology, 10-15 October, Brussels, Belgium, 1995, S98.

20. Estlander, T., Kanerva, L., Kari, O., Jolanki, R. and Mölsä, K., Occupational conjunctivitis associated with type IV allergy to methacrylates, *Allergy*, 51, 56, 1996.

21. Ringenbach, N., Allergies dans l'industrie textile: 4 cas d'hypersensibilite aux colorants (observesen entprise), *Arch. Malad. Prof.*, 46, 219, 1985.

22. Stern, M. A., Occupational asthma from a reactive dye, *Ann. Allergy*, 55, 264, 1985.

23. Estlander, T. and Kanerva, L., Dermatitis and urticaria from reactive dyes. In Abstracts of the 8th International Symposium on Contact Dermatitis. March 20-22, Queens' College, Cambridge, 1986, 048.

24. Jenkins, C. L., Textile dyes are potential hazards, *J. Environ. Health*, 40, 256, 1978.

25. Park, H. S., Kim, J, W. and Hong, C-S., The prevalence of specific IgE and IgG to reactive dye-human serum albmumin conjugate in workers of a dye factory and neighboring factories, *J. Korean Med. Science*, 6, 63, 1991.

26. Kanerva, L., Estlander, T. and Jolanki, R., Skin testing for immediate hypersensitivity in occupational allergology, In *Exogenous Dermatoses: Environmental Dermatitis*, Menne, T. and Maibach, H. I., Eds., CRC Press, Inc., Boca Raton, 1991.

23

Occupational Contact Urticaria Syndrome Due to Rhodium and Platinum

Hideo Nakayama and Tami Ichikawa

CONTENTS

23.1   HYPERSENSITIVITY TO METALS

Metals do not sensitize people, however, metal ions, which have released some of their outermost orbiting electrons, dissolve in water, have a high affinity to epidermal proteins, and therefore, conjugate epidermis becoming contact sensitizers. Nickel, cobalt, mercury, and chromate are common sensitizers while palladium, gold, platinum, indium, and iridium are rare but strong sensitizers. In most cases, ions of these metals provoke contact hypersensitivity. Today, it is believed that the conjugate of numerous metal ions to epidermal protein (presumably and most likely at the sites of –SH and –S=S–) is incorporated in the Langerhans cells and presented to the T lymphocytes.

When the conjugates are recognized as non-self, the effector T cells are initiated, and put into quantity production in the lymph nodes. Later, they enter the blood circulation. When the allergen comes into contact again, such effector T cells, or in another term, killer T cells, go out from the capillaries, attack the site of contact of the epidermis to produce focal cytolysis known as spongiosis. This is an ordinary development in allergic contact dermatitis to metal ions.

On the other hand, immediate allergic reactions to metal are very rare. Only a limited number of the cases of occupational bronchial asthma to platinum have been reported.[1]

The following cases of contact urticaria syndrome due to rhodium and platinum are even more rare. But we have to understand that such cases had been present, and may occur in any country in the future. These cases were reported in 1983, and actually, similar factories are present worldwide.

23.2 THE CASES OF RHODIUM AND PLATINUM HYPERSENSITIVITY

In a big factory manufacturing precious metal accessories and parts for electric and electronic machineries in Chiba Prefecture, Japan, the following symptoms were first observed in 1970:

- Contact urticaria
- Contact dermatitis
- Bronchial asthma
- Rhinitis allergica
- Conjunctivitis allergica

These allergic reactions were slightly improved with the usage of antihistamine and corticosteroid ointments, but the number of the patients gradually increased until 17 (34%) out of 50 workers in a section were involved in 1977. The situation became really critical for this factory.

Management requested the inspection of the factory and a solution to this apparently occupational disaster by the author. On examination of the patients, the above-mentioned symptoms were confirmed (Figure 23.1), and it turned out that most of the patients belonged to the section where palladium, platinum, and rhodium were salvaged from various used metal products. None of the patients indicated that similar symptoms were present among the family members or had been present before they had the job in this factory, therefore, hereditary allergic conditions such as atopy were quickly ruled out.

The procedure of the unit of the factory is shown in Table 23.1. The combination of the symptoms showing type I hypersensitivity, such as urticaria, bronchial asthma, conjunctivitis, and rhinitis, and at the same time type IV hypersensitivity as allergic contact dermatitis was present in the patients who worked in this unit. Urticaria was easily provoked temporarily when the mist of the solution in the unit contacted the skin. Consequently, it was diagnosed as contact urticaria. Coughing, hyperrhinorhea, and epiphora were common complications of the contact urticaria, and asthma frequently attacked the patients not only in the middle of the day but also at dawn, which awakened and greatly harassed some of the patients, suggesting that late responses were also present exceptionally.

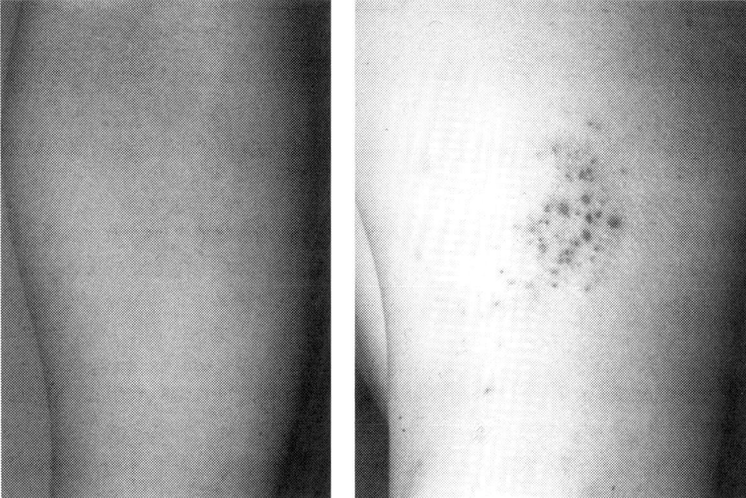

FIGURE 23.1 Contact urticaria (left, provoked by a contact of 0.5% platinum chloride aqueous solution) and allergic contact dermatitis (right) were the skin symptoms of the contact urticaria syndrome patients in this chapter.

Itchy papules were predominantly present on the hands, fingers, arms, and face, and severe cases had generalized eczema, even though they had never suffered from atopic dermatitis-like eruptions before they became workers at this factory.

Based on the chemical substances handled in their units, the causative allergens were investigated, using the metal series patch test allergens (type 5) used at that time. It was just after Finn Chambers were introduced in Japan, and scratch patch tests proposed by Hannuksela were also performed to find out which allergens were provoking contact urticaria and contact dermatitis. At the same time, rhodium and other metals, which had not been known as sensitizers before, were scratch-patch tested and covered with Finn Chambers for 1 hour. The delayed type hypersensitivity was examined on the 2nd, 3rd, and 7th days later (Table 23.2).

23.3 RESULTS OF THE TESTS

Physical diagnosis, mainly auscultation of the chest, pulmonary formation, chest X-ray examination performed by the specialists of pulmonary diseases, and otorhinologists confirmed the diagnosis of bronchial asthma and allergic rhinitis. The application of a single drop of 0.5% platinum chloride in aqueous solution produced a wheal and flare 20 minutes after the application (Figure 23.1), and disappeared a few hours later. Another single drop of the same platinum chloride solution applied on a round filter paper disc 5mm in diameter, and attached on the nasal mucous membrane of one patient instantly produced severe rhinorrhea, sneezing, wheezing, and asthma attack. Therefore, the test was never performed on other patients, because even though it could provoke the immediate allergic reaction, it was considered to be dangerous.

**TABLE 23.1 Process and Chemicals Used
in the Precious Metal Factory**

Process

Dissolution of scraps
(Pt, Au, Rh, Ru, Pd, Ir, etc.)
↓

Neutralization
↓

Filtration
↓

Formation of ammoniated metals
↓

Separation of ammoniated metals

Chemicals used

$H_2PtCl_6 \cdot 6H_2O$
$PdCl_2$
IrO_2
$RhCl_3 \cdot 3H_2O$
$HAuCl_4 \cdot 4H_2O$
Various kinds of ammoniated metals, acids, and bases
Hydrazine
Various kinds of alloys (Pd-Cu, Pd-Cu-Ni, Ru-Al, Fe,
 Au/Ag/Pd-Cu/Ni, Au-Cu/Ni, Ag-Cu/Ni, Pt/Rh-Al_2O_3, etc.)

TABLE 23.2 Investigation of Allergens

1. Patch test
   a. Dental metal series patch test allergens
   b. Special metals
        Rhodium chloride (5% and 2% pet.)
        Ruthenium chloride (5% and 2% pet.)
        Iridium chloride (5% and 2% pet.)
        Hydrazine (10, 5, 2, and 1% pet.)
2. Scratch-patch test using Finn Chambers for one hour (Modified Hannuksela's method)
3. Nasal disc test

Note: 5mm diameter filter paper discs were applied with one drop of 0.5% platinum chloride solution
and used for the nasal disc tests.

There had been no descriptions at that time that rhodium, ruthenium, and iridium
were sensitizers. As the metal ions were highly soluble in water, a RAST test was
not possible. Needless to say, the skin tests were performed carefully. Rhodium
chloride, rutenium chloride, and iridium chloride, at 5 and 2% in petrolatum, were

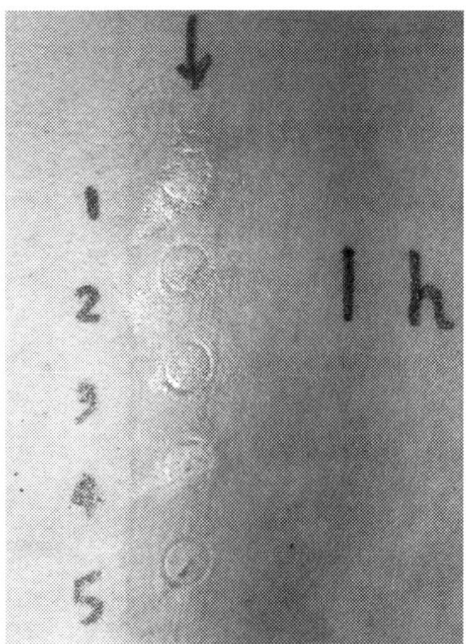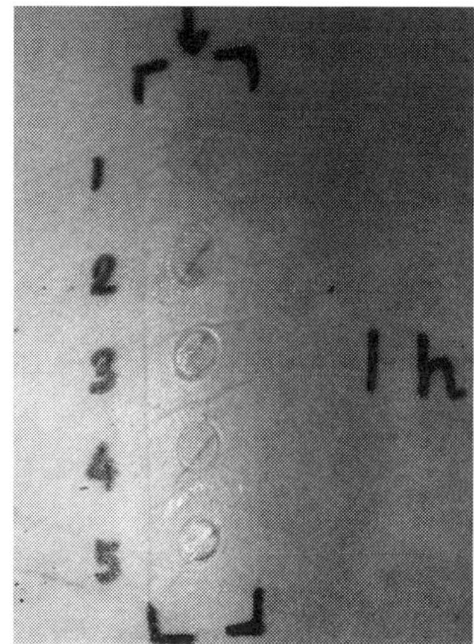

FIGURE 23.2   Scratch patch tests using 2% rhodium chloride in petrolatum (No. 1 of the left) and 0.5% platinum chloride in aqueous solution (No. 4 of the left) provoked strong positive wheal and flare reactions after the application and covering by Finn Chambers for one hour with a patient. The same reagents showed negative reactions on a control (right).

prepared, and scratch patch tested according to Hannuksela's method for one hour. The results showed a strong positive with rhodium chloride (Figure 23.2), showing that it was as strong a sensitizer as platinum. The results of orthodox closed patch test for 2 days produced 4 strong positives with rhodium chloride, 8 strong positives with platinum chloride (Figure 23.3), two positives with mercury bichloride, and one positive with stannic chloride. The positive reactions were composed of erythema, edema, and papules on the second and third days of the patch test. Later they become eczematous, and itching was remarkable. These reactions were considered as delayed type contact hypersensitivity, because normal persons did not produce such strong eczematous reactions.

Curiously, all 12 patients tested showed normal values of serum IgE. Asthma and rhinitis were present in 12 among these 14 patients. Contact urticaria was present in 7 patients among the 12. Contact dermatitis was present in 5 among the 14 patients. The combination of these diseases and the skin test results are shown in Table 23.3. Maximization tests on guinea pigs showed positive results in 4 out of 5 animals tested (80%).

Based on these skin manifestations, symptoms, and the test results, these patients were considered to have suffered from occupational contact urticaria syndrome, proposed by Maibach. These cases were reported in Japan in 1982.[2]

23.4   SOLUTION

Platinum and rhodium were judged as the main sensitizers of this occupational contact urticaria syndrome, and as it was quite clear that the workers were exposed

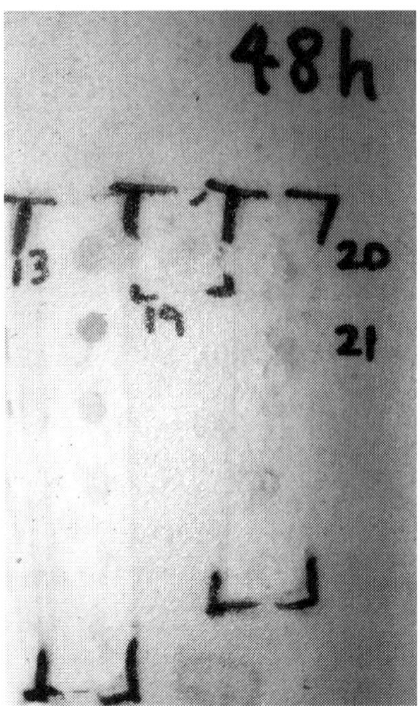

FIGURE 23.3   Positive patch test reactions of a patient to 0.5% platinum chloride in aqueous solution (No. 13), 2% (No. 20) and 5% (No. 21) rhodium chloride in petrolatum respectively are demonstrated. Vesicles with itching were noted.

TABLE 23.3   The Cases Studied

Case	Age	Contact Urticaria	Contact Dermatitis	Asthma or Rhinitis	Positive allergens — Immediate			Positive allergens — Delayed		
1	38	○		○	Pt					
2	38	○		○	Pt	Rh		Pt		
3	58			○	Pt	Rh				
4	23	○	○	○	Pt	Rh		Pt		
5	24	○		○	Pt			Pt		
6	29	○		○	Pt	Rh		Pt		
7	32		○	○	Pt	Rh		Pt	Rh	
8	25	○		○	Pt	Rh			Rh	Hg
9	29	○		○	Pt	Rh				
10	30		○	○				Pt		
11	29		○					Pt	Rh	Hg
12	26		○					Pt	Rh	Sn

Note: Serum level of IgE: normal in all cases. Eosinophilia: not present.

TABLE 23.4 Methods of Solutions

1. Improvement of facilities
   a. Improvement to decrease the leakage of metal containing mist
   b. Elimination of mist and vapor containing the metal ions by aspiration, change of airflow, and installation of double couplings around the pipings
   c. Improvement of protecting clothes
   d. Cooling system to decrease sweating
2. Disposal of leaked allergens by washing with acylglutamate
3. Education of the workers
   a. Education on the mechanism and the causating allergens of the occupational disease
   b. More frequent changing of their working clothes

to the mists containing rhodium and platinum, the authors proposed to make a double covering for the manufacturing process step in question. Those allergens already present on the floor, walls, desks, chairs, and other equipments were washed out using 2% acylglutamate aqueous solution, because it had a chelating effect to catch and eliminate metal ions as rhodium and mercury. The patients were educated with the diseases they had suffered from, in the mechanism, causating allergens, and prevention (Table 23.4). After that, this unique occupational diseases disappeared except for the rare instances of only slight and mild provocation of dermatitis and rhinitis. One serious episode was later reported when two patients, several years after the solution of the disease, had carelessly crawled into the chimney of the factory to clean it. They soon suffered from a severe attack of rhinitis, conjunctivitis, and asthma with breathing difficulty. Fortunately, they managed to escape from the chimney lumen, were sent to a hospital immediately, and were saved. It was considered quite lucky that they did not die of asthma.

23.5 DISCUSSION

Rhodium allergy is rare,[3] but platinum allergy has been rarely reported.[1,4,5] Rhodium is a precious metal, with the atomic number 45, a molecular weight 103, and having outer electron arrangements as illustrated in Table 23.5. Its sensitizing ability to conjugate with carrier proteins is undoubtedly owed to it having 3 fewer electrons at the 4d suborbit in the N orbit. Because nonionized rhodium having these 3 electrons (in total 9 electrons) in the suborbit does not dissolve in water, consequently there is no ability to sensitize. The ionized trivalent rhodium ions, Rh^{3+}, must have conjugated to albumin to produce immediate allergic reactions, such as contact urticaria, bronchial asthma, rhinitis, and conjunctivitis. At the same time, they also conjugated to epidermal proteins to produce allergic contact dermatitis. It must have been a similar case with platinum to have produced tetravalent platinum ions, Pt^{4+}, causing both forms of immediate reaction and contact hypersensitivity.

Curiously, many kinds of ionized metals, such as silver, lead, antimony, iron, manganese, and ruthenium do not sensitize people except on very rare occasions, whereas chromate, nickel, mercury, cobalt, platinum, rhodium, and palladium are

TABLE 23.5 Rhodium

Atomic number	45
Atomic weight	102.905
Melting point	1920°C
Electron arrangements	

	Orbit	Rh	Rh^{3+}
K	(1s)	2	2
L	2s	2	2
	2p	6	6
M	3s	2	2
	3p	6	6
	3d	10	10
N	4s	2	2
	4p	6	6
	4d	9	6

capable of sensitizing people rather easily. The difference between these two metal ion groups lies in the fact that the former has an odd number of electrons such as 1 or 5 in the outermost suborbit except for Ag^+, while the latter have an even number electrons as 0 or 6 or 8 in the outermost suborbit. It means that the loss of active pain electrons in the outmost suborbit may enable the conjugation to host proteins by regaining such paired electrons from the bases of carrier protein.

Contact urticaria syndrome is rarely seen with metals, presumably because ionized metals are haptens which rarely conjugate to serum albumin. Rhodium and platinum ions seem to be exceptions, judging from the presence of the cases described, and other reports on occupational asthma caused by platinum hypersensitivity.

Rhodium hypersensitivity was later reported by Bedello et al.[3] The cases described were ordinary allergic contact dermatitis, and contact urticaria was not described with these cases.

REFERENCES

1. Merget, R., Schultze-Werninghaus, G., Muthorst, T. et al.: Asthma due to the complex salts of platinum. A cross-sectional survey of workers in a platinum refinery, *Clin. Allergy,* 18, 569–580, 1988.
2. Imai, T. and Nakayama, H.: Occupational contact dermatitis complicating bronchial symptomes due to rhodium hypersensitivity, *Hifuka no Rinsho* (Dermatological Clinics), 24, 1033–1041, 1982 (In Japanese).
3. Bedello, P. G., Goitre, M., Roncarolo, G., Bundino, S., and Cane, D.: Contact dermatitis to rhodium, *Contact Dermatitis,* 17, 111–112, 1987.
4. Boggs, P. B.: Platinum allergy, *Cutis,* 35, 318–320, 1985.
5. Murdoch, R. D. and Pepys, J.: Platinum group metal sensitivity: Reactivity to platinum group metal salts in platinum halide salt-sensitive workers, *Ann. Allergy,* 59, 464–469, 1987.

24

Seminal Plasma Hypersensitivity

Jonathan A. Bernstein, David I. Bernstein,
and I. Leonard Bernstein

CONTENTS

24.1   INTRODUCTION

Human seminal plasma (HSP) hypersensitivity was first reported by a Dutch gyne-
cologist, J.L.H. Specken, in 1958.[1] Since that time, numerous well-documented cases
of HSP hypersensitivity have appeared in the literature. Still, there is concern that

HSP reactions are often not readily recognized by the medical community, and therefore this unusual entity may be under reported. Human seminal plasma hypersensitivity is defined as a spectrum of clinical symptoms manifesting as either systemic and/or localized reactions after exposure to specific protein components in seminal plasma.[2] Human seminal plasma hypersensitivity reactions have been categorized as "systemic" and "localized" disorders. Women with systemic HSP hypersensitivity present with symptoms of diffuse urticaria, facial, tongue, lip, and throat angioedema with or without stridor, wheezing with severe dyspnea, pelvic and vulvovaginal pain, nausea, vomiting, diarrhea, general malaise, and in the most extreme circumstance, life-threatening hypotension, loss of consciousness, and complete circulatory failure.[2] These reactions typically occur post-coitally within 30 minutes after exposure to HSP and resolve over a 24-hour period, although urticaria, vaginal pain, and malaise may persist for several days to weeks. Fortunately, there have been no reported fatalities from HSP-induced anaphylaxis in the literature.[2]

Women who present with localized HSP hypersensitivity reactions develop immediate post-coital vulvovaginal burning and pain often associated with formation of vesicles.[2] The severity of pain experienced by these women has been compared to "a thousand needles being injected into the vagina." The localized symptoms may persist for hours, days, or weeks.[1,2]

The "gold standard" required for making a diagnosis of either localized or systemic HSP hypersensitivity is complete prevention of symptoms with a condom.[1,2] Rarely, women with HSP hypersensitivity, who engage in fellatio, have been reported to experience systemic or localized symptoms from oral contact with seminal plasma.[3] Women with HSP hypersensitivity occasionally experience a rash after direct skin contact with HSP.

HSP hypersensitivity leads to a significant amount of stress and anxiety in the affected female and her sexual partner. These reactions often cause deterioration of interpersonal relationships because of the inability of couples to have spontaneous, unimpeded sexual intercourse. Furthermore, these reactions may hinder or delay couples from starting a family because of the inability to have unprotected intercourse. However, some women with this problem have been safely impregnated by direct uterine insemination of separated spermatozoa washed several times in phosphate buffered saline or 10% human serum albumin.[4]

24.2 CONSTITUENTS OF HUMAN SEMINAL PLASMA

The average human ejaculate volume is approximately 3 ml but can range between 2–6 ml. Although the ejaculate is comprised of spermatozoa and seminal plasma, the volume of spermatozoa represents less than 1% of the total ejaculate.[5] Human seminal plasma is formed from the secretions of the epididymis, vas deferens, seminal vesicles, prostate, Cowper's (bulbourethral) gland, and gland of Littre.[5] The major contribution to seminal plasma is from the seminal vesicles (1.5–2 ml), the prostate (0.5 ml), Cowper's gland, and gland of Littre (0.1-0.2 ml). Seminal plasma differs from other body fluids because it contains high concentrations of potassium, zinc, citric acid, fructose, phosphoryl choline, spermine, free amino acids, prostaglandins, and enzymes.[5] The major enzymes in seminal plasma are acid phosphatase, diamine oxidase, β-glucuronidase, lactic dehydrogenase, α-amylase, lysozyme, plasminogen activators, pepsinogen, prostate specific antigens, and other seminal proteinases. Most of these constituents are derived from the prostate.[5]

The major anion in seminal plasma is citrate which originates from the prostate and is a potent binder of metal ions. The seminal plasma concentration of citrate parallels the concentration of divalent metals. Fructose originates from the seminal vesicles and is the major reducing sugar found in HSP. Fructose appears to be both an important anaerobic and aerobic source of energy for spermatozoa.[5]

Polyamines are small positively charged organic molecules that are present in high concentrations in seminal plasma. The role of polyamines is still not entirely clear but they may serve as growth factors for mammalian cells and bacteria and as inhibitors of enzymes such as protein kinases. Polyamines have been speculated to be important in protecting the genitourinary system from infection and for maintaining spermatozoa counts and motility. Spermine is the most abundant of the polyamines. It originates from the prostate and strongly binds to acidic or negatively charged molecules such as phosphate ions, nucleic acid, and phospholipids.[5] Large amounts of phosphoryl choline are also present in the seminal plasma and is predominately derived from the epididymis. It acts as a specific substrate for prostatic acid phosphatase, but its actual function is not understood.[5] Prostaglandins (PG) are present in HSP at a total concentration of approximately 100–300 µl/ml. PG have strong stimulatory and inhibitory effects on smooth muscle. The nomenclature of PG was originally based on the belief that they were synthesized in the prostate, but subsequent investigations have shown that the major source of PG is from the seminal vesicles. PGE compounds are the major PG in the male reproductive tract whereas PGF compounds are the major PG in the female reproductive tract. PG play a role in controlling erection, ejaculation, sperm motility, and sperm transport.[5]

Zinc is found in HSP in large amounts and emanates primarily from the prostate. Zinc binds several different proteins. It may serve as a prostate antibacterial factor since it has exhibited significant bactericidal activity against a variety of gram-positive and gram-negative bacteria.[5]

The three major prostate specific antigens secreted by the prostate into seminal plasma include prostate-specific antigen (PSA, seminin, or γ-seminoprotein), prostatic acid phosphatase (PAP), and prostate-specific protein (PSP-94, β-microseminoprotein, or β-inhibin).[5] PSA is a serine protease with chymotrypsin-like and trypsin-like activity. It is structurally related to the kallikreins which are important proteolytic enzymes involved in cell regulation. PSA may be important in initial clotting and subsequent lysis of clotted ejaculates and is a very important marker for monitoring prostate cancer.[5] Semenogelin is a seminal vesicle secretory protein which serves a substrate for PSA during the ejaculate clot lysis reaction.[5] Acid phosphatase and PSP-94 originate from the prostate, but their biologic functions in seminal plasma are unknown.[5]

HSP contains measurable levels of IgG (7–22 mg/dl) and IgA (0–6 mg/dl). The source of these antibodies is unclear, but they can also be measured in prostatic secretions. Expressed prostatic fluid also contains the C3 component of complement (1.82 mg/dl) which is increased ten-fold in patients with prostatic adenocarcinoma. The function of these proteins in HSP is unknown.[5]

24.3 PREVALENCE OF HSP HYPERSENSITIVITY

Accurate prevalence and incidence data on HSP hypersensitivity disorders are currently not available. Presti et al. performed an extensive world literature search on HSP hypersensitivity and found that 32 cases had been reported between 1958 and 1989.[1] Table 24.1 summarizes major characteristics of these women documented to have HSP hypersensitivity. Most of them were between 20 and 30 years old and had localized vaginal pain associated with systemic symptoms of urticaria and pruritis. Interestingly, 13 of the 32 women experienced symptoms the first time they had intercourse.[1] This information was important in establishing preliminary demographic characteristics of women presenting with HSP hypersensitivity. It also provided clues for determining better insights about the clinical presentation and natural course of HSP hypersensitivity reactions.

Recently, our group has gathered additional information on the prevalence of HSP hypersensitivity among women in North America (U.S. and Canada). We utilized a questionnaire which was validated to have a high positive predictive value for diagnosis of HSP hypersensitivity based on its use as a screening tool in 20 women that we evaluated for this disorder.[6] This survey was conducted in 1073 women who had previously contacted our center for more information regarding the diagnosis of HSP hypersensitivity disorders. The questionnaire elicited information regarding age, race, symptoms (systemic vs. localized), duration of symptoms, number of sexual partners, time to symptom onset after initial exposure to HSP, onset of symptoms with first intercourse, recent gynecologic procedures, history of chronic vaginitis, family or personal history of atopy, and history of food or drug allergy.[6] Of the 1073 questionnaires returned, 266 women were determined to have a "possible" HSP hypersensitivity reaction based on their questionnaire responses. Of these women, 178 were characterized as "possible" systemic HSP hypersensitivity and 88 as "possible" localized HSP hypersensitivity. If the women reported that their symptoms were completely prevented by the use of a condom, they were reclassified as "probable" HSP hypersensitivity.[6] Of the 178 women with "possible" systemic HSP hypersensitivity, 87 were determined to have "probable" disease, and 46 of the 88 women with "possible" localized HSP hypersensitivity were determined to have "probable" localized disease.[6] The demographic characteristics, including the geographic locations in North America of these women, remained unchanged before and after the initial and secondary classifications of "possible" or "probable" HSP hypersensitivity reactors, respectively. Interestingly, women with probable localized seminal HSP hypersensitivity were more likely to experience onset of symptoms after first-time exposure to seminal plasma.[6] Women with probable systemic HSP hypersensitivity were more likely to have a history for food allergy.[6] Although this retrospective survey does not provide definitive prevalence

TABLE 24.1   Presentation of 32 Women with Hypersensitivity to Human Seminal Plasma

Age of onset		Predisposing conditions	
<20	1	First intercourse	13
20–30	18	History of pregnancy	8
31–40	5	Gyn surgery	1
41–50	1	Urological surgery	1
>50	6	Unknown	10
	32		33[a]
Reactions		**Onset, min.**	
Dermatitis/Urticaria/Pruritus	27	<5	12
Edema	15	5–30	2
Dyspnea	7	31–60	1
Local pain	18	>60	7
Anaphylaxis	7	Unknown	10
	32		32
History of atopy		**Family history of atopy**	
Yes	19	Yes	12
No	10	No	4
Unknown	3	Unknown	16
	32		32
Multiple partners		**Prevented by condom**	
Yes	7	Yes	20
No	8	No	0
Unknown	17	Unknown	12
	32		32

[a] One patient with history of pregnancy and urologic surgery in partner.

From Presti, M.P. and Druce, H.M., *Ann. Allergy,* 63, 477, 1989. With permission.

data on HSP hypersensitivity, it does indicate that this disorder may be more common than previously recognized.

24.4   DIFFERENTIAL DIAGNOSIS OF HSP HYPERSENSITIVITY

The diagnosis of HSP hypersensitivity requires the exclusion of other underlying disorders which may have similar presenting symptoms. The differential diagnosis of HSP hypersensitivity is summarized in Table 24.2.[1,2,7]

Involvement of the female genital tract during systemic allergic reactions was first described in 1922 by Cooke who reported two patients who experienced hives, asthma, and uterine bleeding after a systemic reaction to an allergy injection.[8] Subsequently, there were other instances of women who experienced uterine and

TABLE 24.2   Differential Diagnosis of HSP Hypersensitivity

1. Seasonal allergic vulvovaginitis
2. Recurrent allergic *Candida* vulvovaginitis
3. Seminal plasma fluid transfer of a drug or drug metabolite to a drug-sensitive female
4. Seminal plasma transfer of food allergens to a food allergic female
5. Infection
   a. Chronic yeast infections
   b. Sexually transmitted diseases (i.e., *Herpes simplex virus, Cytomegalovirus, Gonorrhea, Syphilis, Trichomonas*)
6. Contact dermatitis secondary to condoms or diaphragms or their constituents, such as lubricants, gels or spermaticides
7. Structural problems (i.e., small vaginal introitus)
8. Physically-induced symptoms (exercise or vibratory angioedema)
9. Reactions secondary to vaginal exposure to chemicals, soaps, scented and/or tinted toilet tissues and sanitary napkins

Adapted from Presti, M.P. and Druce, H.M., *Ann. Allergy,* 63, 477, 1989; Jones, W.R., *Austr. N.Z. J. Obstet. Gynecol.,* 31, 137, 1991; and Witkin, S.S., *Am. J. Reprod. Immunol. Microbiol.,* 15, 34, 1987.

pelvic pain during systemic reactions to immunotherapy. Rosenzweig et al. used the passive transfer assay (the "Prausnitz-Kuestner" [P-K] reaction) to demonstrate that pollen extracts applied to the vaginas of nonatopic volunteers previously injected with serum from atopic patients caused itching, pain, and swelling 1–2 hours after application.[8] Other investigators demonstrated that the vaginal discharge of atopic girls and women during peak pollen seasons was rich in eosinophils.[8] These observations supported the diagnosis of "seasonal allergic vulvovaginitis".[8] These women may experience temporary relief of their localized vulvovaginal symptoms with topical corticosteroid creams or systemic antihistamines. Long-lasting symptomatic improvement in women with seasonal allergic vulvovaginitis has also been achieved using allergen-specific immunotherapy. One study reported significant improvement in 13 out of 16 women with seasonal allergic vulvovaginitis after 3 years of allergen specific immunotherapy.[8]

Foreman and Catterall were the first investigators to suggest that women expressing recurrent vulvovaginal *Candida* infections may have developed localized hypersensitivity reactions to *Candida albicans*.[9] Kudelko empirically treated 70 women diagnosed with recurrent *Candida* vulvovaginitis by *C. albicans* immunotherapy.[10] Women were treated primarily based on a history of recurrent or chronic vaginal yeast infections and confirmatory immediate scratch or intracutaneous skin test reactivity to *C. albicans*. However, not all of the treated women exhibited positive skin test reactivity to *C. albicans*.[10] In this uncontrolled, non-blinded clinical trial, more than 90% of these women responded to *C. albicans* immunotherapy with good to excellent results.[10] Rosedale et al. treated ten women experiencing recurrent *C. albicans* vaginitis with *C. albicans* immunotherapy. Eight of ten women significantly improved after treatment. The average interval between recurrent infections increased from 5.1 to 15.7 months after 18 months of therapy in these women.[9] More recently, Rigg et al. treated 18 women with recurrent allergic *Candida* vulvovaginitis by *C. albicans* immunotherapy.[11] They reported that 16 women responded to treatment with a decrease in the mean number of episodes of vaginitis from 17.2 to 4.3 per year.[11] However, these investigators emphasized the importance of performing a placebo controlled, double-blinded study using a standardized *C. albicans* extract in a homogenous population of women with this disorder before *C. albicans* immunotherapy could be recommended as a standard treatment for recurrent allergic *Candida* vulvovaginitis.[11]

Recurrent allergic *Candida* vaginitis has been postulated to occur as a consequence of either transient inhibition of cell-mediated immunity or mast cell-mediated mediator release, or both.[7,12] Women with this disorder have been demonstrated to have reduced *in vitro* lymphocyte proliferation in response to *C. albicans*. This has been postulated to be a result of a macrophage-driven, increased production of PGE_2 which directly inhibits IL-2 production and subsequent T-cell proliferation.[7,12] Vaginal washings from some of these women contain elevated PGE_2 levels, supporting a role for PGE_2-induced inhibition of cell-mediated immunity and subsequent occurrence resulting in development of localized vaginal allergic responses to *Candida*.[7,12] Previously, it had been demonstrated that PGE_2 levels are also increased in the vaginal washings of females who experience direct vaginal allergic reactions in response to sensitizing agents such as pollens, chemicals in soaps and detergents, sanitary napkins, or contraceptive spermicides.[12] Vaginal washings analyzed for specific IgE antibodies by RAST in such cases during episodes of vaginitis revealed anti-Candida IgE, anti-rye grass IgE, and anti-HSP IgE in 19, 4, and 25%, respectively.[12] Increased levels of specific IgE antibodies to *Candida* were found more frequently in vaginal washings from women with recurrent *Candida* vulvovaginitis than in their peripheral blood.[12]

Seminal plasma transfer of food allergens and drugs and/or their metabolites have been documented to cause localized and systemic reactions in susceptible atopic females.[2] For example, a woman with a known penicillin drug allergy experienced diffuse urticaria within 30 minutes after sexual intercourse. After further probing, it was revealed that her sexual partner had been taking Dicloxacillin for a skin infection.[13] Further reactions were prevented with the use of a condom until he completed the course of antibiotics. Another illustration of transfer allergy concerned a woman with documented contact dermatitis to the periwinkle plant, from which the vinca alkaloid chemotherapeutic agent, Vinblastine, is derived. She experienced severe vaginitis if she had sexual intercourse with her husband 3–4 days after he received Vinblastine for treatment of his Hodgkin's disease.[14] This reaction was completely prevented with the use of a condom. Finally, a woman with documented allergy to walnuts, was reported to experience diffuse urticaria and a sensation of throat swelling within minutes after sexual intercourse. Further history revealed her boyfriend had eaten walnuts shortly before sexual intercourse.[2] These case reports indicate the potential for allergic reactions to occur in response to allergens being transferred to susceptible atopic females by seminal plasma. In some cases the semen has been found to contain high levels of IgE. Presumably, specific IgE in semen could bind to IgE receptors on mast cells or basophils in the female reproductive tract. If the corresponding allergen is also present in the semen, an immediate hypersensitivity reaction could ensue.

Other agents which may potentially elicit localized or systemic symptoms that could simulate HSP hypersensitivity include latex condoms or diaphragms, constituents of condoms, and other barrier contraceptive methods such as spermatocidal gels and lubricants, sanitary napkins, and scented or colored toilet paper.[7] Localized or systemic physical urticaria and/or angioedema can be elicited by the exercise or vibration associated with sexual intercourse. All women with a diagnosis of HSP hypersensitivity should be excluded for common sexually transmitted diseases caused by *Herpes simplex*, *Cytomegalovirus*, *Neisseria gonorrhea*, *Papilloma virus*, *Treponema pallidum,* and *Trichomonas vaginalis* as these infections may present with similar symptomatology. Finally, the size of a woman's vaginal vault must be assessed to exclude trauma associated with sexual intercourse due to a small introitus.

24.5 HISTOPATHOLOGY

Until recently, there has been a paucity of information regarding the histopathology of localized vaginal HSP reactions in women. On gross examination, the external genitalia of these women appear excoriated and erythematous with or without the presence of vesicles. Routine staining of vulvovaginal biopsies obtained from two women with localized HSP hypersensitivity revealed mild to moderate lymphocytic infiltration in the submucosa with generalized dilatation of the blood vessels. On occasion, extravasation of polymorphonuclear cells into the interstitium was observed. There was significant edema in the connective tissue associated with the inflammatory infiltrate. There was no evidence of eosinophilia and special staining for mast cells was unremarkable. In general, these biopsies were consistent with nonspecific inflammation and inconsistent with a typical allergic IgE-mediated reaction. To establish whether specific immunopathologic features are characteristic of this disorder, further vulvovaginal tissue biopsies with immunofluorescence staining are required in cases of localized HSP hypersensitivity (unpublished data).

24.6 IMMUNOSUPPRESSIVE PROPERTIES OF HSP

Early scientific interest in seminal plasma centered about the question of immunological tolerance to spermatozoa. Tung et al. found a high incidence of anti-sperm antibodies present at an early age (1–10 y/o) in both males and females.[15] They speculated that the presence of anti-spermatozoa antibodies in children was the result of immune responses to exogenous antigens such as microorganisms that cross react with human sperm.[15] Investigators have identified immunosuppressive factors that may be important in regulating the production of these anti-sperm antibodies and for distinguishing self and non-self proteins. Lord et al. demonstrated that HSP had a suppressive effect on cellular immunity using the mixed lymphocyte reaction and mitogen-induced lymphocyte blast transformation assays.[16] They determined that HSP contained one or more factors capable of suppressing cell-mediated humoral immune responses. The molecular weight of one of these HSP suppressive factors was greater than 200,000 Da which is similar in size to inhibitory proteins found in bovine seminal plasma.[16] This seminal plasma immunosuppressive factor has been speculated to be important for suppressing local immune responses to spermatozoa in the female reproductive tract.[16]

Marcus et al. performed a series of experiments to investigate the correlation between infertility and anti-sperm antibodies.[17-20] They found that spermatozoal proteins either inhibit or stimulate *in vitro* normal lymphocyte DNA synthesis depending on the dose. In addition, they suppressed mitogen-induced lymphocytic responses in a dose dependent fashion.[17] Pretreatment of spermatozoa with the glycoprotein specific enzymes, neuraminidase, and α-methyl-D-mannoside, abrogated these suppressive effects.[17] Several fractionated HSP proteins were also found to exhibit potent immunosuppressive properties.[18] They found that Sephadex G-100 fractions 1 and 4 inhibited spontaneous blast transformation while fractions 1 and 3 inhibited mitogen-induced blastogenesis.[18] These findings indicated that suppression of lymphocyte proliferation could occur from either spermatozoan or seminal plasma constituents.[18] Both HSP and spermatozoa were also shown to inhibit T-cell associated E-Rosette formation.[19] The inhibitory effect of seminal plasma persisted after repetitive, freeze-thaw cycling but disappeared when these fractions were heated to 100°C.[19] Finally, these investigations demonstrated that inhibition of lymphocyte cultures persisted after a 24-hour incubation period with HSP. Addition of fresh T-lymphocytes but not B-lymphocytes restored the mitogenic activity of lymphocyte cultures previously exposed to HSP.[20] Their findings indicated that HSP was important in regulating T-lymphocyte responses and could suppress lymphocyte responses directed against spermatozoa.[21]

HSP has also been demonstrated to be a potent inhibitor of complement. A seminal plasma factor, called complement cytolysis inhibitor, has been isolated and is capable of suppressing the cytolytic potential of the terminal components, C5b to 7. The presence of a complement cytolysis inhibitor in HSP suggests that it may protect spermatozoa and vaginal epithelial tissues from complement attack.[22,23]

Wasson et al. demonstrated the presence of immunosuppressive factors in seminal plasma obtained from the spouse of a woman with HSP hypersensitivity. A series of experiments were performed to investigate the effect of seminal plasma immunosuppressive factors on peripheral blood mononuclear cell (PBMC) proliferation.[24] They studied target PBMCs of a nonatopic female donor that had a brisk proliferative response to the mitogen, phytohemagglutinin (PHA) but not to HSP. When these PBMCs were pre-incubated with HSP and subsequently stimulated with PHA, proliferation to PHA was significantly suppressed. Similar results were found when her PBMCs were stimulated by HSP from the husband of an HSP hypersensitive female or a normal male.[24] These findings confirmed previous experiments about the immunosuppressive properties of HSP on cell-mediated immune responses.

Fractionated HSP proteins have been shown to contain varying degrees of allergenic activity. Sephadex G-150 fraction 4 has been reported to contain the greatest amount of allergenic activity by one group of investigators.[25] This fraction contained a protein which had a molecular weight and multiple isoelectric forms similar to prostate-specific antigen (PSA) (MW = 30,000 Da; isoelectric forms of pI 6.6, 7.0, and 7.5). RAST inhibition assays comparing G-150 fraction 4 and a partially purified preparation of PSA produced very similar inhibition curves suggesting that PSA may be a major allergen responsible for eliciting reactions in HSP hypersensitive females.[25] However, investigators have identified allergenic activity in response to other Sephadex fractions and most likely more than one HSP protein are involved in this disorder.[26]

24.7 CLINICAL INVESTIGATION OF HSP HYPERSENSITIVITY

Most of the current information about HSP hypersensitivity originates from case reports and limited clinical investigation of these cases. Halpern et al. extensively studied the case of a 29-year-old female with HSP hypersensitivity.[26] The woman experienced severe allergic reactions immediately after sexual intercourse. These episodes occurred after her first exposure to seminal plasma and had become progressively worse with each episode of sexual intercourse.[26] Her symptoms consisted of diffuse urticaria, swelling of her lips, eye lids, tongue, and pharynx, resulting in difficult breathing, severe shortness of breath with chest congestion, pelvic pain, uterine contractions, general malaise, and loss of consciousness.[26] The culmination of these symptoms occurred within 15 to 30 minutes after HSP exposure and resolved over 24 hours. The authors employed several *in vitro* and *in vivo* immunologic assays to characterize the responsible seminal plasma proteins and the underlying mechanism(s) responsible for this reaction, including zone electrophoresis, immunoelectrophoresis, ionic exchange column chromatography, P-K reactions in humans, passive cutaneous anaphylaxis in guinea pigs and primates, passive hemagglutination tests, agglutinating antibody assays, and complement fixation tests.[26] The patient demonstrated skin test sensitivity to whole seminal plasma obtained from her husband and from normal human donors. Skin test reactivity was not elicited in response to spermatozoa. Skin testing was also negative using serum obtained from her husband and semen obtained from rabbit, guinea pig, horse, bull, bovine submaxillary mucin, and bovine testicular hyaluronidase.[26] Therefore, they demonstrated that the responsible allergen(s) were species-specific and originated from the seminal fluid and not spermatozoa. Passive serum transfer assays to normal human skin revealed positive reactions to seminal fluid at serum dilutions of 1:20 to 1:100. These reactions were negative after heating the patient's serum for 4 hours at 56°C prior to injection into naive recipients, indicating that IgE (reaginic) antibody was involved.[26] Passive hemagglutination, agglutinating antibodies, and complement fixation assays were negative. DEAE-cellulose ion exchange chromatography was used to identify the sensitizing antigens in seminal plasma. Three major fractions were eluted. Fraction 2 contained the highest amount of protein and sialic acid and also elicited the greatest skin test reaction in the patient.[26] Zone electrophoresis revealed that the proteins in seminal plasma eliciting the strongest skin test results were basic in pH and migrated between the serum albumin and fast α_2-globulin bands. Precipitation of the patient's serum with specific anti-sera to either IgM or IgA antibodies was utilized to further identify the specific antibody involved in this reaction. Serum devoid of IgA antibody did not transmit the sensitivity to naive recipient volunteers.

This indicated that the responsible antibody was associated with the IgA antibody class.[26] Subsequent experiments by Ishuzaki et al. revealed that IgE antibodies could have been present in IgA antibodies prepared this way. An attempt by these investigators to desensitize this individual using whole seminal plasma was unsuccessful.[26]

Levine et al. reported a case of a 29-year-old atopic female who experienced diffuse hives, swelling, nasal congestion, and sneezing 1 hour after intercourse.[27] These symptoms progressively worsened with each episode of intercourse. Recurrence of symptoms were completely prevented with a condom during sexual intercourse.[27] Seminal plasma hypersensitivity was confirmed by skin testing using her sexual partner's whole HSP. Significant histamine release in response to seven different HSP samples was demonstrated using leucocytes isolated from the patient's whole blood. Fractionation of HSP obtained from donor vasectomized males revealed that 90% of the allergenic activity was present in fraction 4, which corresponded to proteins with a molecular weight of 20,000–30,000 Da. Fraction 4 also elicited the strongest positive skin test reaction in the patient at a dilution as low as 1:100,000.[27]

Schulz et al. reported a 25-year-old female who experienced diffuse urticaria, periorbital swelling, and abdominal cramping immediately after intercourse.[28] The symptoms increased in intensity with repeated sexual intercourse, culminating in complete circulatory collapse. Use of a condom completely prevented her allergic symptoms. Skin testing using her sexual partner's or normal donor HSP at a dilution of 10^{-6} resulted in a significant immediate wheal and flare reaction.[28] Positive passive transfer experiments to naive recipients confirmed that reaginic antibody was involved. Lymphocyte proliferation using the patient's lymphocytes stimulated with diluted HSP was negative.[28] Chromatographic separation of pooled HSP revealed that the seminal plasma protein(s) responsible for eliciting the positive skin reaction had an approximate molecular weight between 14,000–18,000 Da. Isoelectric focusing of pooled HSP followed by skin testing revealed allergenic activity in the fractions with a pH of 8.4 to 8.6.[28]

Chang et al. reported a series of HSP hypersensitivity cases occurring in one family which he referred to as "familial allergic seminal vulvovaginitis."[29] These women all experienced severe discomfort after their first contact to seminal fluid during sexual intercourse. Most of their symptoms were localized consisting of stinging, burning, and pain during or immediately after ejaculation.[29] Skin testing with HSP was positive at a concentration of 1:1000 which was a weaker skin test response compared to those reactions elicited in women with systemic HSP hypersensitivity.[29]

Voorhorst reported a case of a young woman who experienced post-coital vaginal itching prior to the birth of her second child.[30] Her reactions progressively became worse, leading to diffuse urticaria with dyspnea and stridor associated with nausea, diarrhea, and shock on two occasions. She exhibited a very strong positive skin test reaction to her husband's seminal plasma confirmed by RAST testing.[30] A positive P-K reaction was demonstrated and could be ablated by heating her serum for 30 minutes at 56°C. To identify the origin of the allergenic protein in seminal plasma, she was skin tested to extracts made from different male organs obtained from the urogenital tract of a healthy male who had recently died in a motor vehicle accident. Proteins from the prostate yielded the strongest skin test reactions compared to the extracts derived from the seminal vesicle, bladder, epididymis, or testes. From these results, it was concluded that the most probable origin of relevant allergenic seminal plasma proteins was the prostate gland.[30]

A patient with severe atopic dermatitis exhibited severe anaphylactic reactions after unprotected intercourse with her husband.[31] Human seminal plasma hypersensitivity was confirmed by skin testing and specific RAST testing.[31] Significant leukocyte histamine release was demonstrated in response to her husband's serum and HSP, serum from normal male donors but not to serum from female controls. Immunotherapy using her husband's whole seminal plasma after 1 year was unsuccessful.[31]

Freeman reported a case of a woman who was allergic to her husband's seminal plasma and sweat.[32] The patient had a 6-year history of severe itching and flushing of the face and upper extremities 10 minutes after unprotected sexual intercourse with her husband.[32] Skin testing to her husband's sweat and seminal plasma yielded significant positive skin test reactions. Positive skin test reactions were also elicited in response to pooled donor HSP and sweat obtained from her two sons. Interestingly, she had no reaction to her own sweat during exercise. No further investigation was performed to determine whether HSP and sweat share common allergens which could elicit this reaction.[32]

Bernstein et al. studied two women with systemic HSP hypersensitivity and two women with localized HSP hypersensitivity.[33] Both women with systemic HSP hypersensitivity had positive direct skin tests and significant leucocyte histamine release responses to their sexual partners' HSP. One woman also demonstrated cutaneous reactivity to her spouse's spermatozoal extract. Immediate hypersensitivity to spermatozoa in this woman was supported by a positive P-K reaction and leucocyte histamine release.[33] A positive P-K reaction, RAST, and specific RAST inhibition in addition to neutralization of passive transfer antibodies by HSP were demonstrated in one of these women. The woman with localized HSP reactions did not develop humoral antibodies in response to seminal plasma although one patient had significant titers of IgM and IgG sperm agglutinating antibodies to HSP. This woman also demonstrated lymphocyte blast transformation and a migration inhibitory factor response to HSP.[33] All four women and their husbands had histocompatibility leucocyte antigen typing which revealed a marked degree of shared histocompatibility locus antigens between two of the women and their respective spouses.[33] This investigation confirmed that IgE-mediated immune responses were involved in systemic HSP hypersensitivity and provided preliminary evidence that cell-mediated responses might be involved in localized HSP hypersensitivity reactions.[33]

Reactions to seminal plasma have also manifested as fixed cutaneous eruptions. For example, a woman experienced a pruritic, erythematous, macular rash which blistered and progressed to a purpuric, hyperpigmented, macular lesion in the same regions of her body after exposure to seminal plasma.[34] These reactions involved the vulva, vagina, and isolated regions of one finger, ear, hip, and breast and were not associated with other systemic symptoms.[34] Skin testing using HSP obtained from her husband and a vasectomized male donor were negative. Direct immunofluorescence performed on a skin biopsy from the right breast was also unremarkable. The rash was completely prevented with the use of a condom.[34] Interestingly, the reaction was also prevented by 500 mg of the nonsteroidal anti-inflammatory agent, mefenamic acid, if taken before intercourse. Systemic antihistamines were less effective in providing symptomatic relief. These investigators postulated that mefenamic acid was effective in relieving symptoms by inhibition of prostaglandin synthesis since these mediators had been shown to induce redness, swelling, and pain symptoms characteristic of fixed drug eruptions.[34]

24.8 TREATMENT OF SEMINAL PLASMA HYPERSENSITIVITY

A number of different approaches have been attempted for the treatment of women with HSP hypersensitivity. Prophylactic use of antihistamines 30–60 minutes before sexual intercourse has been reported to control localized and systemic symptoms in selected cases.[35] As mentioned earlier, one woman with an HSP fixed drug eruption was successfully pretreated before sexual intercourse with mefenamic acid.[34] Successful treatment of a woman with localized vaginal HSP hypersensitivity has also been reported using an 8% topical cromolyn sodium solution.[36] However, none of these therapeutic approaches have been uniformly successful in the long term treatment of women with either localized or systemic HSP hypersensitivity.

The most effective treatment approach for women with IgE-mediated HSP hypersensitivity has been immunotherapy with their sexual partner's HSP fractions. Several immunotherapy protocols summarized in Table 24.3 have been used with variable success.[37] Halpern et al. tried to desensitize a woman with HSP hypersensitivity using whole HSP.[26] They treated their patient for 2 years using a conventional immunotherapy protocol but were unable to induce tolerance as the patient continued to have systemic reactions after post-coital exposure to HSP.[26]

A rush immunotherapy protocol has been used in women with HSP hypersensitivity, using specific seminal plasma protein fractions isolated from their partner's whole seminal plasma by separative Sephadex G-100 column chromatography.[38-41] Figure 24.1 illustrates two examples of fractionated peaks obtained after column chromatography of whole HSP.[40] These peaks correlate with different molecular weight proteins. Those specific protein fractions which elicited a significant wheal and flare skin test reaction in the HSP hypersensitive female were combined for immunotherapy.[38-41] The patient's sexual partner was used as a negative control for skin testing.[38-41] This protocol differed from other protocols in that the largest molecular weight proteins found in fraction 1 purposely were excluded from the proteins used for immunotherapy. This reasoning was based on previous observations that fraction 1 contained immunosuppressive factors which could potentially interfere with an immunogenic response. This method has been successful in achieving long lasting tolerance to HSP allergens in women with systemic HSP hypersensitivity.[38-41] True desensitization (i.e., loss of skin sensitivity) has been obtained in several of the women treated using this protocol.[40] Ohman et al. treated a woman with systemic HSP hypersensitivity for 10 months using Sephadex G-100 fractionated protein and was also able to demonstrate clinical improvement. Reduction in her

TABLE 24.3   Immunotherapy with Human Seminal Plasma (HSP) Fluid

Author	Protocol	Side Effects	Outcome	Pt. Profile
Halpern et al.	Classic (2 years) Whole HSP	Not stated	Failed	29-year-old woman atopic family
Mathias et al.	Classic (1 year) Whole HSP	Worsening eczema	Failed	26-year-old woman eczema, seasonal AR
Frisch et al.	Rush (5 days) (IT continued for 9 months) Whole HSP	Not stated	Successful	33-year-old woman nonatopic
Friedman et al.	Classic Purified fractions of HSP	Small, local reaction	Successful[a]	46-year-old woman seasonal AR
Mittman et al.	Rush (2 days) (IT continued for 4 months) Purified fractions of HSP	Mild systemic reaction	Successful	24-year-old woman nonatopic
Ohman et al.	Classic (2 years) Purified fraction of HSP	Local swelling at injection site	Some evidence of improvement	20-year-old woman eczema, AR
Boom et al.	Rush (1 day) Whole HSP (maintenance booster given 1st and 2nd week post-desensitization)	Minor systemic reaction	Successful	28-year-old woman eczema
Bernstein et al.	Rush (1 day) Purified fractions of HSP	Not stated	Successful	32-year-old woman eczema, AR, multiple drug allergy
Blair et al.	Classic (18 months) Purified fractions	Not stated	Successful	30-year-old woman asthma, allergy to milk

[a] Experienced dry cough after 2 weeks of sexual abstinence.

AR = Allergic rhinitis.

From Jones, W.R. and Gale, A.E., *Ann. Allergy,* 41, 325, 1978. With permission.

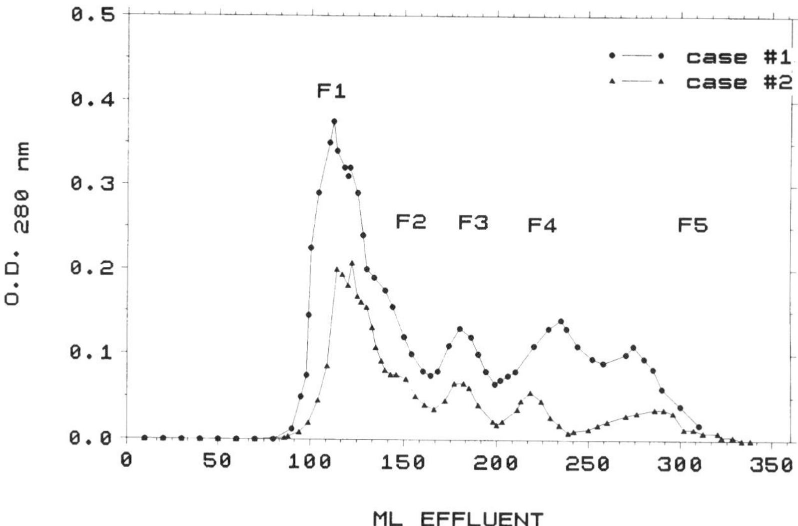

FIGURE 24.1 Fractionated peaks of whole human seminal plasma samples obtained from spouses of two women with seminal plasma hypersensitivity using a Sephadex G-100 column, eluted with 0.05 mol/L phosphate buffer, pH 7.4. (O.D. = optical density.)

clinical symptoms directly correlated with a decline in specific IgE-HSP antibodies and a rise in IgG antibodies.[42]

Until recently, treatment of women with localized HSP hypersensitivity has not been attempted. Previous speculation that these reactions were due to a cell-mediated immune response inhibited the use of immunotherapy in these women.[33] Bernstein et al. reported that three women who presented with a localized vaginal form of HSP hypersensitivity responded to a rapid immunotherapy protocol using their spouse's fractionated HSP proteins.[39] One patient demonstrated evidence of desensitization as she manifested a significant change in her skin test threshold response to fraction 3 post-immunotherapy.[39] Subsequently, two patients conceived and delivered healthy babies.[39] These cases provided the first evidence that localized HSP hypersensitivity may also involve an IgE-mediated mechanism similar to that demonstrated in women with systemic reactions.

Some patients with localized or systemic HSP hypersensitivity reactions may require additional booster injections of specific HSP fractions to enhance their tolerogenic responses. Following rapid immunotherapy, women must maintain their tolerance to HSP by having frequent and regular sexual intercourse with their partner two to three times a week. This has not always been possible since some patients or their spouses may have job-related traveling responsibilities and may not always be able to maintain this schedule. This problem has been averted by freezing pools of fresh semen ejaculates which the patient can instill in her vagina while her spouse is away on business. To date, we have successfully treated over 20 women with localized or systemic HSP hypersensitivity by rapid immunotherapy over the past 12 years and have found that this treatment provides long lasting protection.

24.9 HYPOTHETICAL MECHANISMS

Systemic HSP hypersensitivity has been well documented to occur through IgE-mediated humoral mechanisms, but it is still unclear what male or female factor(s) predispose certain women to develop hypersensitivity to HSP. HSP is rich in a variety of different enzymes, (e.g., acid phosphatase, lactic acid dehydrogenase, lysozyme) and proteins (e.g., polyamines, IgG, IgA, prostate-specific antigen) which are found in other body fluids and in many foods. These proteins or enzymes may be potentially cross-reactive with similar antigenic determinants present in HSP. Once sensitization has occurred, future exposure to relevant proteins leads to mast cell activation, release of bioactive mediators, and the physiologic sequelae characteristic of systemic HSP hypersensitivity.

Local immune dysregulation in the vagina could predispose women to become sensitized to HSP. Increased levels of PGE_2 have been demonstrated in women with chronic nonspecific vaginitis.[7] This prostanoid could inhibit cellular immune responses that are important for regulating IgE-mediated immune responses.

Hypersensitivity reactions may be enhanced by immunosuppressive factors present in HSP. These immunosuppressive factors are capable of inhibiting both cell-mediated immune responses and complement activity *in vitro* and therefore could predispose women to develop HSP hypersensitivity.

It is also possible that males, who are asymptomatic carriers of infectious organisms such as yeast, fungi, bacteria, or viruses may be unknowingly exposing their female sexual partners to these organisms or their byproducts which by virtue of cross reactive epitopes could induce IgE-mediated immune responses.[7] Thus, it is essential that we identify those HSP proteins or byproducts responsible for systemic and localized HSP hypersensitivity in order to elucidate the underlying mechanism(s) of these disorders. As the number of women with these disorders increase, there is a greater likelihood of identifying as yet unknown inherent risk factors in women and their sexual partners for HSP sensitization.

24.10 CONCLUSIONS

Systemic and localized HSP hypersensitivity probably occur more commonly than previously recognized. Although IgE-mediated immune responses seem to be involved in women with systemic reactions and many women with localized reactions, there are still many unanswered questions regarding this disorder. There is still a need to identify female and male risk factors, responsible sensitizing protein(s), and the immunohistopathology of HSP hypersensitivity. The current use of rapid immunotherapy to fractionated seminal plasma proteins has been proven to be a practical and effective treatment of this disorder. Unfortunately, this treatment is time consuming, expensive, and not readily accessible to all women with this problem. Work is in progress to better understand the natural course of this disorder and to develop generally accessible and cost effective methods of treatment.

REFERENCES

1. Presti, M. P. and Druce, H. M., Hypersensitivity reactions to human seminal plasma, *Ann. Allergy,* 63, 477, 1989.
2. Jones, W.R., Allergy to Coitus, *Austr. N.Z. J. Obstetr. Gynecol.,* 31, 137, 1991.
3. Shapiro, S.S., Kooistra, J.B., Schwartz, D., Yunginger, J.W., and Haning, R.V., Induction of pregnancy in a woman with seminal plasma allergy, *Fertil. Steril.,* 36, 405, 1981.
4. Mikkelsen, E. J., Henderson, L. L., Leiferman, K. M., and Gleich, G. J., Allergy to human seminal fluid, *Ann. Allergy,* 34, 239, 1975.
5. Coffey, D. S., The molecular biology, endocrinology, and physiology of the prostate and seminal vesicles, *Campbell's Urology,* 6th edition, 1, Walsh, P. C., Retik, A. B., Stamey, T. A., and Vaughan, E. D., Jr., Eds., W. B. Saunders Company, Philadelphia, 1992, 221.
6. Bernstein, J.A., Sugumaran, R., Bernstein, D.I., and Bernstein, I.L., Prevalence of human seminal plasma hypersensitivity among symptomatic women, *Ann. Allergy,* 78, 54, 1997.
7. Witkin, S. S., Immunology of recurrent vaginitis, *Am. J. Reprod. Immunol. Microbiol.,* 15, 34, 1987.
8. Berman, B. A., Seasonal allergic vulvovaginitis caused by pollen, *Ann. Allergy,* 22, 594, 1964.
9. Rosedale, N. and Browne, K., Hyposensitization in the management of recurring vaginal candidiasis, *Ann. Allergy,* 43, 250, 1979.
10. Kudelko, N. M., Allergy in chronic monilial vaginitis, *Ann. Allergy,* 29, 266, 1971.
11. Rigg, D., Miller, M.M., and Metzer, W.J., Recurrent allergic vulvovaginitis: Treatment with *Candida albicans* allergen immunotherapy, *Am. J. Obstet. Gynecol.,* 2, 332, 1990.
12. Witkin, S. S., Jeremias, J., and Ledger, W. J., A localized vaginal allergic response in women with recurrent vaginitis, *J. Allergy Clin. Immunol.,* 81, 412, 1988.
13. Green, R. L. and Green, M. A., Postcoital urticaria in a penicillin-sensitive patient, (letter) *J. Am. Med. Assoc.,* 254, 531, 1985.
14. Paladine, W. J., Cunningham, T. J., Donavan, M. A., and Dumper, C. W., Possible sensitivity to vinblastine in prostatic or seminal fluid, (letter) *N. Engl. J. Med.,* 29, 52, 1975.
15. Cooke, W. D., McCarty, T. A., and Robitaille, P., Human sperm antigens and anti-sperm antibodies, *Clin. Exp. Immunol.,* 25, 73, 1976.
16. Lord, E. M., Sensabaugh, G. F., and Stites, D. P., Immunosuppressive activity of human seminal plasma, *J. Immunol.,* 118, 1704, 1977.
17. Marcus, Z. H., Herman, J. H., and Hess, E. V., The effect of human spermatozoa on antigen and mitogen induced blastogenesis, *Arch. Androl.,* 1, 89, 1978.
18. Marcus, Z. H., Freisheim, J. H., Houk, J. L., Herman, J. H., and Hess, E.V., *In vitro* studies in reproductive immunology, *Clin. Immunol. Immunopathol.,* 9, 318, 1978.
19. Marcus, Z. H., Hess, E. V., Herman, J. H., Troiano, P., and Freisheim, J., *In vitro* studies in reproductive immunology-2 demonstration of the inhibitory effect of male genital tract constituents of PHA-stimulated mitogenesis and E-rosette formation of human lymphocytes, *J. Reprod. Immunol.,* 1, 97, 1979.
20. Marcus, Z. H. and Hess, E. V., *In vitro* studies in reproductive immunology, 3. Restoration of mitogenic activity of lymphocytes inhibited by seminal plasma in man, *Arch. Androl.,* 6, 67, 1981.

21. Hess, E. V. and Marcus, Z. H., The inhibitors in seminal plasma, *J. Lab. Clin. Med.,* 96, 577, 1980.
22. Jenne, D. E. and Tschopp, J., Molecular structure and functional characterization of a human complement cytolysis inhibitor found in blood and seminal plasma: identity to sulfated glycoprotein 2, a constituent of rat testis fluid, *Proc. Natl. Acad. Sci. U.S.A.,* 86, 7123, 1989.
23. Petersen, B. H., Lammel, C. J., Stites, D. P., and Brooks, G. F., Human seminal plasma inhibition of complement, *J. Lab. Clin. Med.,* 96, 582, 1980.
24. Wasson, A. W., Coy, E. A., Kooistra, J. B., and Yunginger, J. W., Seminal plasma immunosuppressive factors in the spouse of a woman with seminal fluid allergy, *Am. J. Reprod. Immunol. Microbiol.,* 15, 99, 1987.
25. Yunginger, J. W., Jones, R. T., Klee, G. G., and Squillace, D. L., Allergy to human seminal plasma (HSP): identification of prostate specific antigen (PSA) as a major allergen, *J. Allergy Clin. Immunol.,* 87, 343, 1991 (abstract).
26. Halpern, B. N., Ky, T., and Robert, B., Clinical and immunological study of an exceptional case of reaginic type sensitization to human seminal fluid, *Immunology,* 12, 247, 1967.
27. Levine, B. B., Siraganian, R. P., and Schenkein, I, Allergy to human seminal plasma, *N. Engl. J. Med.,* 17, 894, 1973.
28. Schulz, K. H., Schirren, C., and Kueppers, F., Allergy to seminal fluid, (letter) *N. Engl. J. Med.,* 290, 916, 1974.
29. Chang, T-W., Familial allergic seminal vulvovaginitis, *Am. J. Obstet. Gynecol.,* 126, 442, 1976.
30. Voorhorst, R., Female allergy to seminal fluid, (letter) *Ann. Allergy,* 40, 252, 1978.
31. Mathis, G. G. T., Frick, O. L., Caldwell, T. M., Yunginger, J. W., and Maibach, H. I., Immediate hypersensitivity to seminal fluid and atopic dermatitis, *Arch. Dermatol.,* 116, 209, 1980.
32. Freeman, S., Woman allergic to husband's sweat and semen, *Contact Dermatitis,* 14, 110, 1986.
33. Bernstein, I. L., Englander, B. E., Gallagher, J. S., Nathan, P., and Marcus, Z. H., Localized and systemic hypersensitivity reactions to human seminal fluid, *Ann. Int. Med.,* 94, 459, 1981.
34. Best, C. L., Walters, C., and Adelman, D. C., Fixed cutaneous eruptions to seminal-plasma challenge: a case report, *Fertil. Steril.,* 50, 532, 1988.
35. Jones, W. R. and Gale, A. E., Concerning seminal plasma allergy, (letter) *Ann. Allergy,* 41, 325, 1978.
36. Goldenhersh, M.J. and Saxon, A., Seminal fluid hypersensitivity: A new approach, *Ann. Allergy,* 6, 256, 1989.
37. Saca, L. F., Munson, J., and Haddad, Z. H., Systemic anaphylaxis due to seminal fluid allergy in a 50-year old woman, *Immunol. Allergy Pract.,* XV, 170, 1993.
38. Friedman, S.A., Bernstein, I.L., Enrione, M., and Marcus, Z.H., Successful long-term immunotherapy for human seminal plasma anaphylaxis, *J. Am. Med. Assoc.,* 251, 2684, 1984.
39. Bernstein, I.L., Gallagher, J.S., Friedman, S.A., and Marcus, Z.H., Standardized immunotherapy protocol for IgE-mediated anaphylaxis to human seminal plasma, *Contrib. Gynecol. Obstet.,* 14, 151, 1985.
40. Bernstein, J.A., Herd, Z.A., Bernstein, D.I., Korbee, L., and Bernstein, I.L., Evaluation and treatment of localized vaginal immunoglobulin E-mediated hypersensitivity to human seminal plasma, *Obstet. Gynecol.,* 82, 667, 1993.

41. Mittman, R.J., Bernstein, D.I., Adler, T.R., Korbee, L., Nath, V., Gallagher, J.S., and Bernstein, I.L., Selective desensitization to seminal plasma protein fractions after immunotherapy for postcoital anaphylaxis, *J. Allergy Clin. Immunol.*, 86, 954, 1990.
42. Ohman, J.L., Malkiel, S., Lewis, S., and Lorusso, J.R., Allergy to human seminal fluid: characterization of the allergen and experience with immunotherapy, *J. Allergy Clin. Immunol.*, 85, 103, 1990.

25

Contact Urticaria Syndrome and Childhood Atopic Dermatitis

Flora B. de Waard-van der Spek and Arnold P. Oranje

CONTENTS

25.1   INTRODUCTION

Food-induced contact urticaria syndrome (CUS) occurs in more than half of the infants and toddlers with atopic dermatitis (AD).[1] Contact urticaria induced by foods is immunological or nonimmunological of origin.[2-4] Contact urticaria is often observed in young children with AD, but also in adults with AD or contact dermatitis. Urticaria occurs preferably in the eczematous areas, because the skin is more easily penetrated by antigens. The clinical presentation in older children and in adults

**TABLE 25.1 Foods Inducing Contact Urticaria in Infants
and Toddlers with Atopic Dermatitis***

Almonds	Fish (especially codfish)	Pork
Bananas[a]	Hazelnuts	Raw potatoes
Chicken	Kiwi[a]	Sesame
Beef	Nuts (various)	Tomatoes
Cow's milk	Paprika	Wheat
Eggs	Peanuts	

[a] These foods are also natural histamine liberators.

* Based on our own experiences.

differs somewhat and is more restricted to and around the mouth. Then it is called oral allergy syndrome. IgE responses are divided into early, late, and delayed reactions.[4] Most of the IgE responses occur together and often a direct reaction is followed by a late one. This means that an urticarial reaction can be followed by an eczematous eruption.

25.2 DEFINITION

Contact urticaria syndrome can be defined as a direct urticarial reaction after contact with an allergen (for example, food or animal products). We recognize immune-mediated and nonimmune-mediated patterns. In particular is contact urticaria a part of the clinical presentation in infants and toddlers with AD and food allergy.

25.3 FOOD-INDUCING CUS

Many foods can provoke food induced contact urticaria (Table 25.1). Overall the most common allergen is egg, followed by cow's milk and others such as wheat, fish, and peanut. Different other foods may induce CUS. It depends on early exposure to the allergen. For differential diagnostic reasons, one should realize that animal products (saliva, hair) can induce CUS too. Atopic dermatitis is a complicated disease often strongly influenced by flare factors such as contact urticaria, allergic contact dermatitis, and late phase reactions. Contact urticaria can induce eczema by basic immunological mechanisms but also by eliciting of scratching.[4,5]

25.4 CLINICAL SYMPTOMS

Common symptoms of food allergy with the skin as the most prominent target are refusal of foods, vomiting, and urticaria on the hands and around the mouth. These symptoms belong to CUS (Figure 25.1).[1] FA is variable in presentation depending on the organ involved.[4] Symptoms on the skin and the mucous membranes may be the sole manifestations of food allergy (Table 25.2).

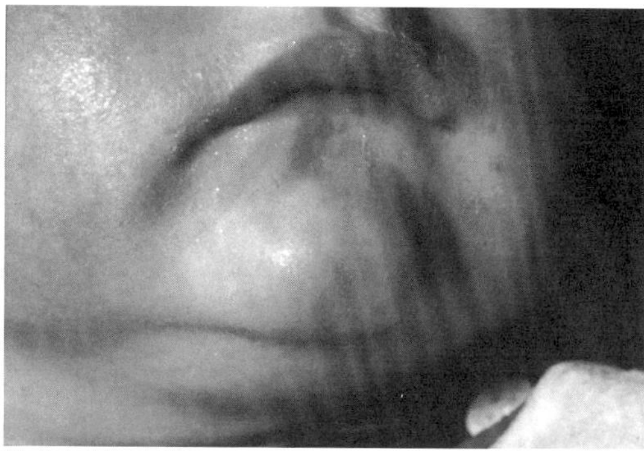

FIGURE 25.1   Urticarial rash on the chin of a child with cow's milk allergy. The cow's milk dropped along the chin.

TABLE 25.2   Common Symptoms of Food Allergy in Children with Atopic Dermatitis [AD], with the Skin as the Main Target

Urticaria
Contact urticaria
Quinckes edema
Flare-ups of AD
Pruritus or pain in the mouth (and swelling)[a]
Perleche, aphthae
Food refusal, vomiting, diarrhea[b]

[a] Oral allergy syndrome.

[b] Common, though instead of other listed symptoms, not of skin and mouth.

25.5 DIAGNOSIS

Based on the mechanism of CUS, imitating provocation tests have been described.[4,6-8] These tests are specially performed in young children with AD suspected from food allergy. Tests available are the open application test, the RUB test, and the SAFT.[6-8] The Skin application food test (SAFT) was developed by the authors.[8] In detail: 2 square cm areas are marked. Finn Chambers (big size, 1 cm^2) containing food (allergen) or control fluid (0.9% Sodium chloride) on filters are applied to the skin area cleansed of fat using 96% alcohol. The foods (0.1 ml or a slice) are fixed to the skin with Finn Chamber Scanlon® plasters (Norgeplaster, A/S Oslo, Norway). Additionally, we examine the patch sites at intervals of 10 minutes. Maximum time of application is 30 minutes. Scores of 0 and 1+ (only redness) are regarded as negative. The reactions 2+ (redness and edema) and 3+ (redness and edema covering 4 cm^2) are regarded as positive (Figure 25.2a and 25.2b). Positive tests correlate well

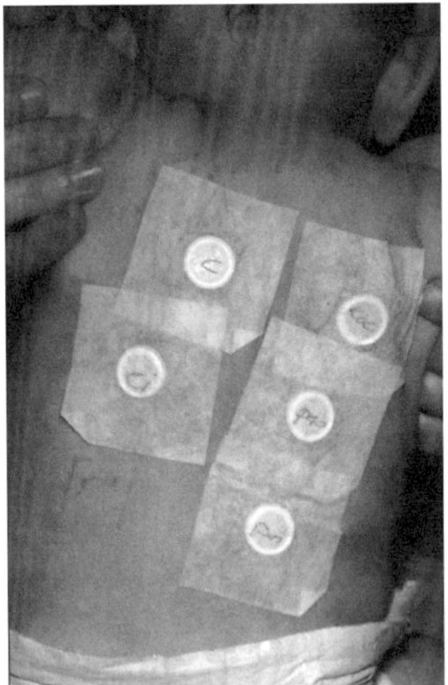

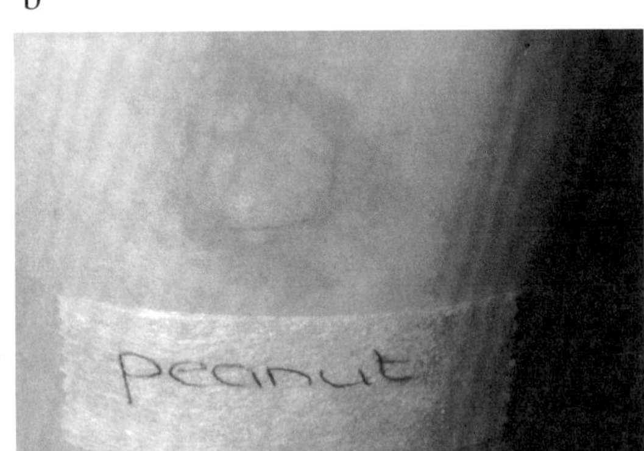

FIGURES 25.2   Infant tested by SAFT with control (NaCL solution), cow's milk, eggwhite and peanut (standard series in our hospital) (Figure 25.2a). Positive SAFT (skin application food test) performed with egg white. The reactions were read as 3+ (Figure 25.2b).

with RAST scores and oral provocations (Waard-van der Spek, de FB, to be published). If the SAFT is negative on normal skin and the suspicion of CUS is high, the SAFT test can be repeated on eczematous skin.[4] We do not practice this last-mentioned method anymore. Another possible solution is to perform a scratch-patch test (Oranje, not published data), however in these cases we now prefer the prick-prick test. In small children aged less than 3 years, the SAFT is considered as adequate in clinical practice. From 3 years on, we use the prick-prick method with pure foods in the way they are consumed.[9] In this technique, the investigator pricks first into the antigen and thereafter into the skin. Screening with the mixed-food RAST is a useful tool to identify the children with atopic immune response to 6 common allergic foods (cow's milk, egg, peanut, soy, cod fish, and wheat). The SAFT correlates well with the RAST scores as published earlier (Tables 25.3 and 25.4).[1]

TABLE 25.3   Results of SAFT and RAST with Cow's Milk and Egg White in 40 Atopic Children with Immediate Contact Reactions

All determinations (n = 95)		SAFT+ RAST+	SAFT+ RAST–	SAFT– RAST+	SAFT– RAST–
Cow's milk and/or	+	51	9	2	0
egg allergy	–	0	0	7	26

Note: RAST class ≥ 2 is considered positive. SAFT and RAST results correlated significantly with cow's milk and/or egg allergy by Fisher's exact test (p = 0.001).

From Oranje et al., *Acta Derm. Venereol.,* 1991; 71:263-6 (1). With permission.

TABLE 25.4 Comparison of Height of Scores of SAFT and RAST

SAFT (classes)	RAST cow's milk and egg (classes)				
	0	**1**	**2**	**3**	**4**
0	18	8	7	7	2
1	0	0	0	0	0
2	2	3	12	12	14
3	1	3	9	9	16

Note: Rank correlation coefficient (Spearman, $r_s = 0.58$, $p < 0.001$).

SAFT = 0 or 1 means negative; 2 and 3 = positive.

RAST ≥ 2 is considered as positive.

From Oranje et al., *Acta Derm. Venereol.*, 1991; 71:263-6 (1). With permission.

25.6 GUIDELINES FOR EXAMINATION

Contact urticaria is very often noticed by the parents, but its exact origin and the history are often not completely clear. The parents do not know exactly which food or other substance is responsible. We observe CUS seldomly in our patients in our out-patient office. CUS has disappeared before the patient visits. Tests for CUS are performed if the history is suspected, in therapy-resistant atopic dermatitis and in doubtful cases with vomiting, diarrhea, or food-refusal.

25.7 MANAGEMENT

AD is a multifactorial inflammatory disease with a variety of triggering factors, such as aeroallergens, foods, and pathologic stress. Dietary restrictions are indicated in selected cases of AD and especially useful in children, aged 0–5 years with AD. The younger the child, the bigger the chance that a diet is helpful in the management of AD. Diagnosis of FA relies on combined interpretation of "weighted" history and of the results of serological and skin tests. Final and ideal proof of FA is achieved by (double-blind) oral provocation. From age 3 years, we perform the DBPCOC, before that age if we do a challenge we perform it open.

Food allergy is not only based on direct IgE mediated, but also delayed reactions are common. Late IgE reactions can be observed by later reading of SAFT.[10] Patch tests for delayed type reactions (atopy patch tests) read after 1 and 2 or after 2 and 3 days add approximately another 10% of patients with food allergy (Figure 25.3).[10]

25.8 PROGNOSIS AND COMPLICATIONS

Contact urticaria syndrome to cow's milk normally disappears in most cases within a period of 3 years. Egg shows less regression. Peanut stays lifelong in 99% of the cases.

The most severe presentations of CUS are a generalized reaction and anaphylaxis. Generalized reactions have occurred after local application of milk or egg containing products.[11,12] Even anaphylaxis have been described.[11]

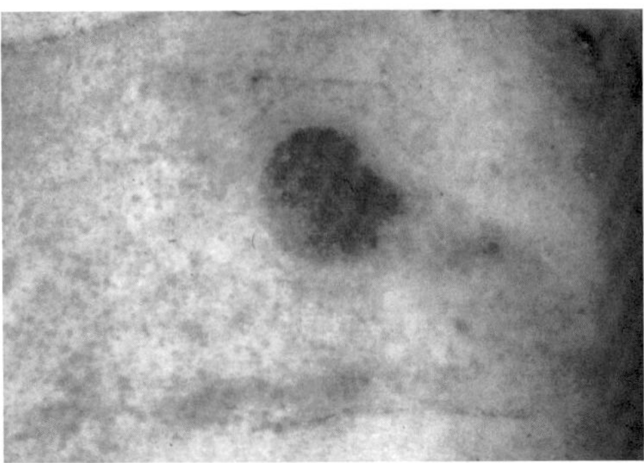

FIGURE 25.3   Positive APT (atopy patch test, delayed type testing) performed with cow's milk in a child with atopic dermatitis. The reaction was read after 48 hours.

REFERENCES

1. Oranje, A.P., Aarsen, R.S.R., and Liefaard, G., Immediate contact reactions to cow's milk and egg in atopic children. *Acta Derm. Venereol. [Stockh.]*, 1991; 71:263-66.
2. Metcalfe, D.D. and Sampson, H.A., Workshop on experimental methodology for clinical studies of adverse reactions to foods and food additives. *J. Allergy Clin. Immunol.*, 1990; 86:421-42.
3. Atherton, D.J., Skin manifestations of food allergy. In Hamburger RN: Food Intolerance in Infancy: *Allergology, Immunology and Gastroenterology*, Los Angeles/Raven Press, Ltd., 1989;145-54.
4. Oranje, A.P., Aarsen, R.S.R., Mulder, P.G.H. et al., Food immediate-contact hypersensitivity and elimination diet in young children with atopic dermatitis. Preliminary results in 107 children. *Acta Derm. Venereol. [Stockh.]*, 1992; 176: 41-4.
5. Dahl, M.V., Flare factors and atopic dermatitis. The role of allergy. *J. Dermatol. Science*, 1990; 1:311-8.
6. Salo, O.P., Mäkinen-Kiljunen, S., and Juntunen, K., Milk causes a rapid urticarial reaction on the skin of children with atopic dermatitis and milk allergy. *Acta Derm. Venereol. [Stockh.]*, 1986;66:438-42.
7. Gronemeyer, W., Fuchs, E., and Bandilla, K., "Reibtest" und RAST. *Z. Hautkr,* 1979; 54: 205-12.
8. Oranje, A.P., Skin provocation test (SAFT) based on contact urticaria: a marker of dermal food allergy. In: Vermeer, J., Ed., *Proceedings of Metabolic Disorders and Nutrition Related to the Skin,* Basel, Karger, 1991, 20:228-31.
9. Dreborg, S., *The Skin Prick Test,* Thesis, Linkoping, 1987.
10. Isolauri, E. and Turjanmaa, K., Combined skin prick and patch testing enhances identification of food allergy in infants with atopic dermatitis. *J. Allergy Clin. Immunol.,* 1996; 97:9-15.
11. Jarmoc, L.M. and Primack, W.A., Anaphylaxis to cutaneous exposure to milk protein. *Clin. Pediatr.,* 1987; 26: 154-5.
12. Court, J. and Lee-May, N.G., Danger of egg white treatment for nappy rash. *Arch. Dis. Child.,* 1984;59: 908.

26

Paronychia

Antonella Tosti and Bianca Maria Piraccini

CONTENTS

26.1   DEFINITION

Chronic paronychia (CP) is a common nail disorder that almost exclusively affects adult women. It is clinically characterized by a chronic inflammation of the proximal nail fold with or without nail plate abnormalities. CP usually has a prolonged course interspersed with recurrent self-limited episodes of acute exacerbations. Although the pathogenesis of CP is still being discussed, accumulating evidence indicates that in most cases the condition represents a clinical variety of contact urticaria.[1,2]

26.2   ANATOMY OF THE PROXIMAL NAIL FOLD

The nail unit consists of four specialized epithelia: the nail matrix, the nail bed, the hyponychium, and the proximal nail fold. The proximal nail fold, which surrounds the proximal nail plate, is a skin fold that consists of a dorsal and a ventral portion (Figure 26.1). The dorsal portion of the proximal nail fold is anatomically similar to the skin of the dorsum of the digit but thinner and devoid of pilosebaceous units. The ventral portion of the proximal nail fold, which can not be seen from the exterior and proximally continues with the germinative matrix, covers approximately one fourth of the nail plate. It closely adheres to the nail plate surface and keratinizes with a granular layer. The limit between the proximal nail fold and the nail matrix can be histologically established at the site of disappearence of the granular layer.

The horny layer of the proximal nail fold forms the cuticle, which is firmly attached to the superficial nail plate and prevents the separation of the nail plate from the proximal nail fold. The integrity of the cuticle is essential for maintaining the homeostasis of this region.

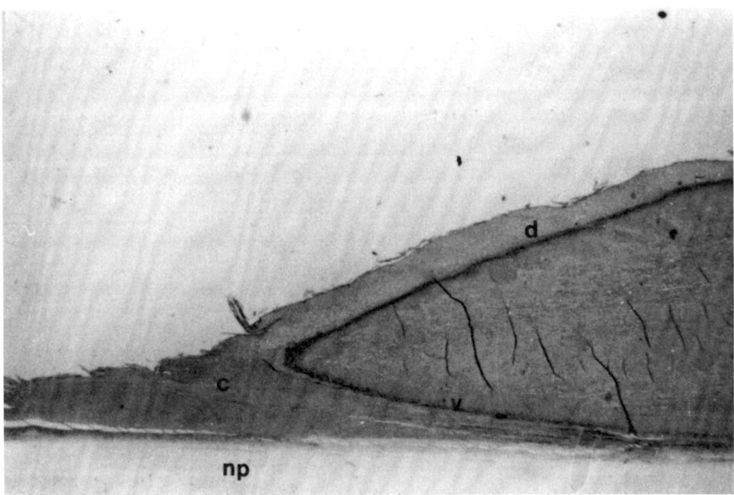

FIGURE 26.1   The proximal nail fold consists of a dorsal (d) and a ventral (v) portion. The horny layer forms the cuticle (c), which closely adheres to the underlying nail plate (np).

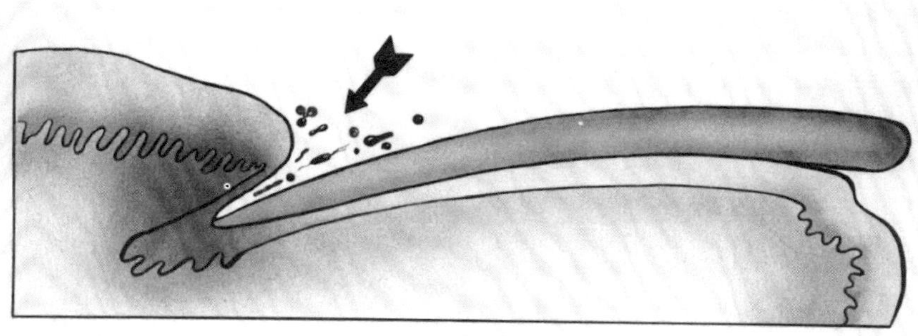

FIGURE 26.2 Schematic drawing of the pathogenesis of chronic paronychia.

26.3 PATHOGENESIS

CP is an environmental disease that results from an impairment of the epidermal barrier of the proximal nail fold. The first step in the development of CP is always a mechanical or chemical trauma that produces cuticle damage.

The cuticle can be injured in several ways including manicuring, occupational trauma, frequent handwashing, continuous exposure to water, and/or irritative compounds. In fact, CP almost exclusively affects housewives and some occupational groups which are exposed to environmental factors that may damage the cuticle. When the cuticle is damaged or lost, the epidermal barrier of the proximal nail fold is destroyed and the proximal nail fold is suddenly exposed to a variety of environmental hazards.

Irritants and allergens may easily penetrate the proximal nail fold and produce an inflammatory reaction of the nail fold and nail matrix, which interferes with the normal nail growth and therefore with the formation of a new cuticle. The proximal nail fold becomes progressively separated from the nail plate by a pocket, which has an important role in maintaining and aggravating CP. In fact, it becomes a receptacle for microorganisms and environmental factors that further promote the chronic inflammation (Figure 26.2).

Candida sp. and bacteria can frequently be isolated from the proximal nail fold of patients with CP. *Candida* and bacteria are responsible for the acute inflammatory exacerbations that occur during the course of the disease (Figure 26.3). CP is therefore a multifactorial condition which can be induced and maintained by several causes. Depending on the major etiological factor, CP can be classified in the following types.

26.3.1 Contact Allergy

CP may occasionally be a consequence of contact sensitization to common allergens. In these patients, CP is due to an acute contact dermatitis of the proximal nail fold (Allergic chronic paronychia) and the cause of sensitization may be disclosed by

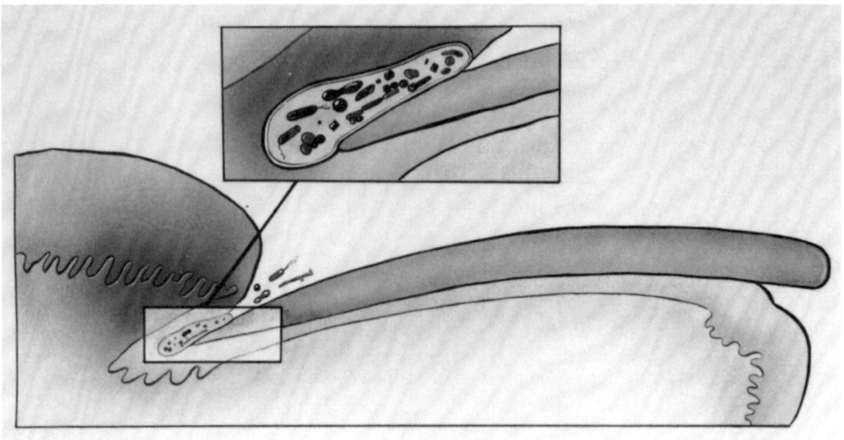

FIGURE 26.3   Schematic drawing of the acute flares of CP.

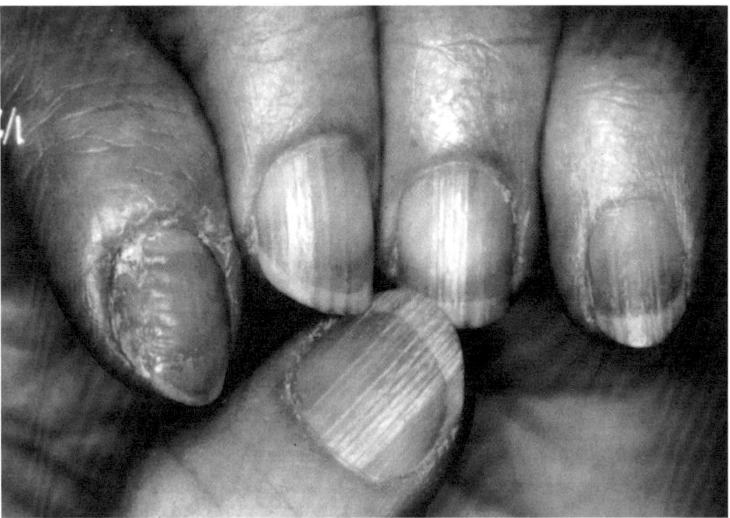

FIGURE 26.4   Allergic CP due to contact allergy to tioconazole contained in a nail solution.

patch testing. In our experience, allergic CP is most commonly caused by topical drug ingredients, rubber compounds, and mineral oil additives (Figure 26.4).

26.3.2   Food Hypersensitivity

CP due to immediate hypersensivity reaction to foods is a variety of immediate contact dermatitis due to foods.[2-4] It is more commonly seen in occupational food handlers but it can also occur in housewives with intense cooking activity. These patients develop an inflammatory reaction of the proximal nail fold associated with itching immediately after handling raw food ingredients.

In our experience, CP due to immediate food hypersensitivity is most commonly caused by tomatoes, garlic, onions, and flour, but other vegetables and fish can occasionally be involved.

The specific foods that are responsible for food hypersensitivity CP may, however, considerably vary in different countries depending on the eating habits of the resident population. Conventional patch tests are not useful for the diagnosis of this type of CP, which can be clearly identified with a provocative test using fresh foods on the proximal nail fold.

Patients with allergic contact paronychia as well as patients with chronic paronychia due to food hypersensitivity frequently harbor *Candida* sp. or bacteria in their proximal nail fold. *Candida* and bacteria colonization, however, is only a secondary phenomenon and treatment with antifungals or antibiotics is not useful.

26.3.3 *Candida* Hypersensitivity

Patients with CP may develop a hypersensitivity to *Candida* antigens. A similar reaction has previously been reported in patients with chronic recurrent vaginitis.[5]

These patients have negative patch tests, negative provocative tests, harbor *Candida* sp. in their proximal nail fold, but do not improve with systemic antifungals. They usually have an immediate reaction to the intradermal skin test with *Candida* and a positive provocative test to crude *Candida* antigen.

26.3.4 Irritative Reaction

Most patients with CP have negative patch tests and negative provocative tests. These patients, who improve with preventive measures and topical steroids, have an irritative dermatitis of the proximal nail fold.

Irritative CP is commonly seen in children who suck their thumbs. Thumb sucking CP results from the repetitive mechanical trauma associated with the maceration and the chemical irritation caused by saliva. In some occupational groups, irritative CP may be complicated by the penetration of small particles of organic or inorganic materials in the proximal nail fold. These include fragments of hair or thorns, metallic dusts, fiberglass particles, etc. Foreign bodies, however, usually only aggravate the inflammatory reaction, granulomatous infiltration being a rare evenience.

Patients with irritative chronic paronychia may subsequently acquire a secondary hypersensitivity and develop allergic chronic paronychia, food hypersensitivity paronychia, or *Candida* hypersensitivity paronychia.

26.3.5 *Candida* Paronychia

This is in our experience very uncommon, except for patients with chronic mucocutaneous candidiasis and HIV infection. In *Candida* paronychia, proximal nail fold inflammation is usually associated with proximal onycholysis (Figure 26.5) or onychomycosis due to *Candida*. *Candida* sp. can be isolated both from the proximal nail fold and clippings of the affected nail plate.

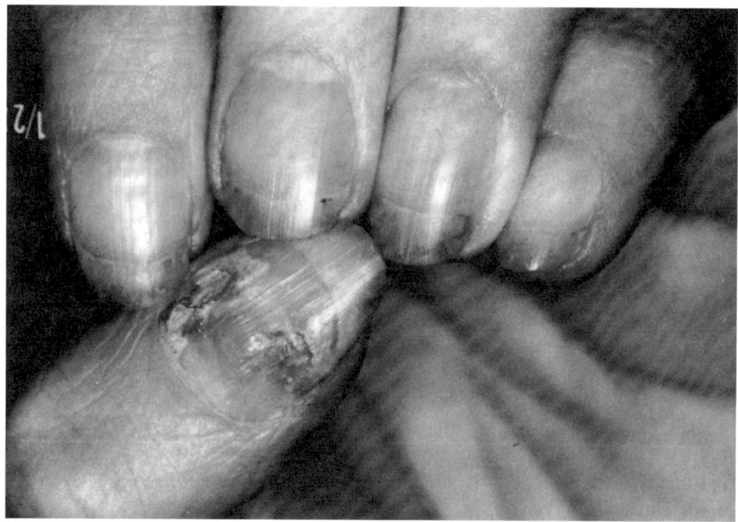

FIGURE 26.5   *Candida* paronychia: the proximal nail fold inflammation is associated with proximal onycholysis due to *Candida*.

Since the isolation of *Candida* sp. from the proximal nail fold is not exclusive to *Candida* paronychia, most cases of CP due to other causes being frequently associated with secondary *Candida* colonization, the diagnosis of *Candida* parony-chia can only be established on the basis of the results of treatment with systemic antifungals.

To summarize, therefore, CP may actually be due to various different conditions. These include allergic contact dermatitis, immediate hypersensitivity, irritative con-tact dermatitis, and, in a minority of cases, a true *Candida* infection.

26.4   CLINICAL FEATURES

CP is a fingernail disease that most frequently affects the second, third, and first digits of the dominant hand. It can involve one or several nails. Clinically, the affected finger shows mild erythema and swelling of the proximal nail fold. The cuticle is absent and the ventral portion of the nail fold is detached from the nail plate. In longlasting cases, the nail fold is retracted, thickened, and rounded.

The course of CP is interspersed with self-limited episodes of painful acute inflammation. Patients complain of worsening of the periungual erythema and puls-ing pain. The acute exacerbations of CP are most frequently due to secondary *Candida* and bacterial infections, with the formation of small abscesses in the space that formed between the proximal nail fold and the nail plate. These microbial abscesses drain spontaneously and this explains why the exacerbations of CP subside without treatment in a few days (Figure 26.3). Acute exacerbations of CP are not only due to microbial colonization, but can also be caused by irritants or allergens that penetrate the proximal nail fold and induce a contact dermatitis.

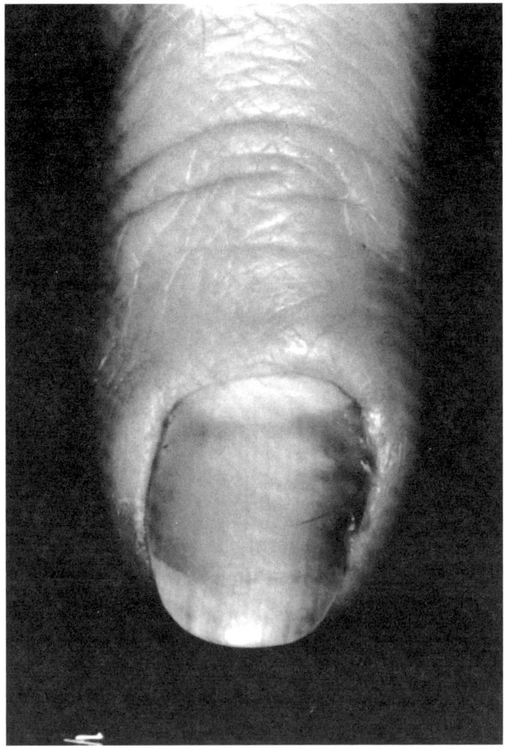

FIGURE 26.6   Green discoloration of the lateral margin of the nail due to *Pseudomonas aeruginosa* colonization.

The nails of patients with CP frequently present secondary nail plate abnormalities. Transverse grooves are retrospective indicators of previous acute flares. Onychomadesis is the result of matrix damage produced by a severe inflammatory exacerbation. Green discoloration of the lateral margins indicates secondary infection due to *Pseudomonas* (Figure 26.6).

26.5 PATHOLOGY

CP is pathologically characterized by eczematous changes of the proximal nail fold.[1] The proximal nail fold epithelium shows focal spongiosis, lymphocytic exocytosis, and parakeratosis. Fungal hyphae may be present in the stratum corneum. The dermis contains a moderately dense mononuclear superficial perivascular infiltrate. The pathological study of the proximal nail fold of patients with food hypersensitivity CP after a positive provocative test reveals marked eczematous changes with vesiculation and evident edema of the papillary dermis (Figure 26.7).

At the immunohistochemical study, an increased number of CD 1a+/CD4+ Langerhans cells are detected within the epidermis and superficial dermis. The

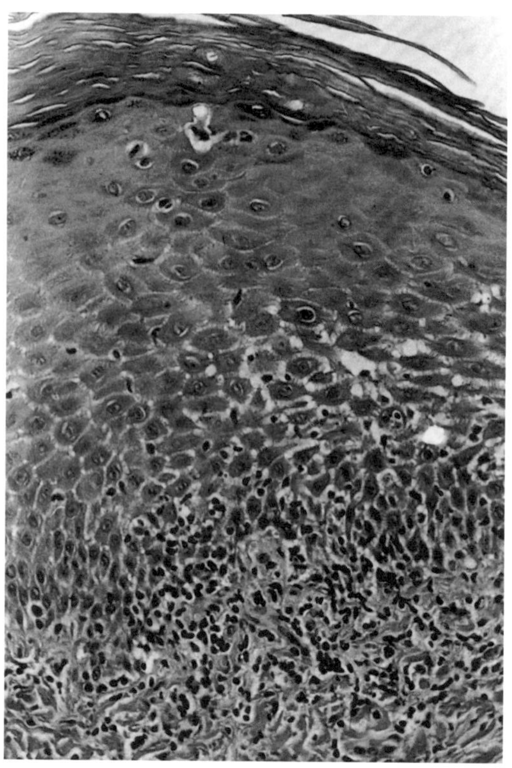

FIGURE 26.7 Pathology of the proximal nail fold after a positive provocative test: the epidermis shows marked spongiosis with vesiculation and lymphocytic exocytosis. A mononuclear inflammatory infiltration is present in the superficial dermis.

mononuclear infiltrate consists of mature T-peripheral lymphocytes (CD2+, CD3+, CD5+) with a CD4/CD8 ratio of 5–6/1.[2]

The pathological and immunohistochemical findings that characterize food hypersensitivity CP may be observed both in irritative contact dermatitis and allergic contact dermatitis and up to now there are no clinical, pathological, or immunological criteria that permit us to establish if this reaction is due to true allergy or to irritation.

26.6 DIAGNOSIS

The different types of CP may be distinguished by a careful clinical history and specific examinations (Table 26.1).

26.6.1 Anamnesis

Occupational and recreational activities should be researched in detail. Patients should be asked whether they have noticed if their condition worsens after handling any particular substance.

TABLE 26.1 Diagnosis of Chronic Paronychia

	Patch Tests	Provocative Tests	*Candida* sp. Isolation	Bacteria Isolation	Response To Systemic Antifungals
Allergic chronic paronychia	+	+/–	+/–	+/–	–
Food hypersensitivity with chronic paronychia	+/–	+	+/–	+/–	–
Candida hypersensitivity with chronic paronychia	–	–	+	+/–	–
Irritative chronic paronychia	–	–	–	–	–
Candida chronic paronychia	–	–	+	+/–	+

26.6.2 Allergological Evaluation

26.6.2.1 Patch Testing

When contact allergy is suspected, closed patch tests should be made with the standard series and additional allergens properly selected according to the patients anamnesis. Results should be read at 48 and 72 hours and, when possible, at day 7.

26.6.2.2 Provocative Tests

In food handlers and patients with a strenuous cooking activity, 20 minute open patch tests should be carried out using the fresh foods suspected of causing the dermatitis on the affected skin of the proximal nail fold.

This test should be performed when the patients are in a stable phase, at least 2 weeks after an acute exacerbation of the disease. Patients with immediate food hypersensitivity develop an immediate erythemato-edematous reaction associated with moderate itching which persists from several hours to a few days (Figure 26.8 and 26.9). In these patients, the same food which gave the positive provocative test may or may not produce a positive reaction when applied under closed or open patch test on the normal back skin or when tested with a scratch chamber test on the volar forearm. Results of prick tests are also variable.

26.6.3 Cultures

Samples should be taken from the affected nail fold using a moistened sterile swab. Nail clippings and subungual debris should also be cultured if proximal onycholysis and onychomycosis are present. In our experience, *Candida* sp. is isolated in about 60% of patients. The isolation of Gram+ or Gram- bacteria is common and only indicates secondary nail colonization.

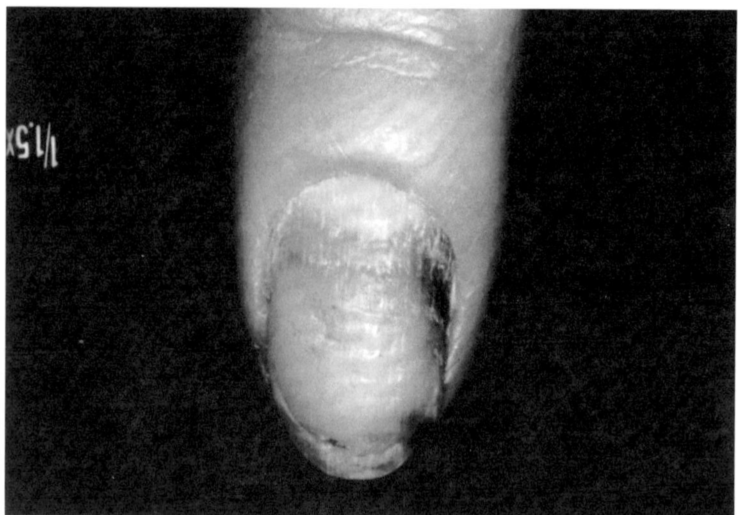

26.8

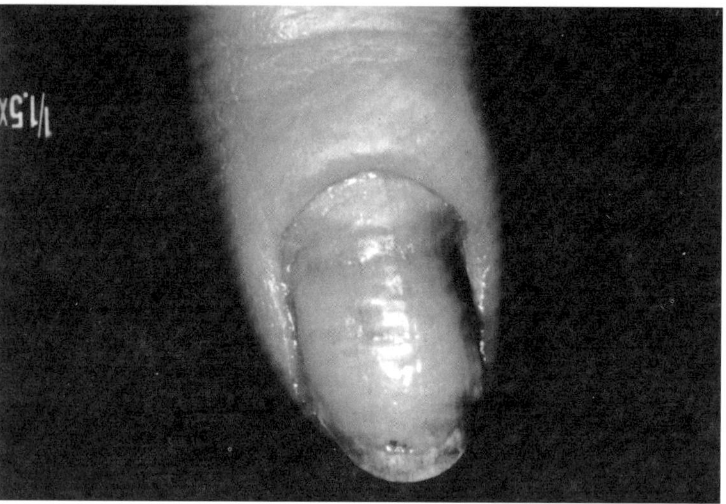

26.9

FIGURE 26.8 and 26.9   Contact hypersensitivity CP before (Figure 26.8) and after a provocative test with tomato. After 20 minutes (Figure 26.9) the proximal nail fold shows erythema and edema associated with intense itching.

26.7   DIFFERENTIAL DIAGNOSIS

Table 26.2 lists a number of conditions which may occasionally involve the proximal nail fold and be misdiagnosed as CP. In our experience, the differential diagnosis of CP mainly includes psoriasis and psoriasiform dermatoses, bullous dermatoses, digital ischemia, and tumors. Psoriasis and psoriasiform conditions may affect the distal digit and produce a CP due to retention of scales under the proximal nail fold. Etretinate treatment may aggravate this phenomenon.

TABLE 26.2	**Differential Diagnosis of Chronic Paronychia**

Acrodermatitis enteropathica
Acute paronychia
Atopic dermatitis
Bazex's syndrome
Chronic mucocutaneous candidiasis
Chronic radiodermatitis
Digital ischemia
Drugs   Retinoids
            Antineoplastics
Erythema multiforme
Frostbite
Granulomas
Metastases
Parakeratosis pustolosa
Pemphigoid
Pemphigus vulgaris
Pernio
Psoriasis
Sarcoidosis
Scytalidium infection
Syphilis (primary)
Tumors
Yellow nail syndrome

Bullous dermatoses, most commonly pemphigus vulgaris, may involve the ventral portion of the proximal nail fold and produce nail fold lesions that are clinically indistinguishable from CP. Digital ischemia frequently causes pseudoinflammatory changes of the periungual tissues with dark erythema and edema. Primary nail tumors and digital metastases can also produce swelling and erythema of the distal digit mimicking a CP.

26.8 TREATMENT

The correct treatment of CP can not be generalized since it requires the identification of different etiological factors that may cause the condition. Patients with CP need precise counseling on the environmental hazards that may elicit their condition, such as exposure to wet environment and microtrauma.

Patients with irritative CP as well as patients with CP due to contact allergy, food hypersensitivity, or *Candida* hypersensitivity greatly improve with the daily application of medium- or high-potency topical steroids. In severe cases, systemic steroids can be given for a few days to obtain a prompt reduction of inflammation and pain. If *Candida* is present, we also prescribe a topical imidazole derivative to be applied in the morning.[6] Systemic antifungals are not useful, except in the case of *Candida* paronychia, which is very uncommon.

CP can be considered cured only when the cuticle has completely regrown indicating that the barrier function of the proximal nail fold has been restored. This usually takes several months. If patients do not interrupt exposure to environmental hazards that may cause proximal nail fold damage, CP frequently relapses.

REFERENCES

1. Zaias, N., Paronychia, in *The Nail in Health and Disease*, 2nd ed., Zaias, N., Ed., Appleton & Lange, Norwalk, 1990, Chap. 13.
2. Tosti, A., Guerra, L., Morelli, R., Bardazzi F., and Fanti, P. A., Role of food in the pathogenesis of chronic paronychia, *J. Am. Acad. Dermatol.*, 27, 706, 1992.
3. Hjorth, N. and Roed-Petersen, J., Occupational protein contact dermatitis in food handlers, *Contact Dermatitis*, 2, 28, 1976.
4. Maibach, H., Immediate hypersensitivity in hand dermatitis, *Arch. Dermatol.*, 112, 1289, 1976.
5. Regulez, P., Garcia Fernandez, J. F., Moragues, M. D., Schneider, J., Quindos, G., and Ponton, J., Detection of anti-Candida albicans IgE antibodies in vaginal washes from patients with acute vulvovaginal candidiasis, *Gynecol. Obstet. Invest.*, 37, 110, 1994.
6. Tosti, A. and Piraccini, B. M., Diseases of the nails, in *Conn's Current Therapy*, Rakel, R. E., Ed., W. B. Saunders Company, 1996, 762.

27

Immediate and Delayed Type Protein Contact Dermatitis

Matti Hannuksela

CONTENTS

27.1   INTRODUCTION

Proteins are thought to cause mainly IgE-mediated immediate allergy manifested as allergic conjunctivitis, rhinitis, asthma, gastrointestinal disturbances, or contact urticaria. Sensitization occurs usually, if not always, via the airway and gastrointestinal mucosa. Antigen-presenting cells (APCs) process the antigens and present them to T-helper cells (Th). For unknown reasons, stimulation with protein allergens usually results in the formation of Th2 cells, B-cells, and humoral immunity. The Th1 subsets are also stimulated, leading to the formation of T-cells (Figure 27.1).[1,2]

High-affinity IgE receptors are found on mast cells, basophils, and Langerhans cells. Low-affinity receptors are found on a number of cells, including Langerhans cells, lymphocytes, macrophages, eosinophils, and platelets.[2] As a consequence of an epidermal challenge with protein allergens, we usually see allergic contact urticaria. It is caused by histamine derived from mast cell granules (Figure 27.2) and

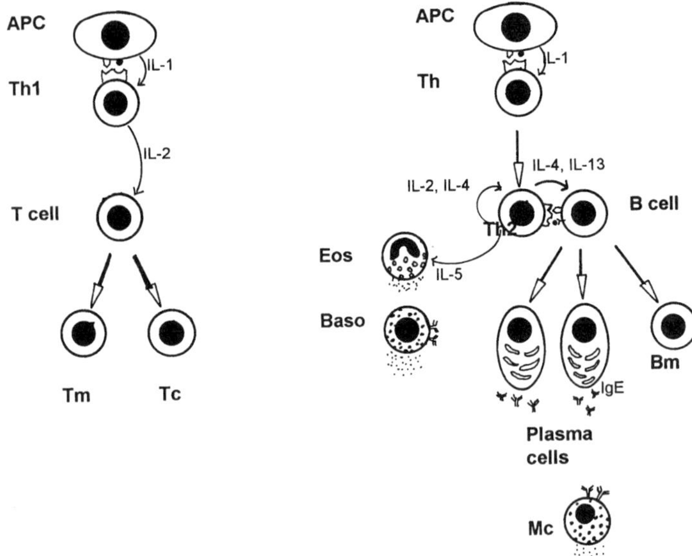

FIGURE 27.1   Simplified presentation of type I and type IV allergies. APC = antigen presenting cell, Th = T helper cell, Eos = eosinophil, Baso = basophil, Mc = mast cell, Bm = B memory cell, Tm = T memory cell, Tc = T cytotoxic (effector) cell, IL = interleukin.

can be prevented by antihistamines. IgE might not be the only immunoglobulin mediating immediate reactions. In the case of an immediate reaction from shiitake mushroom, no specific IgE except anti-shiitake IgG was found in the patient's serum.[3]

Sometimes vesicles resembling those seen in acute eczematous dermatitis appear within 20 minutes after the challenge.[4-6] The mechanism underlying the formation of such immediate vesiculation is unknown. Patients with immediate allergy may also contract real eczematous dermatitis.[3,5,7,8] The mechanism of this type of cutaneous reaction might be either an ordinary type IV allergic reaction or a reaction mediated by IgE bound on the Langerhans cells (Figure 27.2).

27.2   PROTEIN CONTACT DERMATITIS

Protein contact dermatitis was discovered as early as the 1930s. Peck[9] made patch and scratch tests with inhalant allergens and foods in 93 of children with atopic dermatitis. Of the 23 children up to 1 year of age, 9 were patch test positive and 10 scratch test positive. Two infants were patch test positive to wheat, 1 to egg and 1 to fish. Eight infants reacted to inhalant allergens in patch tests (6 to feathers, 1 to cow and sheep hairs, and 1 to dog hair). Out of the remaining 70 children, 18 reacted to inhalant allergens, but only 3 to foods in patch tests. The avoidance of allergens was usually beneficial for inhalants but not for foods.

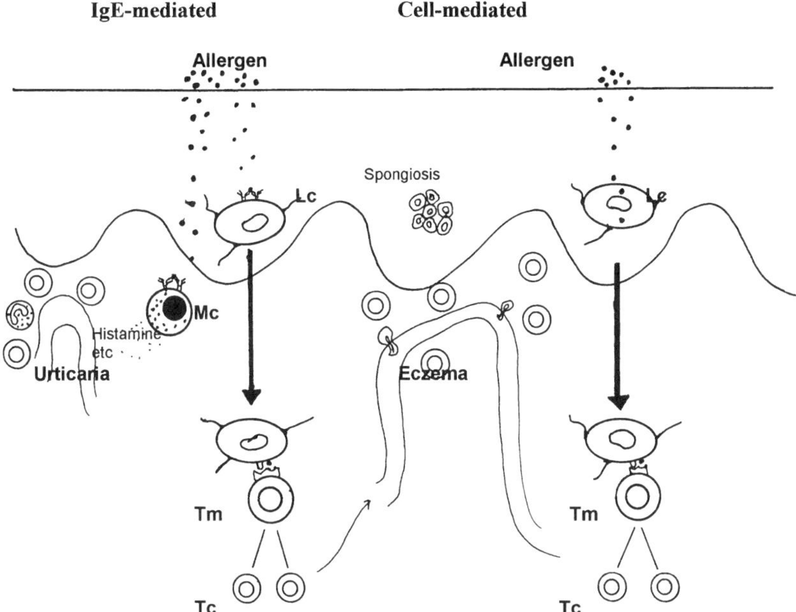

FIGURE 27.2 The IgE-mediated and cell-mediated mechanisms of protein contact dermatitis and urticaria. Lc = Langerhans cell, Mc = mast cell, Tm = T memory cell, Tc = T cytotoxic (effector) cell.

Cow milk also causes both immediate and delayed allergies in infants. Isolauri and Turjanmaa[10] tested 183 small children with moderate or severe atopic dermatitis. Double-blind placebo-controlled peroral challenge (DBPCPC) tests were positive in 54%. Of those reacting positively in the DBPCPC test, 48% reacted to milk in the skin prick test and 61% in the patch test. In the DBPCPC test negative group, the skin prick test was positive in 16% and the patch test in 18%. The sensitivity of the skin prick test alone was 48%, while that of the combination of prick and patch tests was as high as 86%.

In the 1930s and 1940s, a few doctors were interested in proteins as the cause of contact dermatitis,[11-13] but it was not until the 1980s that this interesting type of dermatitis became recognized again. Since then, house dust mite has attracted more attention than the other inhalant allergens as exacerbating contact agents in atopic dermatitis.

The term "protein contact dermatitis" was introduced by Hjorth and Roed-Petersen.[4] They found positive patch test reactions to garlic, onion, cress, carrot, chicory salad, leek, chives, horseradish, various fishes, lobster, and chicken in 1 to 7 of 33 food handlers with hand dermatitis suspected to be occupational.

27.3 PROTEIN CONTACT ALLERGENS IN ATOPIC DERMATITIS

Mite allergen *Der p* I has been shown to be responsible for the delayed patch test reactions in atopic patients with a positive skin prick test reaction to house dust mite[14,15] and also for the T-cell response *in vitro*.[16] When applied repeatedly, house dust mite produced dermatitis in both involved and uninvolved skin of patients with atopic dermatitis.[17] Patch test positivity to house dust mite seems to be connected with atopic dermatitis, but not with respiratory atopy. Palma-Carlos et al.[18] found positive patch test results to house dust mite in 45% of patients with atopic dermatitis only, in 77% of patients with atopic dermatitis and respiratory allergy, but in none of those with respiratory allergy only.

Patch test positivity to the house dust mite does not depend on the level of serum IgE. High serum IgE and positive patch tests to the mite were encountered in 32 out of 130 (25%) patients with atopic dermatitis, and low serum IgE and a positive patch test in 19 of 130 (15%).[19] Five of 16 atopic dermatitis patients with a positive patch test to *Dermatophagoides pteronyssinus* and 2 of 10 patch test positive to *D. farinae*, were RAST-negative.[20] Neither scratch nor intradermal test results showed any correlation with the patch test results.

The other protein contact allergens in atopic dermatitis producing positive patch test reactions include storage mite,[21] birch pollen,[18,22-25] grass pollen, weed pollens, fungi, cockroach, and animal danders[25,26] among others. *Pityrosporum ovale* belongs to the normal flora of the skin and can cause immediate allergy. In a chamber scarification patch test, it produced a positive response in 64% of patients with atopic dermatitis, but in only 3% of healthy volunteers.[27] Immediate hypersensitivity reactions were detected in skin prick tests, but no correlation was seen between the results of these two tests.

27.4 OCCUPATIONAL PROTEIN CONTACT DERMATITIS

Delayed allergic-type scratch chamber test and patch test results from a number of foodstuffs have been seen in food handlers.[4,5] Rub tests made in 7 food handlers with hand dermatitis and with positive delayed scratch chamber test results produced an eczematous reaction in 5 of them in 1–4 days: carrot, celeriac, orange peel, clove, and Jamaica pepper, each in 1 patient.[5] Positive patch tests to allspice, clove, cinnamon, ginger, paprika, almond, garlic, and iceberg lettuce were reported by Kanerva et al.[28] The authors used spices and other foods as is for patch testing, but considered testing with dilution series more informative. Of 70 spice factory workers, 36 reported skin symptoms, most commonly dry skin and itching.[29] Allergic contact dermatitis was diagnosed in 6 of them, and irritant contact dermatitis in 4. Cinnamic aldehyde and cinnamic alcohol produced positive patch tests, and cinnamic aldehyde positive skin prick tests. The test reactions were difficult to evaluate.

A cosmetician contracted severe hand dermatitis from a calf placenta extract, and in a scratch chamber test, dissolved extracts elicited positive reactions in 1 day and undissolved extracts in 2 days.[30] Cow dander is another animal protein to cause immediate and delayed contact allergies.[31] Susitaival et al.[32] examined 41 dairy farmers with hand dermatitis. Skin prick tests were done with a commercial cow dander extract. They were also subjected to scratch tests, a 20 min patch test and a 24 h patch test with dander from the patients' own cows. Fifteen patients showed immediate allergy only, 13 delayed allergy only, and 13 both immediate and delayed allergies. Seven of the 15 patients with immediate allergy alone reacted in the skin prick test only, 6 in the 20 min patch test only, and 2 in both. This result suggests that there might be two types of immediate allergic reactions, and a skin prick test is not sufficient to detect them both. The finding should be confirmed.

Shiitake mushroom (*Lentinus edodes*)[3,33] and flours[34] are further causes of both immediate and delayed allergies. Both allergies can be manifested as contact dermatitis.[34,35] Xylanase and cellulase have been reported to cause both allergic contact urticaria and delayed allergic contact dermatitis in one case each.[36] Alpha-amylase, a flour additive, showed an immediate response in a skin prick test or a scratch chamber test in 7 out of 32 bakers with baker's dermatitis.[35] Two of them showed a delayed response in the scratch chamber test. *Verbena* plants[37] and pearl oysters[38] are further examples of proteinaceous agents producing both immediate and delayed type occupational allergies.

Natural rubber latex allergy is usually mediated by IgE and can be detected by skin prick testing and RAST. There is some evidence but no definite proof that delayed type hypersensitivity with or without immediate allergy to latex proteins also occurs.[39-41]

27.5 MECHANISMS OF PROTEIN CONTACT DERMATITIS

Protein contact dermatitis has several possible mechanisms (Table 27.1). Irritation is obviously the most common, but is the least well known among them. Many housewives and other food handlers have noticed that tomato and sometimes also paprika irritate the skin.

TABLE 27.1   Types of Protein Contact Dermatitis (PCD) and Their Mediators and Possible Mechanisms

Type of PCD	Mediators and possible mediators
1. Irritation	Unknown.
2. Nonimmunologic CU	Prostaglandins. Mostly unknown.
3. Immunologic CU	a. IgE on mast cells. Histamine etc. are released.
	b. IgG(?) on mast cells.
	c. Unknown.
4. Eczematous dermatitis	a. Cell mediated T cell reaction.
	b. IgE on Langerhans cells.
	c. Prolonged or repeated CU.
5. Erythema multiforme	IgE-mediated?

Note: CU = contact urticaria.

Nonimmunologic contact urticaria from cinnamon is obviously caused by cinnamic alcohol, but the causative agents in other spices, e.g., in mustard, are unknown. The reaction may be only redness and itching, but real contact urticaria occurs in some cases and contact dermatitis in some others.

Immediate allergic contact dermatitis appearing as tiny vesicles, redness, and later also scaling is usually mediated by IgE, sometimes possibly by IgG. Skin prick testing might not always be sufficient to detect immediate allergy. There are some results to suggest that the 20 min patch test may be positive, while the prick test is negative.[32]

Erythema multiforme-like eruption may develop from epicutaneous exposure to chemicals and proteins. It is rare and its pathomechanism remains unclear.[42] *Thuja* essential oil,[42] capsicum,[43] and rubber latex[44] are examples of allergens that have caused, through skin contact, an eruption resembling erythema multiforme.

The results of concomitant skin prick and patch testing suggest that delayed allergic contact dermatitis may be mediated by IgE on Langerhans cells and by classical T-cell mediated contact allergy. There is some evidence to show that Th2 type cytokines play a role in a subclass of delayed type hypersensitivity.[45-47] This type of reactivity has been shown in contact allergy to nickel,[46] budesonide,[47] and tuberculin.[48]

The concentrations of allergens in test materials used for patch testing with proteins have ranged from that used in skin prick testing to 10,000 times this level.[9,15,23,49,50] Stripping may enhance the penetration of protein allergens into the skin,[49] but it may also increase the number of irritant reactions.[50] In individual cases, scratch chamber testing seems to be superior to patch testing in detecting contact allergy to proteins.[51] It is possible that a delayed type patch test reaction is nothing but an expression of normal immunity in part of the positive cases. Little is known about the clinical significance of positive patch test results.

In conclusion, protein contact dermatitis is a special form of contact dermatitis which has many mechanisms. These mechanisms are, so far, poorly known. Much work on this fascinating phenomenon should be done in the future. The optimal patch test concentration and the vehicle as well as the appropriate test procedure for a use test should be determined for each individual allergen. The cellular events, the mediators, and the influence of various exogenous factors in various types of protein contact dermatitis also remain to be clarified.

REFERENCES

1. Frew, A. J., The immunology of respiratory allergies. *Toxicol. Lett.* 1996: 86: 65-72.
2. Mygind, N., Dahl, R., Pedersen, S., and Thestrup-Petersen, K., *Essential Allergy.* Second edition. Oxford: Blackwell Science 1996: 12–55.
3. Tarvainen, K., Salonen, J.-P., Kanerva, L., Estlander, T., Keskinen, H., and Rantanen, T., Allergy and toxicodermia from shiitake mushrooms. *J. Am. Acad. Dermatol.* 1991: 24: 64–66.
4. Hjorth, N. and Roed-Petersen, J., Occupational protein contact dermatitis in food handlers. *Contact Dermatitis* 1976: 2: 28–42.

5. Niinimäki, A., Scratch-chamber tests in food handler dermatitis. *Contact Dermatitis* 1987: 16: 11–20.

6. Roger, A., Guspi, R., Garcia-Patos, V., Barriga, A., Rubira, N., Nogueiras, C., Castells, A., and Cadahia, A., Occupational protein contact dermatitis in a veterinary surgeon. *Contact Dermatitis* 1995: 32: 248–249.

7. Acciai, M.C., Brusi, C., Francalanci, S., Gola, M., and Sertoli, A., Skin tests with fresh foods. *Contact Dermatitis* 1991: 24: 67–68.

8. Pigatto, P.D., Riva, F., Altomare, G.F., and Parotelli, R., Short-term anaphylactic antibodies in contact urticaria and generalized anaphylaxis to apple. *Contact Dermatitis* 1983: 9: 511.

9. Peck, S.M., Eczema of infancy and childhood. *N.Y. State J. M.* 1934: 24: 957–964.

10. Isolauri, E. and Turjanmaa, K., Combined skin prick and patch testing enhances identification of food allergy in infants with atopic dermatitis. *J. Allergy Clin. Immunol.* 1996: 97: 9–15.

11. Taub, S.J. and Zakon, S.J., Neurodermatitis due to protein sensitization. *J. Allergy* 1933: 4: 53–59.

12. Hill, L.W., The classification of eczematoid eruptions in children with especial reference to contact dermatitis. *J. Ped.* 1942: 20: 537–548.

13. Epstein, S., Milker's eczema. *J. Allergy* 1948: 19: 333–341.

14. Mitchell, E.B., Crow, J., Chapman, M.D., Jouhal, S.S., Pope, F.M., and Platts-Mills, T.A.E., Basophils in allergen-induced patch test sites in atopic dermatitis. *Lancet* 1982: i: 127–130.

15. Platts-Mills, T.A.E., Mitchell, E.B., Rowntree, S., Chapman, M.D., and Wilkins, W.R., The role of dust mite allergens in atopic dermatitis. *Clin. Exp. Dermatol.* 1983: 8: 233–247.

16. Rawle, F.C., Mitchell, E.B., and Platts-Mills, T.A.E., T cell responses to the major allergen from the house dust mite Dermatophagoides pteronyssinus antigen P1: comparison of patients with asthma, atopic dermatitis, and perennial rhinitis. *J. Immunol.* 1984: 133: 195–201.

17. Norris, P.G., Schofield, O., and Camp, R.D.R., A study of the role of house dust mite in atopic dermatitis. *Br. J. Dermatol.* 1988: 118: 435–440.

18. Palma-Carlos, A.G., Palma-Carlos, M.L., and Caiado, E., Delayed skin reactivity to airborne allergens in atopic dermatitis. *Allergy* 1993: 48: Suppl.16: 18.

19. Imayama, S., Hashizume, T., Miyahara, H., Tanahashi, T., Takeishi, M., Kubota, Y., Koga, T., Hori, Y., and Fukuda, H., Combination of patch test and IgE for dust mite antigens differentiates 130 patients with atopic dermatitis into four groups. *J. Am. Acad. Dermatol.* 1992: 27: 531–538.

20. Kuwano, A., Sugai, T., Shoji, A., Katoh, J., Nagareda, T., and Teramae, K., Patch testing with *dermatophagoides* antigens prepared by Hollister-Stier in atopic dermatitis patients. *Environ. Dermatol.* 1994: 1: 34–41.

21. Vieluf, D., Przybilla, B., Baur, X., and Ring, J., Respiratory allergy and atopic eczema in thatcher due to storage and house dust mite allergy. *Allergy* 1993: 48: 212–214.

22. Reitamo, S., Visa, K., Kähönen, K., Käyhkö, K., Stubb, S., and Salo, O.P., Eczematous reactions in atopic patients caused by epicutaneous testing with inhalant allergens. *Br. J. Dermatol.* 1986: 114: 303–309.

23. Reitamo, S., Visa, K., Kähönen, K., Käyhkö, K., Lauerma, A.I., Stubb, S., and Salo, O.P., Patch test reactions to inhalant allergens in atopic dermatitis. *Acta. Derm. Venereol. (Stockh.)* 1989: Suppl 144: 119–121.

24. Räsänen, L., Reunala, T., Lehto, M., Virtanen, E., and Arvilommi, H., Immediate and delayed hypersensitivity reactions to birch pollen in patients with atopic dermatitis. *Acta Derm. Venereol. (Stockh.)* 1992: 72: 193–196.

25. Clark, R.A.F. and Adinoff, A.D., Aeroallergen skin prick testing and patch testing with patients with atopic dermatitis. *J. Allergy Clin. Immunol.*, 1990: 85: 206.

26. Langeland, T., Braathen, L.B., and Borch, M., Studies of atopic patch tests. *Acta Derm. Venereol. (Stockh.)* 1989: Suppl 144: 105–109.

27. Rokugo, M., Tagami, H., Usuba, Y., and Tomita, Y., Contact sensitivity to Pityrosporum ovale in patients with atopic dermatitis. *Arch. Dermatol.* 1990: 126: 627–632.

28. Kanerva, L., Estlander, T., and Jolanki, R., Occupational allergic dermatitis from spices. *Contact Dermatitis* 1996: 35: 157–162.

29. Meding, B., Skin symptoms among workers in a spice factory. *Contact Dermatitis* 1993: 29: 202–205.

30. von den Driesch, P., Fartasch, M., Diepgen, T.L., and Peters, K.P., Protein contact dermatitis from calf placenta extracts. *Contact Dermatitis* 1993: 28:46–47.

31. Schneider, W., Coppenrath, R., and Ruther, H., Über Tierhaar-Allergie. *Berufsdermatosen* 1960: 8: 1–13.

32. Susitaival, P., Husman, L., Hollmén, A., Horsmanheimo, M., Husman, K., and Hannuksela, M., Hand eczema in Finnish farmers. A questionnaire based clinical study. *Contact Dermatitis* 1995: 32: 150–155.

33. Salonen, J.-P., Tarvainen, K., Kanerva, L., Keskinen, H., Valta, R., and Kotimaa, M., Ruokasienten tuotannossa syntyvät allergiat. *Suom Lääkäril* 1990: 45: 2441–2445.

34. Pigatto, P.D., Polenghi, M.M., and Altomare, G.F., Occupational dermatitis in bakers a clue for atopic contact dermatitis. *Contact Dermatitis* 1987: 16: 263–271.

35. Morren, M.-A., Janssens, V., Dooms-Goossens, A., van Hoyeveld, E., Cornelis, A., de Wolf-Peeters, C., and Heremanns, A., Alpha-Amylase, a flour additive: An important cause of protein contact dermatitis in bakers. *J. Am. Acad. Dermatol.* 1993: 29: 723–728.

36. Kanerva, L. and Tarvainen, K., Allergic contact dermatitis and contact urticaria from cellulolytic enzymes. *Amer. J. Contact Dermatitis* 1990: 1: 244–245.

37. Potter, P.C., Mather, S., Lockey, P., Knottenbelt, J.D., Paulsen, E., Skov, P.S., and Andersen, K.E., Immediate and delayed contact hypersensitivity to verbena plants. *Contact Dermatitis* 1995: 33: 343–346.

38. Nakamori, M., Matsuo, I., and Ohkido, M., Coexistence of contact urticaria and contact dermatitis due to pearl oysters in an atopic dermatitis patient. *Contact Dermatitis* 1996: 34: 438.

39. Lezaun, A., Marcos, C., Martín, J.A., Quirce, S., and Díez Gómez, M.L., Contact dermatitis from natural latex. *Contact Dermatitis* 1992: 27: 334–335.

40. Wyss, M., Elsner, P., Wütrich, B., and Burg, G., Allergic contact urticaria from natural latex without contact urticaria. *Contact Dermatitis* 1993: 28: 154–156.

41. Placucci, F., Vincenzi, C., Ghedini, G., Piana, G., and Tosti, A., Coexistence of type I and IV allergy to rubber latex. *Contact Dermatitis* 1996: 34: 76.

42. Puig, L., Fernández-Figueras, M.-T., Montero, M.-A., Ferrándiz, C., and Alomar, A., Erythema-multiforme-like eruption due to topical contactants: expression of adhesion molecules and their ligands and characterization of the infiltrate. *Contact Dermatitis* 1995: 33: 329–332.

43. Raccagni, A.A., Bardazzi, F., Baldari, U., and Righini, M.G., Erythema-multiforme-like contact dermatitis due to capsicum. *Contact Dermatitis* 1995: 33: 353–354.

44. Bourrain, J.-L., Woodward, C., Dumas, V., Caperan, D., Beani, J.-C., and Amblard, P., Natural rubber latex contact dermatitis with features of erythema multiforme. *Contact Dermatitis* 1996: 35: 55–56.

45. Marcinkiewicz, J. and Chain, B.M., Regulation of *in vitro* release of Th2 type cytokines (IL-4, IL-6) in the T cell response to the trinitrophenyl (TNP) hapten. *Cell. Immunol.* 1993: 146: 406–411.

46. Probst, P., Küntzlin, D., and Fleischer, B., Th2-type infiltrating T cells in nickel induced contact dermatitis. *Cell. Immunol.* 1995: 165: 134–140.

47. Koga, T., Fujimura, T., Imayama, S., Katsuoka, K., Toshitani, S., and Hori, Y., The expression of Th1 and Th2 type cytokines in a lesion of allergic contact dermatitis. *Contact Dermatitis* 1996: 35: 105–106.

48. Ohmen, J.D. et al., Overexpression of IL-10 in atopic dermatitis. Contrasting cytokine patterns with delayed-type hypersensitivity reactions. *J. Immunol.* 1995: 154: 1956–1963.

49. Langeweld-Wildschut, E.G., Thepen, T., and Bruynzeel-Koomen, C.A.F.M., The atopy patch test; its sensitivity and specificity and a comparison of different methods. *Allergy* 1993: 48: Suppl 16: 18.

50. van Voorst Vader, P.C., Coenraads, P.J., Nater, J.P., Lier, J.G., and Worst, T.E., Atopic dermatitis: methodology of patch tests with house dust mite allergens. *Br. J. Dermatol.* 1990: 123: 675–676.

51. el Sayed, F. and Bazex, J., Scratch-chamber tests in meat handler's dermatitis. *Contact Dermatitis* 1994: 30: 256.

28

The Oral Allergy Syndrome

Ronald van Ree

CONTENTS

28.1 INTRODUCTION

The Oral Allergy Syndrome (OAS) can be regarded as a special form of the Contact Urticaria Syndrome, localized in mouth and throat. When food-related allergic symptoms are diagnosed as OAS, we are generally referring to an IgE-mediated type I allergic response. This syndrome is most frequently observed in pollen-allergic subjects.[1-5] Probably the best known example of pollen-related OAS is allergy to fruits of the family of the *Rosaceae* (apple, peach, pear, etc.) in patients suffering from birch pollinosis.[6-8] It is now well accepted, that crossreactivity of IgE antibodies is the explanation of such linked allergies.[6,9] Several related structures in pollen and fruits were identified over the past decade.[10,11] At first, their close resemblance was shown by means of *in vitro* methods like RAST-inhibition. More recently, the introduction of recombinant technology has resulted in the actual demonstration of structural homology between pollen and food allergens.[12-15] The close relationship between pollen-allergy and OAS was recently illustrated in a very special way: ceremonial consumption of corn pollen by Navajo Indians induces OAS.[16]

28.2 CLINICAL PRESENTATION

Symptoms related to OAS are (usually) of the immediate type, occurring within minutes after oral contact with the food in question. They include oralpharyngeal pruritis (itching of mouth, palate, and throat), angioedema (swelling) of lips, tongue, and palate, and hoarseness. The immediate character of the reactions, in combination with the presence of specific IgE antibodies, confirms an IgE-mediated mechanism.

The oral symptoms are not always isolated, but can be accompanied by reactions in the gastrointestinal tract or by systemic reactions like urticaria, rhinitis, asthma, or anaphylactic shock.[1,2] Whether reactions remain restricted to mouth and throat is, at least partly, dependent on the allergen source. OAS caused by pollen-related allergy to fruits like apple and peach is hardly ever accompanied by gastrointestinal or systemic reactions. In contrast, oral symptoms caused by, for example, consumption of celery can often give systemic reactions like anaphylactic shock.[2,17,18]

Whether symptoms remain limited to mouth and throat or not seems to be (at least partly) determined by the stability of the allergens involved. It is well-known that allergens in extracts from fruits, like, e.g., apple, are very labile.[19,20] Consequently, *in vivo* diagnostics (skin prick testing) is only possible with material directly derived from fresh fruit.[21] The major apple allergen, Mal d 1,[13,22] is a protein closely related to the major birch pollen allergen Bet v 1.[12,23] Recently, Vieths et al. reported that Bet v 1 is, indeed, a highly heat-labile and protease-sensitive structure (Eighth International Paul-Ehrlich-Seminar, March 11–13 1996, Bethesda, U.S.). Shrimp is a food that frequently causes more systemic reactions (e.g., anaphylactic shock), in combination with OAS. The major allergen from shrimp has been identified as a muscle protein, tropomyosin.[24-26] This structure is, in contrast to Bet v 1-like proteins, very heat-stabile.[27]

Food allergens capable of reaching other organs than mouth and throat seem to affect, predominantly, those organs that are already involved in allergic reactions caused by inhalant allergens. In other words, the "weak links in the chain" are most likely to be affected. Housedust-mite allergic subjects can develop allergy to foods of invertebrate animal origin, like crustaceans and mollusks. Like in the case of pollen and vegetable foods, crossreactive IgE antibodies are the explanation of this phenomenon.[28-30] In a group of 28 patients with mite-related asthma and food allergy to snails, all subjects demonstrated asthmatic episodes after consumption of snails.[30]

28.3 OAS NOT RELATED TO INHALANT ALLERGENS

As mentioned, OAS is usually observed in patients with respiratory allergies. In these cases, sensitization is caused by the inhalant allergen. The observation that the onset of respiratory allergies preceeds that of the food-related OAS supports this mechanism of "cross-sensitization."[1,31] Furthermore, several RAST- and blot-inhibition studies have demonstrated that IgE-binding to food allergens is completely inhibited by the crossreactive inhalant allergen, whereas in the opposite case hardly any inhibition is observed.[29,30,32-36]

Not all patients with OAS suffer from respiratory allergies. Several foods have been shown to induce OAS, independent from inhalant allergens. A clear example is peanut allergy, recently reviewed by Loza et al.[37] Two major allergens indicated in peanut allergy are Ara h 1 and Ara h 2. These allergens do not have their related homologues in pollen. Several fruits were also reported to cause OAS without pollinosis.[38-41] Not much is known about the allergens involved in this "pure" fruit allergy. A 30 kD allergen and an 8–10 kD allergen were suggested to be important.[38,40] Symptomatology in fruit-allergic patients without pollinosis seems to be more severe, including anaphylactic shock[38] (Dr. M. Fernández Rivas, personal communication). Again, this might indicate that the responsible allergens are more stable than the classical OAS-inducing allergens, like Mal d 1. Sensitization probably occurs in the gastrointestinal tract, OAS being just one of the resulting symptoms.

28.4 DIAGNOSIS OF OAS

The quality of both *in vivo* and *in vitro* diagnostic products for OAS is rather poor. As mentioned, allergens in food extracts are frequently labile resulting in false negative diagnoses. On the other hand, a positive diagnosis is not always supported by clinical symptoms. Patients with a positive RAST or skin prick test for a group of different cross-reactive vegetable foods often only demonstrate symptoms to a selection of these foods.[4,42,43] In some cases, a positive diagnostic test is not at all accompanied by symptoms. To date, the most reliable form of diagnosis of food allergy seems to be the double-blind placebo-controlled food challenge.[44] The identification of individual structures in food extracts, responsible for the allergic response, might change this.

28.5 POLLEN-RELATED OAS: WHICH ALLERGENS ARE INVOLVED?

Three IgE binding structures involved in pollen-vegetable food crossreactivity were identified over the past decade: Bet v 1-related proteins, profilin, and carbohydrate determinants on glycoproteins.[10,11] For Bet v 1, it is beyond discussion that its homologues in fruits can cause OAS. Profilin was more recently identified as a cross-reactive allergen.[45,46] Profilin is present in all eukaryotic cells, resulting in a very broad spectrum of IgE cross-reactivity.

IgE antibodies of some patients recognize vegetable foods largely on the basis of profilin.[11,46] This is illustrated for two sera in Figure 28.1. Depletion of these sera of their anti-profilin IgE resulted in an almost complete loss of IgE-reactivity with several foods. One of these patients reported OAS related to vegetable foods (Figure 28.1B), the other suffered from generalized urticaria (Figure 28.1A). For

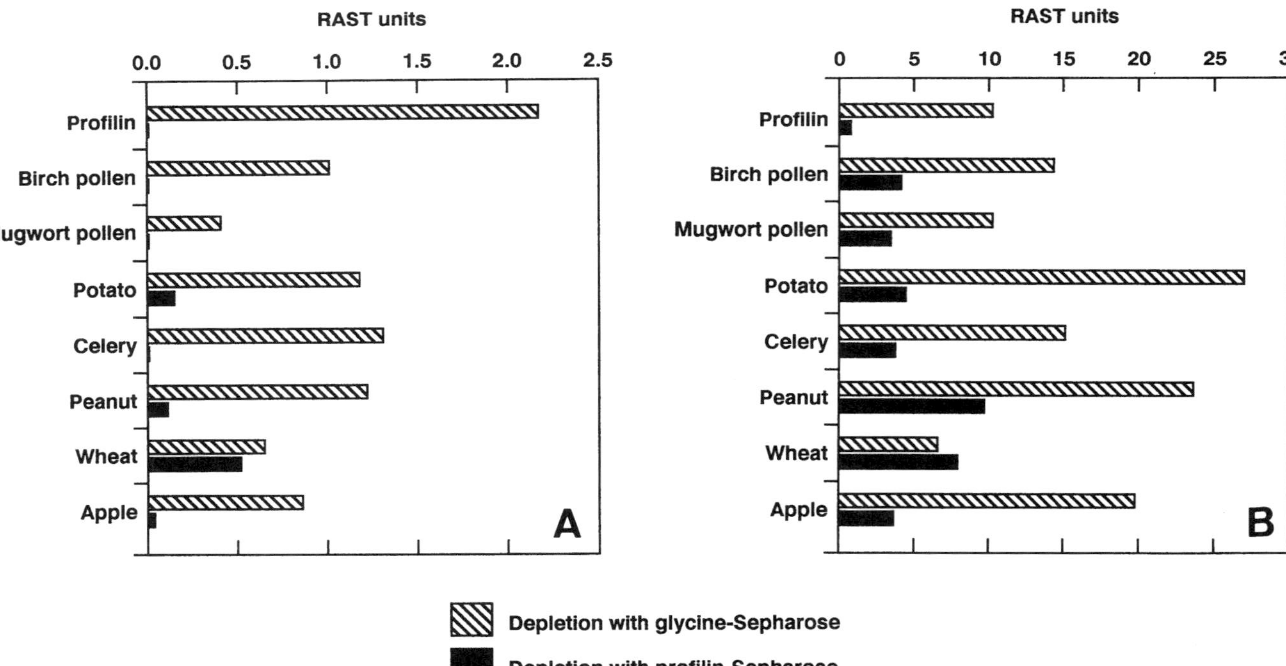

FIGURE 28.1 Depletion of anti-profilin IgE. Anti-profilin IgE was removed from two sera (Figure 28.1A and 28.1B) by incubation with Sepharose-coupled profilin from *Lolium perenne* grass pollen.[34] As a negative control, glycine-inactivated Sepharose was used. The depleted sera were, subsequently tested in a RAST[49] for profilin (efficiency of depletion), 2 pollen and 5 vegetable foods. Only the reactivity with wheat flour is unaffected.

patients from Mediterranean countries, with OAS caused by *Rosaceae* fruits like peach and apple, profilin was reported to be an important allergen.[34] In this case, the sensitizing pollen was grass pollen instead of birch pollen (Bet v 1), the latter being virtually absent in the Mediterranean climate zone.

As they did for Bet v 1, Vieths et al. investigated the stability of profilin. They reported a higher stability than found for Bet v 1 (Eighth International Paul-Ehrlich-Seminar, March 11–13 1996, Bethesda, U.S.). This perhaps explains why profilin, in some cases, was linked to more systemic reactions.[46,47]

Patients with IgE antibodies directed to carbohydrate determinants (N-linked glycans) have a very similar spectrum of crossreactivity as observed in the case of profilin (Figure 28.2). The basic structure recognized by these IgE antibodies is a N-glycan of the complex type (Figure 28.3). Their immunogenicity in mammals is determined by the presence of a fucose, $\alpha(1,3)$-linked to the proximal GlcNAc, and a xylose, $\beta(1,2)$-linked to the core mannose.[48] These structures are also found in N-glycans of invertebrate animals. For this reason, sera with N-glycan specific IgE often also bind to seafoods and insect venoms.[49] Patients with IgE antibodies directed to carbohydrate determinants usually do not demonstrate OAS or any other symptoms upon contact with the foods, recognized by their IgE. The identification and isolation of the three structures involved in pollen-vegetable food cross-reactivity facilitates discrimination between clinically relevant (e.g., giving OAS) and irrelevant structures.

28.6 BIOLOGICALLY ACTIVE VS. INACTIVE IgE ANTIBODIES?

Subjects with food-specific IgE antibodies do not always have food allergy, as was shown in the case of carbohydrate-specific IgE. In addition, not all patients with birch pollinosis and crossreactive IgE antibodies to Bet v 1 and its homologue in apple (Mal d 1) demonstrate OAS upon contact with apples.[12] What is the explanation for this? Of course, the titer of crossreactive IgE is important. It has been reported that birch pollen-related OAS is more severe during the birch pollen season, when IgE titers tend to increase.[12,32,50] This, however, cannot be the full explanation. Patients with high titers of food-specific IgE can be completely symptom-free.

A possible explanation might be the number of cross-reactive epitopes that is recognized on a food allergen. Cross-linking of mast cell-bound IgE is only possible when at least 2 epitopes are recognized. Most glycoproteins in the molecular weight range of allergens (10–70 kD) contain a single N-glycan.[51-54] If cross-reactivity between pollen and vegetable foods is purely based on N-glycans, these foods will not be able crosslink IgE and cause histamine release. Similarly, cross-reactivity between pollen and foods, linked to Bet v 1 or profilin, can be single- or multi-epitope based. This hypothesis is illustrated in Figure 28.4.

28.7 IMMUNOTHERAPY AS A TREATMENT OF OAS?

Pollinosis can be successfully treated by immunotherapy. How does immunotherapy affect the related OAS? Only a limited number of studies have addressed this

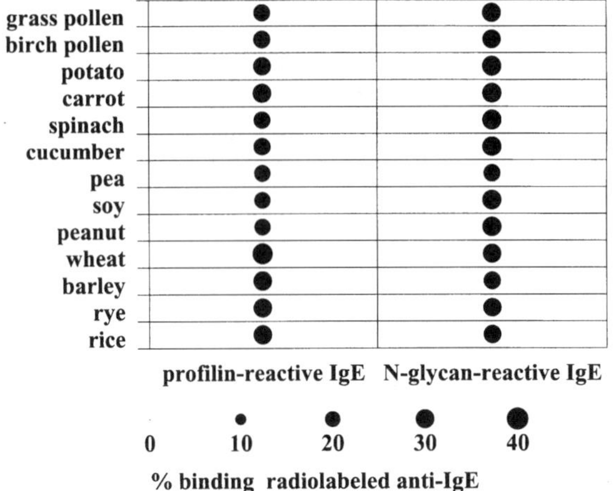

FIGURE 28.2   Sera with a broad spectrum of crossreactivity. RAST results are shown for two sera with pollen and vegetable foods. The serum on the left is profilin-reactive, the one on the right is carbohydrate-reactive. Serologically both patients are indistinguishable. Only the profilin-reactive serum has food-related symptoms.

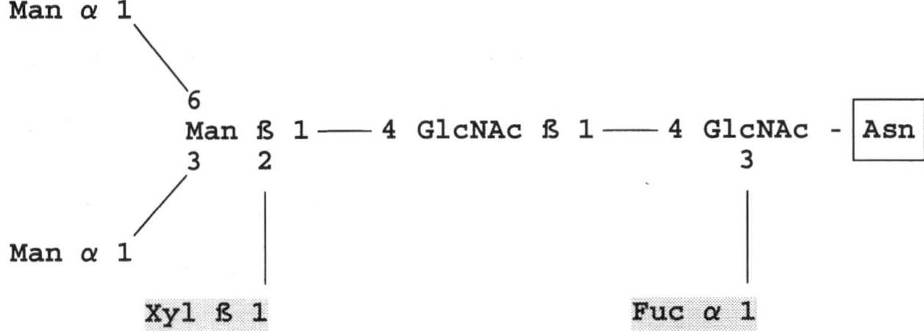

FIGURE 28.3   Basic structure of plant-derived complex N-glycans. N-glycans are attached to an asparagine (Asn) of a glycoprotein. The plant-specific monosaccharides in the structure are shaded. Man: mannose, GlcNAc: N-acetyl-glucosamine, Fuc: fucose and Xyl: xylose.

question,[55-57] but not in a double-blind placebo-controlled way. The consensus of these papers is that birch pollen immunotherapy probably has some beneficial effect on the food allergy.

In contrast, housedust mite immunotherapy was suggested to induce OAS occasionally.[58] In the course of therapy, IgE antibodies against snails and shrimps were induced. For one patient, it was demonstrated that these new IgE antibodies were directed to tropomyosin in mites, and were cross-reactive with tropomyosin in snail and shrimp. The patient reported a strong increase in oral allergic symptoms upon consumption of shrimps. Tropomyosin is the major allergen of shrimp.[24,25]

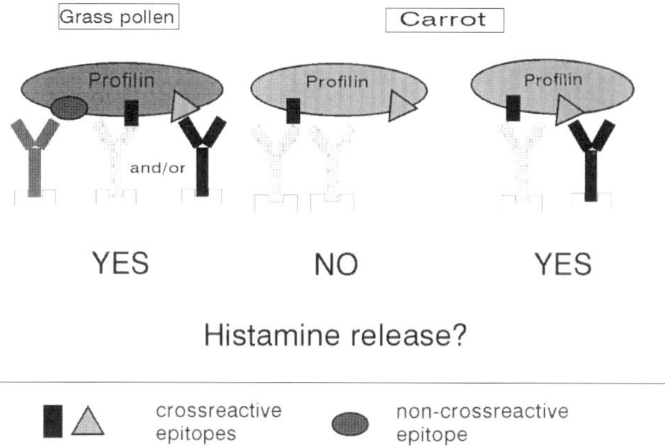

FIGURE 28.4   One or two crossreactive epitopes? A hypothetical explanation for the observation that not all patients with crossreactive IgE to profilin have food-related symptoms. As an example profilin from grass pollen and from carrot are depicted. When only one cross-reactive epitope is recognized, no histamine release can be induced by carrot profilin.

Both possible beneficial and detrimental effects of immunotherapy on OAS deserve attention. Clear answers will only be obtained in well-designed double-blind placebo-controlled trials.

28.8 CONCLUDING REMARKS

- The oral allergy syndrome is, in most cases, a result of the development of respiratory allergies. When not linked to inhalant allergens, OAS seems to be more frequently accompanied by severe symptoms (anaphylactic shock).
- The identification and isolation of cross-reactive allergens involved in OAS (Bet v 1 and profilin) enables the improvement of diagnostic products for this type of food allergy. So far, the golden standard still is the double-blind placebo-controlled food challenge.
- The presence of high titers of specific IgE in the absence of symptoms might be explained by a too limited number of (cross-reactive) epitopes recognized.
- The potential of immunotherapy for the treatment of OAS remains to be determined. Both improvement and induction of OAS have been indicated.

REFERENCES

1. Ortolani, C., Ispano, M., Pastorello, E. A., Bigi, A., and Ansaloni, R. The oral allergy syndrome, *Ann. Allergy*, 61, 47, 1988.
2. Ortolani, C., Pastorello, E. A., Farioli, L., Ispano, M., Pravettoni, V., Berti, C., Incorvaia, C., and Zanussi, C., IgE-mediated allergy from vegetable allergens, *Ann. Allergy*, 71, 470, 1993.

3. Boccafogli, A., Vicentini, L., Camerani, A., Cogliati, P., D'Ambrosi, A., and Scolozzi, R., Adverse food reactions in patients with grass pollen allergic respiratory disease, *Ann. Allergy*, 73, 301, 1994.

4. Bernhisel-Broadbent, J., Allergenic cross-reactivity of foods and characterization of food allergens and extracts, *Ann. Allergy, Asthma Immunol.*, 75, 295, 1995.

5. Pastorello, E. A., Incorvaia, C., and Ortolani, C., Atlas on mechanisms in adverse reactions to food. The mouth and pharynx, *Allergy*, 50 (Suppl. 20), 41, 1995.

6. Lahti, A., Björksten, F., and Hannuksela, M., Allergy to birch pollen and apple, and crossreactivity of the allergens studied with the RAST, *Allergy*, 35, 297, 1980.

7. Löwenstein, H. and Eriksson, N. E., Hypersensitivity to foods among birch pollen-allergic patients, *Allergy*, 38, 577, 1983.

8. Dreborg, S. and Foucard, T., Allergy to apple, carrot and potato in children with birch pollen allergy, *Allergy*, 38, 167, 1983.

9. Halmepuro, L., Vuontela, K., Kalimo, K., and Björksten, F., Cross-reactivity of IgE antibodies with allergens in birch pollen, fruits and vegetables, *Int. Arch. Allergy Appl. Immunol.*, 74, 235, 1984.

10. Calkhoven, P. G., Aalbers, M., Koshte, V. L., Pos, O., Oei, H. D., and Aalberse, R. C., Cross-reactivity among birch pollen, vegetables and fruits as detected by IgE antibodies is due to at least three distinct cross-reactive structures, *Allergy*, 42, 382, 1987.

11. Van Ree, R. and Aalberse, R. C., Pollen-vegetable food crossreactivity: serological and clinical relevance of crossreactive IgE, *J. Clin. Immunoassay*, 16, 124, 1993.

12. Ebner, C., Birkner, T., Valenta, R., Rumpold H., Breitenbach, M., Scheiner, O., and Kraft, D., Common epitopes of birch and apples- Studies by Western and Northern blotting, *J. Allergy Clin. Immunol.*, 88, 588, 1991.

13. Vanek-Krebitz, M., Hoffmann-Somergruber, K., Laimer da Camara Machado, M., Susani, M., Ebner, C., Kraft, D., Scheiner, O., and Breiteneder, H., Cloning and sequencing of Mal d 1, the major allergen from apple (*Malus domestica*), and its immunological relationship to Bet v 1, the major birch pollen allergens, *Biochem. Biophys. Res. Comm.*, 214, 538, 1995.

14. Breiteneder, H., Hoffmann-Sommergruber, K., O'Riordain, G., Susani, M., Ahorn, H., Ebner C., Kraft, D., and Scheiner, O., Molecular characterization of Api g 1, the major allergen of celery (*Apium graveolens*), and its immunological relationships to a group of 17-kDa tree pollen allergens, *Eur. J. Biochem.*, 233, 484, 1995.

15. Rihs, H. P., Rozynek, P., May-Taube, K., Welticke, B., and Baur, X., Polymerase chain reaction based cDNA cloning of wheat profilin: A potential plant allergen, *Int Arch. Allergy Immunol.*, 105, 190, 1994.

16. Freeman, G. L., Oral corn pollen hypersensitivity in Arizona Native Americans: some sociologic aspects of allergy practice, *Ann. Allergy*, 72, 415, 1994.

17. Pauli, G., Bessot, J. C., Dietemann-Molard, A., Braun, P. A., and Thierry, R., Celery sensitivity: clinical and immunological correlations with pollen allergy, *Clin. Allergy*, 15, 273, 1985.

18. Wütrich, B., Stägter, J., and Johansson, S. G. O., Celery allergy associated with birch and mugwort pollinosis, *Allergy*, 45, 566, 1990.

19. Björksten, F., Halmepuro, L., Hannuksela, M., and Lahti, A., Extraction and properties of apple allergens, *Allergy*, 35, 671, 1980.

20. Rudeschko, O., Fahlbusch, B., Henzgen, M., Schlenvoigt, G., Herrmann, D., Vieths, S., and Jäger, L., Investigation of the stability of apple allergen extracts, *Allergy*, 50, 575, 1995.

21. Rosen, J. P., Selcow, J. E., Mendelson, L. M., Grodofsky, M. P., Factor, J. M., and Sampson, H. A., Skin testing with natural foods in patients suspected of having food allergies: is it a necessity?, *J. Allergy Clin. Immunol.*, 93, 1068, 1994.

22. Vieths, S., Janek, K., Aulepp, H., and Petersen, A., Isolation and characterization of the 18-kDa major apple allergen and comparison with the major birch pollen allergen *(Bet v I)*, *Allergy*, 50, 421, 1995.

23. Breiteneder, H., Pettenburger, K., Bito, A., Valenta, R., Kraft, D., Rumpold, H., Scheiner, O., and Breitenbach, M., The gene coding for the major birch pollen allergen *BetvI*, is highly homologous to a pea disease resistence response gene, *EMBO J.*, 8, 1935, 1989.

24. Shanti, K. N., Martin, B. M., Nagpal, S., Metcalfe, D. D., and Rao, P. V., Identification of tropomyosin as the major shrimp allergen and characterization of its IgE-binding epitopes, *J. Immunol.*, 151, 5354, 1993.

25. Daul, C. B., Slattery, M., Reese, G., and Lehrer, S. B., Identification of the major brown shrimp (*Penaeus aztecus*) allergen as the muscle protein tropomyosin, *Int. Arch. Allergy Immunol.*, 105,49, 1994.

26. Leung, P. S. C., Chu, K. H., Chow, W. K., Ansari, A., Bamdea, C. I., Kwan, H. S., Nagy, S. M., and Gershwin, M. E., Cloning, expression, and primary structure of *Metapenaeus ensis* tropomyosin, the major heat-stable shrimp allergen, *J. Allergy Clin. Immunol.*, 94, 882, 1994.

27. Lehrer, S. B., Ibanez, M. D., McCants, M. L., Daul, C. B., and Morgan, J. E., Characterization of water-soluble shrimp allergens released during boiling, *J. Allergy Clin. Immunol.*, 85, 1005, 1990.

28. Witteman, A. M., Akkerdaas, J. H., Van Leeuwen, J., Van der Zee, J. S., and Aalberse, R. C., Identification of a cross-reactive allergen (presumably tropomyosin) in shrimp, mite and insects, *Int. Arch. Allergy Immunol.*, 105, 56, 1994.

29. De Maat-Bleeker, F., Akkerdaas, J. H., Van Ree, R., and Aalberse, R. C., Vineyard snail allergy possibly induced by sensitization to house-dust mite (*Dermatophagoides pteronyssinus*), *Allergy*, 50, 438, 1995.

30. Van Ree, R., Antonicelli, L., Akkerdaas, J. H., Pajno, G. T. B., Barberio, G., Corbetta, L., Ferro, G., Zambito, M., Garritani, M. S., Aalberse, R. C., and Bonifazi, F., Asthma after consumption of snails in house-dust-mite-allergic patients: a case of IgE cross-reactivity, *Allergy*, 56, 387, 1996.

31. Asero, R., Massironi, F., and Velati, C., Detection of prognostic factors for oral allergy syndrome in patients with birch pollen hypersensitivity, *J. Allergy Clin. Immunol.*, 97, 611, 1996.

32. Hirschwehr, R., Valenta, R., Ebner, C., Ferreira, F., Sperr, W. R., Valent, P., Rohac, M., Rumpold, H., Scheiner, O., and Kraft, D., Identification of common allergenic structures in hazel pollen and hazelnuts: a possible explanation for sensitivity to hazelnuts in patients allergic to tree pollen, *J. Allergy Clin. Immunol.*, 90, 927, 1992.

33. Akkerdaas, J. H., Van Ree, R., Aalbers, M., Stapel, S. O., and Aalberse, R. C., Multiplicity of crossreactive epitopes on *Bet v I* as detected with monoclonal antibodies and human IgE, *Allergy*, 50, 215, 1995.

34. Van Ree, R., Fernández Rivas, M., Cuevas, M., Van Wijngaarden, M., and Aalberse, R. C., Pollen-related allergy to peach and apple: an important role for profilin, *J. Allergy Clin. Immunol.*, 95, 726, 1995.

35. Ebner, C., Hirschwehr, R., Bauer, L., Breiteneder, H., Valenta, R., Ebner, H., Kraft, D., and Scheiner, O., Identification of allergens in fruits and vegetables: IgE cross-reactivities with the important birch pollen allergens Bet v 1 and Bet v 2 (birch profilin), *J. Allergy Clin. Immunol.*, 95, 962, 1995.

36. Valenta, R. and Kraft, D., Type I allergic reactions to plant-derived food: a consequence of primary sensitization to pollen allergens, *J. Allergy Clin. Immunol.*, 97, 893, 1996.
37. Loza, C. and Brostoff J., Peanut allergy, *Clin. Exp. Allergy*, 25, 493, 1995.
38. Wadee, A. A., Boting, L. A., and Rabson A. R., Fruit allergy: demonstration of IgE antibodies to a 30 kd protein in several fruits, *J. Allergy Clin. Immunol.*, 85, 801, 1990.
39. Antico, A., Sindrome orale allergica da monosensibilizzazione al kiwi (*Actinidia chinensis*), *Folia Allergol. Immunol, Clin.*, 37, 273, 1990.
40. Lleonart, R., Cisteró, A., Carreira, J., Batista, A., and Moscoso del Prado, J., Food allergy: identification of the major IgE-binding component of peach (*Prunus persica*), *Ann. Allergy*, 69, 128, 1992.
41. Antico, A., Oral allergy syndrome induced by chestnut (*Castanea sativa*), *Ann. Allergy*, 76, 37, 1996.
42. Wütrich, B. and Dietschi, R., Das "Sellerie-Karotten-Beifuss-Gewürz-Syndrom": Hauttest- und RAST-ergebnisse, *Schweiz. Med. Wochenschr.*, 115, 258, 1985.
43. Bircher, A. J., Van Melle, G., Haller, E., Curty, B., and Frei, P. C., IgE to food allergens are highly prevalent in patients allergic to pollens, with and without symptoms of food allergy, *Clin. Exp. Allergy*, 24, 367, 1994.
44. Bock, S. A., *Intestinal Immunology and Food Allergy*, Nestlé Nutrition Workshops Series, Vol. 34, Raven Press, New York, 1995, 105.
45. Valenta, R., Duchene, M., Ebner, C., Valent, P., Sillaber, C., Deviller, P., Ferreira, F., Tejkl, M., Edelmann, H., Kraft, D., and Scheiner, O., Profilins constitute a novel family of functional plant pan-allergens, *J. Exp. Med.*, 175, 377, 1992.
46. Van Ree, R., Voitenko, V., Van Leeuwen, W. A., and Aalberse, R. C., Profilin is a cross-reactive allergen in pollen and vegetable foods, *Int. Arch. Allergy Immunol.*, 98, 97, 1992.
47. Fäh, J., Wütrich, B., and Vieths, S., Anaphylactic reaction to lychee fruit: evidence for sensitization to profilin, *Clin. Exp. Allergy*, 25, 1018, 1995.
48. Faye, L. and Chrispeels, M.J., Common antigenic determinants in the glycoproteins of plants, molluscs and insects, *Glycoconjugate J.*, 5, 245, 1988.
49. Aalberse, R. C., Koshte, V., and Clemens, J. G. J., Immunoglobulin E antibodies that crossreact with vegetable foods, pollen, and Hymenoptera venom, *J. Allergy Clin. Immunol.*, 68, 356, 1981.
50. Foglé-Hansson, M. and Bende, M., The significance of hypersensitivity to nuts in patients with birch pollen allergy, *Allergy*, 48, 282, 1993.
51. Perez, M., Ishioka, G. Y., Walker, L. E., and Chesnut, R. W., cDNA cloning and immunological characterization of the rye grass allergen *Lol p* I, *J. Biol. Chem.*, 265, 16210, 1990.
52. Petersen, A., Becker, W. M., Moll, H., Blümke M., and Schlaak, M., Studies on the carbohydrate moieties of the timothy grass pollen allergen *Phl p* I, *Electrophoresis*, 16, 869, 1995.
53. Van Ree, R., Hoffman, D., Van Dijk, W., Brodard, V., Mahieu, K., Koeleman, C. A. M., Grande M., Van Leeuwen, W. A., and Aalberse, R. C., Lol p 11, a new major grass pollen allergen is a member of a family of soybean trypsin inhibitor-related proteins, *J. Allergy Clin. Immunol.*, 95, 970, 1995.
54. Batanero, E., Villalba, M., and Rodríguez, R., Glycosylation of the major allergen from olive tree pollen. Allergenic implications of the carbohydrate moiety, *Mol. Immunol.*, 31, 31, 1994.

55. Henzgen, M., Schlenvoigt, G., Diener, C., and Jäger, L., Nahrungsmittelallergie bei Frühblüherpollinosis und deren Beeinflussung mittels Hyposensibilisierung, *Allergologie*, 14, 90, 1991.
56. Pauli, G., De Blay, F., Bessot, J. C., and Dietemann, A., The association between respiratory allergies and food hypersensitivities, *Allergy Clin. Immunol. News*, 4, 43, 1992.
57. Kelso, J. M., Jones, R. T., Tellez, R., and Yunginger, J. W., Oral allergy syndrome successfully treated with pollen immunotherapy, *Ann. Allergy Asthma Immunol.*, 74, 391, 1995.
58. Van Ree, R., Antonicelli, L., Akkerdaas, J. H., Garritani, M. S., Aalberse, R. C., and Bonifazi, F., Possible induction of food allergy during mite immunotherapy, *Allergy*, 51, 108, 1996.

29

Combined Skin Prick and Patch Testing Enhances Identification of Food Allergy in Infants with Atopic Dermatitis*

Erika Isolauri and Kristiina Turjanmaa

CONTENTS

29.1   BACKGROUND

Evidence for causal linkage between atopic dermatitis and food allergy stems from therapeutic benefit after exclusion of dietary allergens,[1] and the dermatologic outcome seems to be more favorable if the patient loses the food hypersensitivity.[2-5]

---

* From *J. Allergy Clin. Immunol.*, 1996; 97:9–15. With permission.

Demonstration that certain foods can cause or exacerbate atopic dermatitis is laborious, particularly in infancy, when these conditions are most prevalent.[6]

Most food allergies involve an IgE-mediated hypersensitivity reaction, and patients with atopic dermatitis very often show immediate reactions in skin tests with foods.[7-9] Positive skin prick test responses with dietary allergens, however, do not necessarily imply a role for these allergens in the pathogenesis of atopic dermatitis.[10] Double-blind, placebo-controlled food challenges demonstrated acute-onset clinical reactions consisting of urticaria, pruritus, and erythema in a subset of patients with atopic dermatitis,[7,8,11] whereas others had delayed-onset eczematous reactions.[9,11-13] No relationship has been established between reactivity in skin prick tests and delayed-onset clinical reactions.[6]

The aim of this study was to delineate diagnostic methods of food allergy in infants. For this purpose patients with atopic dermatitis were randomized to double-blind, placebo-controlled, and open cow milk challenges to compare and characterize respective clinical reactions. Skin tests were performed before challenge. Specifically, we aimed to determine whether patch tests eliciting delayed-type hypersensitivity reaction[14] in combination with skin prick tests giving IgE-mediated hypersensitivity reaction could provide an indicator of allergy to cow milk in infants with atopic dermatitis.

29.2 METHODS

29.2.1 Patients

The study comprised 183 children ranging in age from 2 to 36 months (mean 14 months) and fulfilling the Hanifin criteria[15] of atopic dermatitis in children. They had been referred to a teaching pediatric or dermatologic clinic for evaluation of atopic dermatitis and were not selected on the basis of suspected allergy to cow milk. The mean age (95% confidence interval, [CI]) at onset of dermatitis was 4 months (95% CI, 3.5 to 5 months), and the duration of breast-feeding, exclusively and totally, was 3.5 months (95% CI, 3 to 4 months) and 6 months (95% CI, 5 to 7 months), respectively. Gastrointestinal disturbance such as loose stools, vomiting, or diarrhea and respiratory symptoms such as wheezing were seen in 61 and six patients, respectively. There was a family history of atopic disorders in 128 (70%) of the cases.

For 4 weeks before oral milk challenges the patients were given no cow milk. Instead they received breast milk (11%) or a tolerated formula (soy milk 39%, an extensively hydrolyzed whey protein formula 24%, or an amino acid-derived formula 26%). Based on the clinical history, previous skin testing, and/or RAST, the diet additionally excluded egg in most of the cases, cereals, wheat, barley, rye, and oat in 13%, and various fruits and vegetables in 19%. No patient was receiving systemic corticosteroid therapy.

Antihistamine medication was discontinued for periods of 3 days to 6 weeks before skin testing depending on the drug's duration of action. Skin tests were performed during the cow milk elimination period, always by the same person, and were scored (K. T.) before the result of oral milk challenge was known. The total IgE concentration in serum was measured, and RAST was performed to detect circulating cow milk-specific IgE antibodies before the challenge.

The patients were randomized to double-blind, placebo-controlled or open cow milk challenge to compare the respective rates of positive clinical reactions. The diet of the patients remained unaltered during the challenge period. Informed consent was obtained from the parents. The study was reviewed and approved by the Ethical Committee of Tampere University Hospital.

29.2.2 Double-Blind, Placebo-Controlled, Cow Milk Challenge Protocol

On the first day of the challenge, rising doses of the allocated placebo or test formula (1, 5, 10, 50, and 100 ml) were given at approximate 30-minute intervals until milk intake appropriate for the age was reached. The placebo formula was the amino acid-derived Neocate (SHS Int. Ltd., Liverpool, U.K.), and the test formula consisted of Neocate and 10 gm skimmed cow milk powder/100 ml. The concentration of β-lactoglobulin in the placebo preparation was 0.24 µg/L,[16] and the β-lactoglobulin concentration in the test formula was comparable to that in cow milk, 4,000,000 µg/L.[17] The placebo and the test formula preparations looked and smelled alike. A computerized randomization scheme was used to fix the sequence of the challenges so that the nursing staff, attending pediatricians, parents, and investigators were unaware of the administered formula's nature.

The challenge period was 1 week for both the placebo and the test formula. The challenge was begun in the hospital and after the first day was continued in the patient's home. The formulas were prepared under code in the hospital's milk bank for daily administration in age-appropriate doses. For 7 days after commencement of challenge with the placebo or the test formula, the parents recorded any clinical symptoms, specifically skin eruptions and pruritus, vomiting, and irritability. They also noted all stools, describing them as solid, loose, or watery. When a clinical reaction appeared, the challenge was stopped and the patients examined in the hospital. Onset of reaction was defined as the time between the latest dose and the specific symptom and from the start of the challenge. In like manner, the dose eliciting the symptom and the cumulated dose from the start of the challenge were determined. All patients were examined on day 7 and on day 14 of the challenge, and the code was thereafter opened.

29.2.3 Open Cow Milk Challenge Protocol

The open challenges were made with a ready-to-use infant formula containing 192,000 µg/L β-lactoglobulin (Mäkinen-Kiljunen S., unpublished data). The challenge period was 1 week. The challenge was started in the hospital when rising doses of the infant formula were given in the same way as in the blinded challenges. The challenge then continued in the patient's home, and the parents recorded the symptoms of the child. The patients were reviewed in the hospital at the time of any adverse reaction. The challenge was discontinued when a clinical reaction was noticed. All patients were examined on day 7 of the challenge.

Cow milk allergy was defined as an unequivocal adverse reaction to challenge. To judge long-term tolerance and reveal any false-negative result of challenge, all patients negative to challenge continued to consume cow milk. All patients were seen 1 month after commencement of challenge, when the diagnosis was confirmed for both challenge types by the same investigator (E. I.).

29.2.4 Skin Testing

Prick testing was done on the volar aspect of the forearm with a commercially available cow milk allergen, ALK (Allergologisk Laboratorium A/S, Horsholm, Denmark), and a milk powder diluted to normal feed concentration. A 1 mm, one-peak lancet with shoulder to prevent deeper penetration (ALK) was used, and 10 mg/ml histamine dihydrochloride (ALK) was used as positive control. Reactions were read at 15 minutes, and half of the histamine reaction size was recorded as positive (2+).

In patch testing 20 mg humidified skimmed cow milk powder containing 450 µg β-lactoglobulin was applied on uninvolved skin to the patient's back with aluminium cups (Finn Chamber, Epitest Ltd., Hyrylä, Finland) and Scanpore tape. In the morning of the test day, 300 mg of the milk powder was mixed with 0.2 ml of isotonic saline solution to make a "porridge" that remains on the test cup. The same stock was used for several tests during the same day. The occlusion time was 48 hours, and the results were read 15 minutes after removal of the cups and then at 72 hours. Reactions were classified as negative, irritation (IR), significant erythema (?+), and erythema with edema or eczema (+). Microcrystalline cellulose was used as negative control. In a preliminary study patch testing with cow milk was performed on eight nonatopic infants ranging in age from 11 to 32 months with no sign of cow milk allergy. All these tests were negative.

In addition to skin testing with cow milk, prick and patch tests were done for a long list of dietary antigens.

29.2.5 Statistics

The results of the double-blind, placebo-controlled, and open cow milk challenges are given separately and also when the indexes of sensitivity, specificity, and likelihood ratios of positive and negative results for prick and patch tests are calculated alone or in combination (parallel and serial testing). Because of skewed distribution of serum total IgE concentration, logarithmic (ln) transformation was used. Student's two-tailed independent t test and chi square test were used in statistical comparisons. Concordance of prick and patch test results and the concordance of skin prick testing with the commercially available cow milk allergen (ALK) or a milk powder diluted to normal feed concentration were estimated by the Cohen's κ statistic. The McNemar test was used to evaluate the usefulness of parallel and serial skin testing with prick and patch tests compared with that of either test alone.

29.3 RESULTS

Of the total 183 cow milk challenges, 99 (54%) gave results interpreted as positive. The mean (95% CI) age of the patients was 14 months (12 to 16 months) in the positive and 14 months (13 to 16 months) in the negative group; $t = 0.24$, $p = 0.81$. The mean serum IgE concentration was higher in the positive group than in the negative group, viz. 45 kU/L (95% CI, 30 to 67 kU/L) versus 23 kU/L (95% CI, 14 to 37 kU/L); $t = 2.16$, $p = 0.03$. Cow milk-specific IgE antibodies, RAST ≥ 0.4 kU/L, were detected in 55% and 25% of the respective groups; chi square test = 12.61, $p = 0.0004$.

29.3.1 Clinical Reactions to Cow Milk Challenge

There was a 54% positive reaction rate in the 118 patients with double-blind, placebo-controlled challenge and also in the 65 openly challenged patients. In eight cases (blinded challenge three cases and open challenge five cases) the challenge was repeated because of a concomitant viral infection. All placebo challenges were negative. In one case a negative blinded challenge was followed by clinical reactions to open cow milk feeding, making a 1% rate of false-negative challenge.

Of the 99 positive responses to challenge, 49 involved acute-onset pruritus, urticaria, and/or ex anthema, and the other 50 involved delayed-onset reactions of eczematous type (Table 29.1). The symptoms were confined to the skin in 68 of the 99 patients. Vomiting and diarrhea occurred in seven patients with acute-onset reactions, and loose stools or diarrhea occurred in 24 patients with delayed-onset reactions. Respiratory symptoms including wheezing and sneezing occurred in two patients with acute-onset reactions to the challenge.

TABLE 29.1   Reaction Onset Time and Dose, Mean (95% CI), Eliciting the Specific Reaction to Double-Blind, Placebo-Controlled and Open Cow Milk Challenge in Patients with Atopic Dermatitis

	Challenge type	Acute reaction	Delayed reaction
Reaction onset (hr)			
From the last dose	Double-blind	0.1 (0.1–0.2)	5 (4–7)[a]
	Open	0.2 (0.1–0.2)	6 (4–9)[a]
From the start of challenge	Double-blind	1.0 (0.7–1.3)	34 (25–44)[a]
	Open	0.9 (0.6–1.2)	34 (21–46)[a]
Dose eliciting the symptom (ml)			
Last dose	Double-blind	11 (6–16)	87 (78–96)[a]
	Open	9 (3–14)	88 (77–99)[a]
Cumulated dose	Double-blind	21 (10–33)	250 (200–300)[a]
	Open	25 (5–45)	269 (201–337)[a]

[a] Differences statistically significant (Student's t test: $p = 0.0001$) compared with acute-onset reactions.

TABLE 29.2   Skin Prick and Patch Tests for Cow Milk Allergy in Relation to Result of Double-Blind, Placebo-Controlled Cow Milk Challenge (Open Challenge)[a] in Patients with Atopic Dermatitis

| | Double-blind, placebo-controlled challenge (Open challenge) | |
Skin tests	Percent positive $n = 64$ (35)	Percent negative $n = 54$ (30)
Prick		
Positive	48 (47)	14 (17)
Negative	52 (53)	86 (83)
Patch		
Positive	61 (59)	19 (17)
Negative	39 (41)	81 (83)

[a] The results are given separately for double-blind, placebo-controlled, cow milk challenge and (open challenge in parentheses).

29.3.2   Relationship Between Clinical Response and Skin Test Reactivity

Combined prick and patch testing could be performed in the scheduled elimination period in 143 patients, whereas in 40 of 183 cases persistent eczema did not allow skin testing. Of these patients 65 (45%) had multiple food allergies. There were no differences in the family history of atopy between multisensitized and monosensitized patients, but the patients with multiple food allergies showed atopic dermatitis earlier, at 2.8 (95% CI 2.3 to 3.3) months of age compared with the monosensitized patients, at 5.0 (4.1 to 5.9) months; $t = 3.87$, $p = 0.0002$. The patients with multiple food allergies were more frequently (69%) positive to the cow milk challenge than were the monosensitized patients (46%); chi square test = 9.30, $p = 0.002$. The clinical reaction to the cow milk challenge was more frequently confined to the skin (82%) in the multisensitized patients compared with the monosensitized patients (57%); chi square test = 7.03, $p = 0.008$, and a reaction of acute-onset type to low volumes of milk was seen in 64% and 37% of the respective subgroups; chi square test = 7.38, $p = 0.007$. Altogether 13 (15%) patients with negative reaction to cow milk challenges had clinically significant skin test reactivity to egg, cereals, wheat, barley, rye, or oat.

Prick testing with the commercially available cow milk allergen ALK and the milk powder diluted to normal feed concentration gave comparable results: Cohen's κ statistic for concordance was 0.86, with 95% CI 0.77 to 0.95.

Table 29.2 presents the skin test results in relation to the response to blinded and open cow milk challenge. Skin test reactivity was proportionally similar in double-blind, placebo-controlled, and open challenge. Positive prick and patch test responses were associated with negative oral challenge in 14% to 19% of cases (Table 29.2). False-negative skin test results, however, were much more common, which was attributable to the high rate of inappropriately negative prick test results in patients with delayed-onset clinical reactions, whereas patch test results tended to be negative

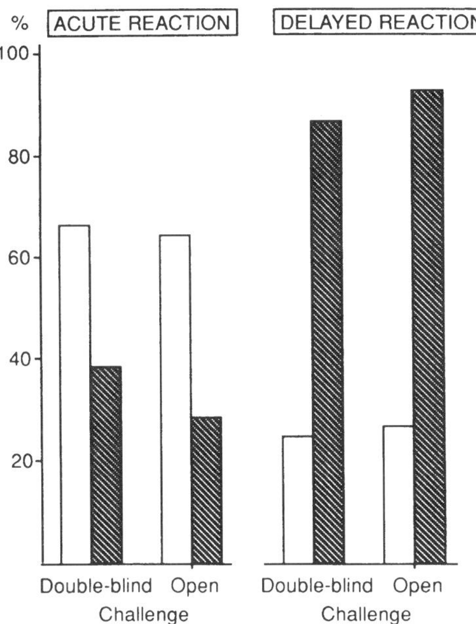

FIGURE 29.1   Correlation of skin test reactivity to cow milk in patients with atopic dermatitis showing acute (n = 49) or delayed (n = 50) clinical reaction to cow milk challenge. *Open bars* denote percent of patients with positive prick test results and *hatched bars* denote percent with positive patch test results. Results are given separately for double-blind, placebo-controlled and open cow milk challenges.

in patients with acute-onset clinical reactions (Figure 29.1). On the other hand, when the results of both challenge types are considered together, prick test results were positive in 67% of the patients with acute reactions, and patch test results were positive in 89% of those with delayed-onset reactions. Parallel testing (prick or patch test positive results) results were positive in 78% of the patients with acute-onset reactions (sensitivity 0.78) and 92% of those with delayed-onset reactions (sensitivity 0.92). Serial testing (prick and patch test positive results) results were positive in 24% of the patients with acute-onset and delayed-onset reactions (sensitivity 0.24). The test responses were jointly positive or negative in only 15% and 38% of cases, respectively. Cohen's κ statistic for concordance of prick and patch test was 0.03, with 95% CI −0.13 to 0.19, indicating that no agreement better than chance exists between the two tests and that the two tests give discrepant values. In calculating values for sensitivity, specificity, and likelihood ratios of a positive and a negative test result for prick and patch testing singly or combined, we considered the results of the double-blind, placebo-controlled challenges and open challenges separately. The skin test reactivity was similar in both challenge types (Table 29.3). Parallel prick and patch testing resulted in heightening of sensitivity with only marginal decrease of specificity when compared with use of either test alone. Serial prick and patch testing resulted in significantly decreased sensitivity and increased specificity

**TABLE 29.3   Sensitivity, Specificity, and Likelihood Ratios of a Positive and a Negative
Result for Skin Prick and Patch Tests, Separately and Combined, in
Diagnosing Cow Milk Allergy in Patients with Atopic Dermatitis[a]**

	Prick	Skin testing patch	Parallel[b]	Serial[c]
Sensitivity	0.48 (0.47)	0.61 (0.59)	0.86 (0.81)	0.24 (0.25)
Specificity	0.86 (0.83)	0.81 (0.83)	0.72 (0.65)	0.94 (1.00)
Likelihood ratio of				
Positive test result	3.46 (2.70)	3.13 (3.41)	3.11 (2.34)	4.24 (undefined)
Negative test result	0.60 (0.64)	0.49 (0.49)	0.19 (0.29)	0.81 (0.75)

Note: Sensitivity (Se) = probability of a true positive test result.

Specificity (Sp) = probability of a true negative test result.

Likelihood ratio of a positive test result = Se/(1 − Sp).

Likelihood ratio of a negative test result = (1 − Se)/Sp.

[a] The results are given separately for double-blind, placebo-controlled, cow milk challenge and (open challenge in parentheses).

[b] Prick or patch test positive results.

[c] Prick and patch test positive results.

compared with use of either test alone. In patients with atopic dermatitis the probability of detecting cow milk allergy was significantly higher with parallel skin testing than with only prick test (McNemar test: chi square = 8.17, p = 0.004) or only patch test (McNemar test: chi square = 6.25, p = 0.01).

29.4   DISCUSSION

Atopic dermatitis is a common and complex, chronically relapsing skin disorder of infancy and childhood. Immunologically it is characterized by increased, mainly allergen-specific, IgE production. Because elevated specific IgE can be demonstrated by skin prick testing, these tests are widely used to disclose food allergy in patients with atopic dermatitis.[7-9] The results in our study support previous findings that T cell-mediated reactions can be distinguished in atopic dermatitis[18-21] and extend these observations to enhance the diagnostic accuracy of skin testing in infants with atopic dermatitis.

Hypersensitivity reactions to allergens have been contemplated in the pathogenesis of atopic dermatitis.[3] In infancy, diet is probably the most important single environmental allergen. Hypersensitivity reactions to dietary allergens may induce dysfunction in the intestine's mucosal barrier,[22] disturb the physiological protein transfer,[23] and consequently lead to excessive permeation of intact proteins.[24,25] The way the antigen is transported across the small intestinal mucosa has a profound effect on the initiation of immune response.[23] Aberrant antigen absorption may lead to exaggeration of immune response, thereby broadening the sensitivity.[23,26] Therefore early identification of patients who would profit from strict avoidance of dietary allergens is important for several reasons: (1) to avoid unnecessary elimination diets involving risk of growth retardation in early life, (2) to ameliorate the clinical course of atopic dermatitis, and (3) as secondary prevention of the development of multiple food allergies.

Double-blind, placebo-controlled oral challenges have demonstrated clinical food hypersensitivity in 30 to 60% of patients with mild to severe atopic dermatitis, with egg and milk accounting for most of the positive clinical reactions.[2,7,8,11] In our study population of infants and young children with atopic dermatitis, the chance of having food allergy was 69%. The prevalence of cow milk allergy was 54%, which is significantly higher than in previous studies in older children.[2,7] This difference is most likely explained by the fact that cow milk allergy frequently is the first manifestation of an allergic diathesis because of the important nutritional role of milk and milk products and less varied diet in early childhood.[2,4,5,10] We therefore suggest that children in whom atopic dermatitis does not improve despite meticulous routine treatment with emollients and topical corticosteroids should be tested for allergy to foods, in particular cow milk.

Cow milk allergy is diagnosed by clinical response to withdrawal and subsequent challenge with cow milk. Children with positive clinical reaction to such oral cow milk challenges have been divided into subgroups according to the reaction onset time: immediate or delayed-onset reactions.[5,9,12,13] The diagnosis is seldom difficult for patients who manifest allergic reaction immediately after cow milk ingestion but may be complex in those with delayed reactions. We detected indistinguishable rates of positive reactions in double-blind, placebo-controlled, and open challenges. In like manner skin test reactivity was proportionally similar in both challenge types. These results would suggest that in this age group an open challenge and careful follow-up may be adequate for practical clinical purposes, also enabling diagnosis of delayed reactions. However, double-blind, placebo-controlled challenges clearly are the gold standard for objective diagnosis of specific food allergies in all age groups.

There is considerable discrepancy as to the estimated value of skin testing in diagnosing food allergy. We chose to investigate unselected patients with atopic dermatitis in an age group with peak prevalence of food allergy and reputedly poor diagnostic reliability of skin testing.[6,10] No direct comparison can be made with previous studies in older children or in patients with clinical history suggestive of food allergy.[7-9,11] However, our results lend support to observations in older children[7] that skin prick testing is an acceptable means of excluding immediate food allergy and of indicating clinical hypersensitivity. Our study demonstrated that many patients with negative prick test results but delayed-onset clinical reactions could be identified by patch testing. Such heterogeneity in response to skin prick and patch tests was previously observed in adults with atopic dermatitis with dust-mite allergen.[19] Skin prick and patch tests thus may distinctly indicate cow milk allergy in infants with atopic dermatitis. However, the methods used for patch testing with foods is so far unstandardized. Also, the vehicle used for testing must be further standardized. With a casein used as allergen in patch testing, the sensitivity was only 0.33 in patients allergic to cow milk, which shows that crude milk powder might be preferable.[27]

Regarding skin prick testing, the commercially available milk allergen (ALK) seems to give results comparable to those with milk powder used in normal feed concentration.

Taken together, our results indicate that parallel prick and patch testing will increase the probability of early detection of food allergy in infants with atopic dermatitis. Accurate and objective demonstration of a causal relationship between the dietary allergen and exacerbation of the infant's atopic dermatitis may be a prerequisite for the compliance of the family to the treatment. Confirmation of the diagnosis is essential in patients with positive skin test results, and for this purpose the most accurate method is double-blind, placebo-controlled food challenge followed by open challenge.

We thank SHS Int. Ltd., Liverpool, U.K., for providing Neocate, and Valio Ltd., Helsinki, Finland, for providing the whey hydrolysate formula for this investigation.

REFERENCES

1. Hide DW, Matthews S, Matthews L. et al., Effect of allergen avoidance in infancy on allergic manifestations at age two years. *J. Allergy Clin. Immunol.*, 1994;93:842–6.

2. Sampson HA and McCaskill CC. Food hypersensitivity and atopic dermatitis: evaluation of 113 patients. *J. Pediatr.* 1985;107:669–75.

3. Sampson HA and Scanlon SM. Natural history of food hypersensitivity in children with atopic dermatitis. *J. Pediatr.* 1989;115:23–7.

4. Bishop JM, Hill DJ, and Hosking CS. Natural history of cow milk allergy: clinical outcome. *J. Pediatr.* 1990;116:862–7.

5. Isolauri E, Suomalainen H, Kaila M et al. Local immune response in patients with cow milk allergy — follow-up of patients retaining allergy or becoming tolerant. *J. Pediatr.* 1992;120:9–15.

6. Zeiger RS. Atopy in infancy and early childhood: Natural history and role of skin testing. *J. Allergy Clin. Immunol.* 1985;75:633–9.

7. Sampson HA and Albergo R. Comparison of results of skin tests, RAST, and double-blind, placebo-controlled food challenges in children with atopic dermatitis. *J. Allergy Clin. Immunol.* 1984;74:26–33.

8. Burks AW, Mallory SB, Williams LW, and Shirrell MA. Atopic dermatitis: clinical relevance of food hypersensitivity reactions. *J. Pediatr.* 1988;113:447–51.

9. Hill DJ, Duke AM, Hosking CS, and Hudson IL. Clinical manifestations of cows' milk allergy in childhood. II. The diagnostic value of skin tests and RAST. *Clin. Allergy* 1988;18:481–90.

10. Sampson HA, Bernhisel-Broadbent J, Yang E, and Scanlon SM. Safety of casein hydrolysate formula in children with cow milk allergy. *J. Pediatr.* 1991;118:520–5.

11. Bock SA and Atkins FM. Patterns of food hypersensitivity during sixteen years of double-blind, placebo-controlled food challenges. *J. Pediatr.* 1990;117:561–7.

12. Hill DJ, Firer MA, Shelton MJ, and Hosking CS. Manifestations of milk allergy in infancy: clinical and immunologic findings. *J. Pediatr.* 1986;109:270–6.

13. Isolauri E, Virtanen E, Jalonen T, and Arvilommi H. Local immune response measured in blood lymphocytes reflects the clinical reactivity of children with cow's milk allergy. *Pediatr. Res.* 1990;28:582–6.

14. Reitamo S, Visa K, Kähnönen K, Käyhkö K, Stubb S, and Salo OP. Eczematous reactions in atopic patients caused by epicutaneous testing with inhalant allergens. *Br. J. Dermatol.* 1986;114:303–9.

15. Hanifin JM. Epidemiology of atopic dermatitis. *Monogr. Allergy* 1987;21:116–31.

16. Isolauri E, Sütas Y, Mäkinen-Kiljunen S, Oja SS, Isosomppi R, and Turjanmaa K. Efficacy and safety of hydrolyzed cow milk and amino acid-derived formulas in infants with cow milk allergy. *J. Pediatr.* 1995;127:550.

17. Mäkinen-Kiljunen S and Sorva R. Bovine β-lactoglobulin levels in hydrolysed protein formulas for infant feeding. *Clin. Exp. Allergy* 1993;23:287–91.

18. Mitchell EB, Crow J, Chapman MD, Jouhal SS, Pope FM, and Platts-Mills TAE. Basophils in allergens-induced patch test sites with atopic dermatitis. *Lancet* 1982;1:127–30.

19. Imayama S, Hashizume T, Miyahara H et al. Combination of patch test and IgE for dust mite antigens differentiates 130 patients with atopic dermatitis into four groups. *J. Am. Acad. Dermatol.* 1992;27:531–8.

20. van der Heijden FL, Wierenga EA, Bos JD, and Kapsenberg ML. High frequency of IL-4-producing CD4$^+$ allergen-specific T lymphocytes in atopic dermatitis lesional skin. *J. Invest. Dermatol.* 1991;97:389–94.

21. Kondo N, Fukutomi O, Agata H et al. The role of T lymphocytes in patients with food-sensitive atopic dermatitis. *J. Allergy Clin. Immunol.* 1993;91:658–68.

22. Jalongen T. Identical intestinal permeability changes in children with different clinical manifestations of cow's milk allergy. *J. Allergy Clin. Immunol.* 1991;88:737–42.

23. Sanderson IR and Walker WA. Uptake and transport of macromolecules by the intestine: possible role in clinical disorders (an update). *Gastroenterology* 1993;104:622–39.

24. Heyman M, Grasset E, Ducroc R, and Desjeux JF. Antigen absorption by the jejunal epithelium of children with cow's milk allergy. *Pediatr. Res.* 1988;24:197–202.

25. Heyman M, Andriantsoa M., Crain-Denoyelle AM, and Desjeux JF. Effect of oral or parenteral sensitization to cow's milk on mucosal permeability in guinea pigs. *Int. Arch. Allergy Appl. Immunol.* 1990;92:242–6.

26. Suomalainen H, Isolauri E, Kaila M, Virtanen E, and Arvilommi H. Cow's milk provocation induces an immune response to unrelated dietary antigens. *Gut* 1992;23:1179–83.

27. Räsänen L, Lehto M, and Reunala T. Diagnostic value of skin and laboratory tests in cow's milk allergy/intolerance. *Clin. Exp. Allergy* 1992;22:385–90.

Index

A

Abietic acid, 16, 35, 120, 123
Acarus siro, 66
ACD. *See* Allergic contact dermatitis
Acetic acid, 35, 66
Acetones, 18, 121, 162–163
Acetyl choline, 198
Acetylsalicylic acid (aspirin), 6–7, 15, 35, 81–84, 120
Acid anhydrides, 46, 49–50
Acrodermatitis enteropathica, 277
Acrylates, 37
Acrylic acid, 35, 124
Acrylics, 18, 121, 167
Actinic keratoses, 112
Acylase, 131–132
Adhesives, 198
Aerogen, 174
Agglutinating antibody assays, 250
Agricultural chemicals, 89–92
Albendazole, 35
Albumin, 28
Alcalase, 130
Alcohols, 18, 35, 132, 163. *See also individual alcohols*
Algae, 16, 120
Alkaline phosphatase, 132
Allantoin, 114
Allergic contact dermatitis (ACD)
   agricultural chemicals and, 90
   capsaicin and, 73
   enzymes and, 132, 133–135
   epoxy resins and, 146
   low-molecular-weight chemicals and, 33, 38–39
   metals and, 191, 194, 196, 199–200, 204, 239
   nomenclature of, 57
   organic acid anhydrides and, 220–221
   paronychia, 274
   proteins and, 282, 284
   substance P and, 73
Allergic contact paronychia, 269–271, 275

Allspice, 122, 282
Almonds, 262, 282
Aloe gel, 114
Alternaria, 138
p-Aminodiphenylamine, 35
Aminophenazone, 16, 35, 120–121, 123
p-Aminophenols, 161
N′N′-bis-(4-aminophenyl)-2,5-diamino-1,4-quinonediimine, 159, 162
Aminothiazole, 18, 35, 121
Ammonia, 18, 35, 121, 162, 168
Ammonium persulfate
   immunologic contact urticaria and, 18, 35, 37
   occupational contact urticaria from, 66, 121, 159, 161, 165
   scratch tests using, 158
Amniotic fluid, 12, 14, 91, 96–97
Amoxycillin, 15, 108
Ampicillin, 15, 91, 108, 120
Amyl alcohol, 120
Amylase, 130–135
α-Amylase, 65, 131, 133–134, 136–138, 243, 283
Anaphylaxis
   from agricultural chemicals, 90
   from antibiotics, 107, 109
   from corn-starch glove powder, 123
   from cosmetics and hair products, 111, 158, 162
   from dairy products, 214
   from dental products, 125
   from dyes, 230
   from food allergies, 150–151, 265, 290–291
   from human seminal plasma, 242, 245, 250–252
   immunologic contact urticaria and, 2, 11
   from low-molecular-weight chemicals, 34
   from metals, 195, 199, 202
   from natural rubber latex, 12, 174, 176, 178
   oral allergy syndrome and, 290–291
Anchovies, 100–101
Anemia, hemolytic, 195
Angioedema
   antibiotics and, 107, 109